The NHS: Beginning, Middle and End?
The autobiography of Dr John Marks

JOHN MARKS

Foreword by
NICHOLAS TIMMINS
Public Policy Editor
Financial Times

Radcliffe Publishing
Oxford • New York

Radcliffe Publishing Ltd
18 Marcham Road
Abingdon
Oxon OX14 1AA
United Kingdom

www.radcliffe-oxford.com
Electronic catalogue and worldwide online ordering facility.

British Library Cataloguing in Publication Data

A catalogue record for this book is available from the British Library.

ISBN-13: 978 184619 272 2

Typeset by Pindar New Zealand (Egan Reid), Auckland, New Zealand
Printed and bound by TJI Digital, Padstow, Cornwall, UK

Contents

Foreword   vii

Acknowledgements   ix

CHAPTER 1   1925–1943 My childhood and life as an evacuee   1

CHAPTER 2   University and the army   13

CHAPTER 3   From lorry driver to principal in general practice   33

CHAPTER 4   My involvement in abortion law reform   43

CHAPTER 5   I get further involved in medical politics   50

CHAPTER 6   I get started in medical politics at the national level 57

CHAPTER 7   A Royal College, an academic approach and a doctorate   70

CHAPTER 8   Early attempts at NHS reform and heart transplants   78

CHAPTER 9   An outdated constitution and Sir Paul Chambers' report   83

CHAPTER 10   I become involved in national negotiations   90

CHAPTER 11   I appear before a disciplinary body and I lose some
             friends   101

CHAPTER 12   I represent the profession at home and abroad   108

CHAPTER 13   AIDS and the BMA   117

CHAPTER 14   A Royal sesquicentennial year   124

CHAPTER 15   International problems and political speculation   133

CHAPTER 16   Two crises and one election   139

CHAPTER 17   Princess Diana opens the library and I have a rough
             ARM   153

CHAPTER 18   The approaching storm   166

CHAPTER 19   A storm breaks: The White Paper   178

CHAPTER 20   The profession rejects the Reforms   189

CHAPTER 21   The campaign continues   203

CHAPTER 22   The Bill and reactions to it   211

CHAPTER 23   The campaign continues: mysterious faxes and
             the Oxford debate   215

CHAPTER 24   My last few months in the chair   222

CHAPTER 25   I am a past Chairman   230

CHAPTER 26   A variety of activities including boxing and lecturing
             and a disputed SRM   238

CHAPTER 27   *Doctors in the Dock*   251

CHAPTER 28   A quiet retirement, a general election and a
             question mark   260

             Index   267

Foreword

JOHN MARKS IS SOMETHING OF A NATIONAL TREASURE. WARM, FUNNY, passionate, opinionated and occasionally contrary, he is a man whose life for more than forty years marched in beat with that of the National Health Service.

The son of a publican – like John Moore, a Conservative secretary of state for health with whom he was later to tangle – he qualified as a doctor on 'vesting day': July 5 1948, the day the NHS started.

It was a fitting joint incarnation. For over the next 40 years and more, John Marks lived through the NHS's history, from its earliest days when patients came in demanding wigs and cotton wool now that the service was free, through his rise in medical politics, to become chairman of council of the British Medical Association – and arguably one of its most successful ones.

There is scarcely a medical issue or controversy – whether ones which purely affected the BMA or others that were played out on the national stage in the full beam of the media spotlight – in which John Marks was not involved.

Abortion law reform, the doctors' 1970s revolt against the General Medical Council, the foundation of the Royal College of General Practitioners, countless NHS reorganisations, and the bloody battle over NHS pay beds and the pay of junior doctors – which saw medics take industrial action for the first time – are just a sample.

Then there was the fierce, principled battle over how the medical profession and the public should respond to the terror of a new disease – AIDS. And the great war that was fought over the Conservatives introduction of market forces into the NHS in the late 1980s and early 1990s – an approach to running the

NHS that lives on, reincarnated, under the current Labour government.

In all of these John Marks played more than a walk-on part. In many he was a principal actor.

For anyone wanting fully to understand the BMA's role in all this, this book is thus required reading. But it is much more than just a dry history of times past. It is laced with anecdote, from the horrifying – the level of some of the training and medical practice 50 and more years ago – to the hilarious, and on to high politics.

Through it all John Marks' effervescent personality and his commitment to the NHS shine through – even if both of those were to lead him into conflict with others, such as Kenneth Clarke, the Conservative Health Secretary, who would claim with equal passion that they too shared the same ideals.

Ken Clarke once observed that the BMA is 'just another trade union, and actually one of the nastiest I have ever dealt with'. Others will make their own assessment of that judgement. But John Marks' account of his life and times provides a contrary view – the tale of a warm, human, liberal and occasionally buccaneering man whose passion for life and causes leaves even those who do not always agree with him eager to count him among their friends.

Nicholas Timmins
Public Policy Editor, *Financial Times*
March 2008

Acknowledgements

MANY YEARS AGO THE THEN EDITOR OF THE *British Medical Journal* (*BMJ*), Stephen Lock, said everyone should write their own obituary. In line with that advice I did so in 2006. My wife Shirley suggested that I should expand it into a short history of my life for my family. Once I started writing and researching I realised that I had committed myself to producing a full book. Gordon MacPherson, a former deputy editor of the *BMJ* and medico-political commentator under his nom de plume of 'Scrutator', and Tim Albert, a former editor of *BMA News Review*, both gave me helpful advice.

At a chance meeting with Ian Black, President of the Men's Health Forum, at a rally in support of junior hospital doctors in February 2007, he suggested that Radcliffe Publishing might be interested in my book and later in the year I contacted Gillian Nineham. She and her colleagues have been very helpful and supportive to me.

However, unbeknown to him, one man is directly responsible for the writing of this book. At the time of my election as Chairman of Council of the British Medical Association (BMA), a long-standing friend David Podro was the owner of International Press Cutting Bureau. Within days of my taking office I started receiving huge numbers of free press cuttings relating to my activities. Those I selected to keep filled 17 scrapbooks. This gift continued until my replacement by Jeremy Lee-Potter and it provided a wonderful source of concrete evidence for statements in the book. I am deeply grateful for his kindness and generosity.

I am grateful to the following for allowing me to quote extracts from their publications: HarperCollins Publishers Ltd, Victor Gollancz, an imprint of The Orion Publishing Group, Times Series Newspapers, *Daily Mail*, *The House*

Magazine, General Practitioner, Doctor, Guardian and *BMA News.*

© The Economist Newspaper Ltd London. 'Britain – Dangerous Doctors', p.9 and 'Still in search of a cure', p. 16, 19/8/89

I also thank Tony Bourne, Chief Executive/Secretary of the British Medical Association for permission to publish a large number of photographs and extracts from the Special Report by the Association's Council on the Government's White Paper, *Working for Patients*, 13 April 1989 (SRM2).

Lastly I am deeply grateful for the help and support I received from my wife Shirley, in this, and everything else that I have done in the last 54 years.

CHAPTER 1

1925–1943 My childhood
and life as an evacuee

AS A YOUNG CHILD I REMEMBER HAVING THREE GRANDPARENTS, Grandpa and Grandma Goldbaum and Grandpa Marks. My mother's parents, Julius Goldbaum (probably Judah) and his wife Binya, escaped from Poland around 1880. It was not until years after they were both dead that we discovered his real name was Reznick and that they had used her maiden name because they were petrified that the Russian secret police would find him in England. He was a small, dapper, grey-haired man with a moustache and a neat beard. He spoke English with a thick Polish accent. The 'parlour' of their modest house in Shoreditch was covered with certificates testifying to his active support for the local Liberal party. Binya was even smaller than her husband. She always wore a black dress and was completely subjugated by Grandpa.

Grandpa Goldbaum had been a tailor and on a pittance he raised a large family in a reasonably comfortable environment. Jenny, his eldest daughter firmly controlled the other children. Next came three sons – Morris, Leslie and Solomon. Soloman died from rheumatic fever while serving in the Royal Flying Corps. Aunt Esther was older than my mother Rose, but after my mother married she became 'older' than her single sister. Rebecca was born in 1900 and changed her name to Irena Gee. The youngest daughter Bertha had a pretty face and shining red hair. At the age of six, dressed in a green satin suit, top hat and cane, I was a pageboy at her wedding to Sam Cohen, who looked rather like Clark Gable.

My father's parents came from Byalistok. Grandfather Marks was a kosher poulterer who always wore the same scruffy cap, ill-fitting black suits, and sported a beard and moustache. His wife Jane (Hanna) died of diabetes in 1924,

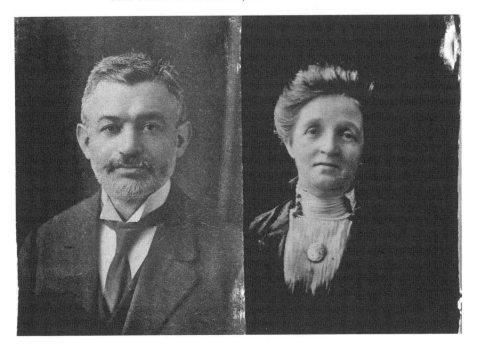

FIGURE 1.1 My maternal grandparents, Julius and Binya Goldbaum.

before my mother met my father. Rebecca (Becky), my father's only sister, ruled the family. Next in seniority was brother Jack who was never spoken about because he had died in Texas after being shot by a local sheriff in mysterious circumstances.

My father, Lewis Myer Kitchinsky was born in London on 30 June 1893. His name was changed by deed poll to Lewis Myer Marks in 1923. He told me that his father used his leather belt often and vigorously on his children. As a result of that my father revolted against corporal punishment and only hit me once in my lifetime. He was very good at school and I always felt it was a tragedy that he had to leave school at 14 to work with Becky and his father. They went to country markets and bought chickens, ducks, geese and turkeys, which they took to London and killed in the kosher tradition to sell to kosher butchers. Late in life he told me that his greatest day was when his father bought a donkey to pull the barrow instead of him.

Solly, the youngest surviving child joined the business in due course. He was a car-mad playboy with countless girlfriends. I remember his Alvis sports coupé, which I was allowed to sit in and which I left in gear one day with disastrous consequences when he started the engine without checking. My father was devoted to his brother and sister and often put their interests ahead of my

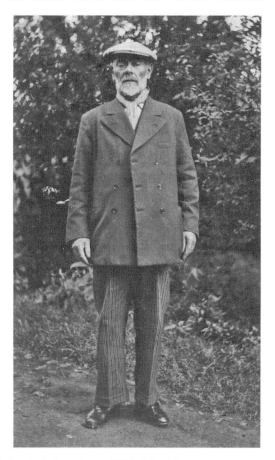

FIGURE 1.2 My father's father, Mottel Kitchinski.

mother's. This played a large part in the Marks family history, as my father spent a great deal of his time with chickens and not at the pub he owned.

My mother's sister Aunt Jenny married an ex-regular soldier called John (Jack) Isaacs. They bought a public house in Islington and one of their customers was the good looking, and relatively wealthy, Lew Marks. Jenny introduced her unmarried sister Rose to this potential husband. Rose worked as a photographer's assistant – serving customers, developing and printing film, and acting as a fully clothed model. She smoked and could do the Charleston.

After a short courtship they were married on 17 August 1924 at Philpot Street Synagogue, in spite of the hostility of Becky, who refused to share her brothers with anyone. Ironically, she balanced her intense dislike of my mother by doting on me. She was my wealthy aunty from whom I got almost anything I asked. For example, at Broad Street station, the terminus of the North London

Railway, there was a model tanker locomotive about 3 feet long. I wanted her to buy it for me. She summoned the station master who said it was not for sale. Neither Becky nor I were pleased. Over the years that memory stayed with me, but as I grew older I began to wonder if it was all a figment of my imagination. My relief was intense when, in my seventh decade, I saw that same model sitting at the Railway Museum in York.

After their wedding Rose and Lew moved to Hackney and he continued to work as a poulterer. This involved early rising, to catch trains to the markets, and late returns. Following my birth on 30 May 1925, my mother found that lifestyle unacceptable. When I was ten months old Jack Isaacs and my father went into partnership and bought a public house, the Grand Junction Arms in Acton Lane, Harlesden. Although they were good friends, their attitudes to work, money and gambling were completely incompatible. Finally my father bought Jack out.

In our garden we had chickens, geese, ducks, rabbits and a goat, as well as an Alsatian dog and a Fox Terrier. Our garden was popular with my cousins and the local kids, but not my mother. Its east side was separated by a wall and some allotments from Waxlow Road, where McVitie and Price had their bakery – one of a very few factories that were functioning at the height of the slump. Sitting on our garden wall I could watch the workers, predominately women, going to and returning from work. In particular I remember a one-legged man busking the workers and singing the popular song, *Wagon wheels*.[1] It was a pitiful sight.

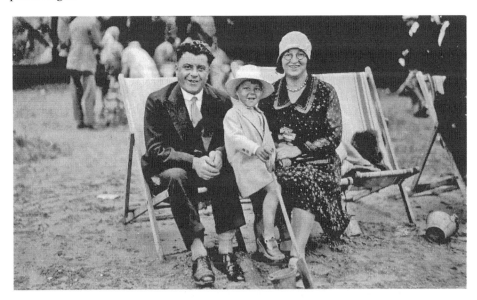

FIGURE 1.3 With my parents, Margate 1929.

The depression was at its height, but we were relatively wealthy. The first school I attended was the state school in Lower Place. My mother made a habit of inviting my school friends, poorly dressed and inadequately shod, for tea. It was probably their best meal in a week.

My parents decided that Lower Place was not suitable and I was sent to Roundwood College, a dame school run by a Miss Templar. Frank, my father's cellarman drove me to school most days, or sometimes my nanny took me on the bus and we walked the last bit.

There was a small Jewish community in Harlesden. Father and a few others founded the West Willesden Synagogue in a hut in Stonebridge Park. One of the other founders was Henry Filer, who had a jeweller's shop in High Street. He and his wife Rose at that time had one child, Roy, who was six months younger than me. We became lifelong friends at Roundwood College.

My brother Vincent was born at home on 10 June 1930. He became my mother's favourite and remained so for the rest of her life. He had knock-knees and a 'children's specialist' recommended that he be fitted with full-length splints, which the poor child wore for about five years. Vincent had a foul temper and I was frequently at the receiving end of it, but because he was 'crippled' retaliation was forbidden. Years later it was recognised that if left alone knock-knees straighten up themselves. My sister Sheila was also born at home on 20 May 1934. As a treat I had been sent to stay with Aunty Becky for a while and when I returned home I found this girl, a sister that I did not want and would not accept. More on that later.

At the age of eleven I sat the entrance examination for grammar school – those who did not pass were sent to the local central school. I passed, and in the autumn of 1936 I started at Willesden County School, one of the excellent coeducational Middlesex County grammar schools. Even at that age I had the ability to remember maps and diagrams and my first geography teacher, 'Pop' Newton, encouraged me and I was top in geography examinations throughout my entire school life. I did reasonably well all round that year, but in my second year things went very wrong. My geography teacher was Mr Small, nicknamed 'Piggy' because he looked and acted like one. I absolutely refused to do his set homework and then nearly every other teacher's homework.[2] When I came top of the geography examination list he accused me of cheating. I did not need to.

My father's pub was in a tough, hard-drinking, working class area. He knew that his staff pocketed some of the pub's takings. What was left over was more than enough to make the business a very lucrative one. Most men would have ignored the problem, but my father became obsessed with it. He decided to sell the business and retire at the age of 51, rather than live comfortably without actually working. He became extremely depressed as soon as he stopped work and attempted to buy other pubs, but he never completed the transactions and lost numerous deposits, money in legal fees and other expenses along the way. He picked at his scalp until it bled and his robust figure wasted away. Life for my mother and the three of us became an absolute nightmare.

We moved to a tiny flat in Harlesden near to my school. My father bought another pub in South Norwood and Vincent and Sheila were sent away to boarding school, while I stayed with the family of a school friend, Maurice Jay. That did not work out for me, and so for the best part of a term I commuted daily from Norwood via tram, the Bakerloo tube, and a long walk from Willesden Junction station. At that time no one considered that was a dangerous or unusual thing for a 12-year-old boy to do on his own.

My father sold the pub in Norwood and bought the Seven Sisters Hotel in South Tottenham. Almost miraculously his mental state returned to normal, as did his physical strength. The business was a 'better class' and my parents formed friendships with many local business people. However, I had a problem. I had been so idle and difficult at school that I was due for a most terrible report and I would certainly have been demoted to a slower stream. Fortunately, Willesden County School posted reports to parents and mine, sent on my directions to a non-existent address in Tottenham, never arrived. However, when my mother took me to Tottenham County School to enrol the excellent headmaster, Dr Thomas – nicknamed 'Bert' after the well-known cartoonist in the *Evening Standard* – wanted to discuss my school record. Somehow I managed to convince him that I was capable of doing School Certificate in four years and I was put into an appropriate class. My form mistress, Mary Taylor, was a new young teacher who taught my strongest and favourite subject. Life became worthwhile again, but throughout my school life I went to great lengths to avoid doing homework.

In 1938 I reached the age of 13 and I had my bar mitzvah. We were members of the small South Tottenham Synagogue but my paternal grandfather was a member of the prestigious Duke's Place Synagogue in the City, the equivalent in the United Synagogue to Canterbury Cathedral. As the few orthodox members of the family would not have been able to attend a synagogue outside of central London because their religion forbade them from travelling on the Sabbath, arrangements were made for me to have my bar mitzvah at Duke's Place.

The bar mitzvah is a great ordeal for a 13-year-old child. He is expected to read from a scroll a portion of the Torah written in Hebrew. In reality, the child has to learn the thing by heart. In addition he has to sing Hebrew blessings – both before and after the reading – and he then has to sing the appropriate lesson from the Prophets with even more blessings. I had a reasonably good soprano voice and made no mistakes, so everyone was happy. I was presented with a book on Jewish festivals which I still have.[3]

On the Sunday following the ceremony I had my bar mitzvah party in the large function room at the Seven Sisters Hotel. Neither my siblings nor any other children were present. Thank goodness things have changed since then and the normal bar mitzvah party now includes a considerable number of the celebrant's friends – of both sexes – who have a great time dancing and singing while elderly grandparents look on in amazement.

During 1939 we saw air raid shelters being dug in parks and peoples' gardens. We were issued with gas masks and leaflets explaining how to make our houses safer. It was decided that young children should be evacuated from the large cities if war broke out and when a German invasion of Poland seemed imminent the plans were activated. On Friday 1 September 1939, along with most of the children at Tottenham County School, I was marched to Seven Sisters Station to board a train. The general rule was that elder children were responsible for their younger siblings. To my lasting shame I refused to take my five-year-old sister Sheila with me. I was prepared to have Vincent, but he refused to come with me, and acting bravely as the elder brother he went with Sheila.

We discovered that our train was going to March, in Cambridgeshire. I was the only person on the train who had heard of it because it had a poultry market and I had been there with my father. Only a British Government could send children to a town that was a strategic railway centre with a huge marshalling yard, Whitemore (now a prison) built by the same engineers that had built the one at Hamm, Germany.

We arrived at March to find they were expecting small children from an infants school. We were lined up and marched through the town; billeting officers allocated us houses along the way. I was in one of the last groups to be settled, and I was billeted with a railway porter's family. On Sunday 3 September we gathered in Market Square to hear Neville Chamberlain's declaration of war speech. It was a scorching hot day and at that time the River Nene, which flowed through the town, was an open sewer. The stench was unbelievable.

Many books have been written about the lives of evacuees and their hosts. I was not treated badly, but many others were. Some evacuees took to bed-wetting and other destructive behaviour. In general, the people of March – particularly the children – loathed and resented 'them Tottenhams'. Once again, I was lucky. Due to my family's poultry business I knew a local chicken merchant, Sid Harwin, and his very large family. They included Sylvia, who was my age, beautiful, and my first serious girlfriend.

March had a boys' grammar school, which dated back to Tudor times, and a girls' high school, Tottenham County, was co-educational, which caused a few problems. In an attempt to give both the locals and the evacuees some form of education, the locals went to school in the mornings and we evacuees attended during the afternoons. To keep us occupied in the mornings we enjoyed free viewings at the local cinemas. March had two cinemas and they changed programmers on Mondays and Thursdays. We saw a lot of films.

A few weeks after arriving in March I decided to run away and go home so that if my parents were killed I would be killed too and not be left an orphan. On the way I called in at the Northern Polytechnic in Holloway Road and enrolled in its matric course. I went home and greeted my parents with these facts. My father reacted most sensibly and without anger. He took me back to March and to Bert Thomas. Bert smiled benevolently, a rare occurrence indeed, and said, 'Boy how would you like to come to school here and go home every night? We will arrange a half fare season ticket for you.' Brilliant. Dad brought the ticket and my commuting started.

I got up at about 5.30 a.m. and walked a mile to Tottenham Hale station. I changed at Broxbourne, and then again at Cambridge or Ely or St Neots, arriving at school at around 9.00 a.m. After school I returned to Tottenham by rail, but due to 'wartime exigencies' I sometimes had to go through to the Liverpool Street terminus and get the 649 trolleybus north to Tottenham. I kept that up for about two weeks and then decided I would become a weekend commuter. After a few weeks of that I surrendered and became a full-time evacuee again. Dad and Bert had won a total victory.

After a few weeks with my first foster-family I moved across the road to an elderly widow, whose simple son was the local milkman. The walls of the terraced houses were like cardboard and another evacuee Audrey Abel and I sang duets through them from our respective tin baths in the kitchens. That billet did not last long either and I was sent to live with Mr and Mrs George Campbell. Mr Campbell was a train driver. I was joined there by Ken Gover, another 'Tottenham' and we became close friends.

After a few months Mrs Campbell took a dislike to Ken and asked him to leave. I was not prepared to stay alone and so we both moved to the Northfield house in Station Road. Mr Northfield was a guard and Mrs Northfield was a kindly woman who treated us well. They had a daughter, Doreen, who was about three years older than we were. We worshipped her as our 'grown-up sister'. She was an usherette at the Hippodrome and we were let in via the back door as often as we wanted.

In the summer of 1940 we sat the General Schools Certificate examinations, colloquially known as 'The Matric'. I got my expected distinction in Geography and had credits in every other subject except English Literature. That was in no small measure the result of my relationship with the woman who taught me

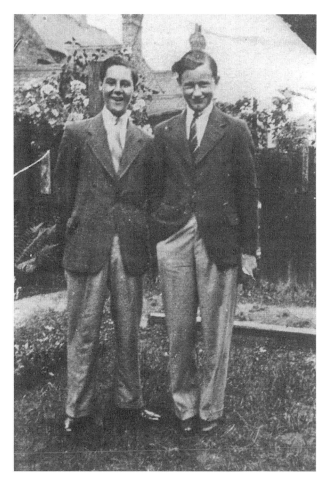

FIGURE 1.4 Two evacuees – Ken Gover and John Marks in the Northfields' garden, March 1942.

English, Mrs Bedding. Married women teachers were very rare in those days, and Mrs Bedding, like most of them, was a First World War widow. She loathed me and made my life hell. In latter years, when I was making public speeches and broadcasts, or being paid to write articles, I mentally cursed her for depriving me of many years appreciation of our beautiful language.

I joined the March Squadron Number 1220 of the Air Training Corps (ATC), which still exists. Apart from drills, aircraft recognition, etcetera, we did quite a lot of flying from the RAF Training Station at Upwood, near Ramsey, then in Huntingdonshire. We went there by coach at the weekend in a state of great excitement, singing *The Yellow Rose of Texas* and other patriotic songs. I remember at least three flights. One took us over the Fens, another to Stratford-

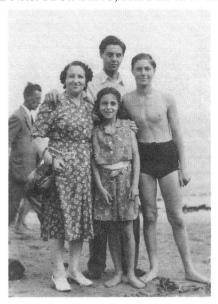

FIGURE 1.5 Rose Marks with her three children, Bournemouth 1947.

upon-Avon – a fair distance from Ramsey. My most memorable trip was in a Westland Lysander, during which we pretended to be a fighter attacking a Blenheim bomber. Everything was recorded by camera guns on the aircraft and later used for analysis and training.

During the summer holidays of 1942, we sixth formers volunteered to help with getting in the harvest and we were sent to a farm in Stony Stratford, Buckinghamshire, where we learnt to stook corn, load wagons, and build hay and wheat stacks. We had a great social life and I met Eileen Bloomfield, a buxom pretty girl who, despite her name, was definitely not Jewish. Our attachment persisted until after I went off to university and it caused my mother a great deal of anxiety.

My Higher School Certificate result in the autumn of 1942 was reasonably good, with passes in Geography, Botany and Zoology, and a distinction in Chemistry. As the situation in London improved and bombing became less intensive, most of the school returned to Tottenham. Then, someone made a decision that because I was just 17 I should do a third year in the sixth form to improve my grades and maybe get a State Scholarship. Our Chemistry master, 'Eggy' Ware – his nickname came from his experiments with hydrogen sulphide, which smells of rotten eggs – was a brilliant teacher. Like many other secondary school teachers he was a first class honours graduate who could not get any other job.

Young men of 18 were liable to conscription. As a member of the ATC I looked forward to joining the RAF. I was persuaded to apply for an engineering cadetship, which meant that I would go to college at the RAF's expense and then be commissioned in its engineering section. At the interview I was asked how could I possibly do engineering with my academic background and with supreme arrogance I said that I could do anything that I had set my mind to. I was offered a place at a technical college in Ealing.

Bert Thomas sent for me and told me, as I already knew, that my parents would like me to do medicine. I completely rejected the idea. Bert then said 'Boy, no medical school would take you.' As in the season ticket encounter, he knew his pupils, and me, very well. I immediately set about applying for places in medical schools. In those days each university, and each London medical school, had its own admission arrangements. I was by then a very late applicant. I applied for a scholarship at St Mary's Hospital, which was allocated solely on the basis of an interview with the Dean. He examined my rugby playing career and very little else. I did not get the place. I also applied to the Westminster Hospital, where my interview consisted of a slanging match between me and the Dean as to why 'people like you' – young Jewish men – should be exempted from conscription. Medical students were deferred from military service as long as they passed their examinations because it was accepted that doctors were required for the Armed Forces, for dealing with civilian casualties and sickness, and for treating people in a normal, post-war society.

Unusually for a London schoolboy, I applied for admission to the Faculty of Medicine at the University of Edinburgh. I had decided by then that I would like a career in Forensic Medicine, and Edinburgh had a world-renowned department headed by Professor Sidney Smith. I had read his textbook of Forensic Medicine,[4] and also the book by Professor Glaister and Professor Brash about the infamous Dr Buck Ruxton, who had murdered his wife and their nanny and dumped the body parts in the Lake District.[5] The university accepted medical students solely on their academic record and their headmaster's report. I was accepted subject to passing the pre-registration examination (about English matric standard) in Physics. As a great concession they exempted me from the Chemistry examination because of my distinction in higher schools.

When I went to Edinburgh in June to sit my pre-registration exams it was British Double Summer time, two hours ahead of the sun. I arrived in Edinburgh in the early afternoon, walked towards Leith, found a cheap hotel, and went to sleep. I awoke in broad daylight to find it was 8.30 a.m. – the exam was at nine in the Old Quadrangle and I had no idea where that was. I rushed out, and asked a group of children what day it was. Accustomed as I was to anti-Semitism I met a new phenomenon of 'anti-Englishism'. The kids in Leith mocked my London accent and were singularly unhelpful. They looked at me as if I were mad and explained to me that in the north the sunset was very late, that it was still the evening of the same day, and not the next morning. I found the examination room, sat the exam on time and passed. I was accepted as a medical student to start in October 1943.

FOOTNOTES AND REFERENCES
1 The original *Wagon Wheels*, music by Peter DeRose and lyrics by Billy Hill, was first sung in the Ziegfeld Follies of 1934.
2 My son and a least one of my grandsons had the same problem.
3 Lehrman SM. *The Jewish Festivals*. London: Shapiro, Valentine; 1938.
4 Smith S. *Forensic Medicine*. London: J & A Churchill; 1957.
5 Glaister J, Brash J. *Medico Legal Aspects of the Ruxton Case*. London: E & S Livingston; 1937.

CHAPTER 2

University
and the army

WHEN I WENT TO EDINBURGH TO START MY DEGREE COURSE IN
September 1943, I found digs in Marchmont with a woman who had another
lodger – first year medical student Michael Miles, who came from Birmingham.
Even by the standards of Marchmont landladies ours was mean and unfriendly. I
did not stay there for very long as I had become friendly with a young veterinary
surgeon who arranged for me to move into digs opposite the Royal (Dick)
Veterinary College. When the landlady discovered she had a medical viper in
the nest I was thrown out.

In Edinburgh medical students spent their first year studying Chemistry,
Physics and Biology for the First Professional Examination, and began the two-
year course in Anatomy. With my scientific background I had more than enough
time for Anatomy. The Head of the Department was Professor Brash, but the
backbone of the department was the Senior Lecturer (in age and standing) Dr
EB Jamieson – Jimmy. He had been in the department since time immemorial
and was, to put it mildly, an eccentric. He always wore a long white coat and a
small black skullcap with a tassel. He spoke slowly, had a phenomenal memory,
and would often greet new students with reminiscences of their fathers. He was
also a misogynist.

His course each year opened with the words, 'The abdomen is divided into
two parts . . .' and continued in the same vein, so that each year students who
had finished the course sold typewritten notes to the 'freshers' who were starting
it. The teaching was based on dissection, and 'Jimmy's Diagrams'. These were
originally blackboard drawings that were published as a loose-leaf book in
1934. We used the seventh edition – a colour edition![1] With my visual memory

I could recall each and every diagram and I did well earning a First Class Merit Certificate, which later secured for me a paid post as an undergraduate demonstrator in Anatomy.

Bodies were dissected by groups of students, who did a different 'part' each term. I started on an upper limb. The other members of the group were Jimmy Harkess, from the notable Edinburgh family of undertakers; Bill Graham, the youngest student in the year and son of a naval engineer from Dunfermline; Dave Atkinson, the eldest son of a chemical engineer at the ICI works in Billingham; and Norrie Bremner, also of Edinburgh. We became friends the first day and remained close for our entire student lives and to a considerable degree throughout our adult lives. In view of my cockney accent, I was immediately nicknamed Jock Marks, which I am still known as by some to this day.

As work was not a problem I devoted a large part of my leisure time to ballroom dancing, at the Palais and elsewhere. The Student's Union had a Saturday night hop and there was a considerable influx of women from the Athol Crescent School of Domestic Science. These 'doughgirls' were in great demand, as women medical students, who comprised about 30 per cent of our year, were conspicuous by their absence from the dances. The band was made up of students from all faculties and made a very acceptable noise.

After I was thrown out of my 'vet' digs, the outlook looked bleak. Jimmy Harkess lived with his mother Kit and father James in Easter Road on the ground floor of a tenement. Above, at number 17, lived an elderly and very prim and proper widow, Mrs Williamson. She had never taken students but somehow Kit persuaded her to take me in. She made two stipulations – no girls and no alcohol. Smoking was permitted.

Mrs Williamson had two sons in the forces who did not give her the love and attention she deserved. She began to mother me and I must have eaten half of her meagre rations in addition to my own. Her real feelings became apparent in May 1946 – my twenty-first birthday – when I arranged a skittles party in Leith. A drunken mob left the skittle alley and gathered outside Mrs Williamson's apartment screaming at the top of their voices, 'Mrs Williamson – Jock is drunk – throw him out'. They could be heard in Holyrood Palace, but not in 17 Easter Road. The matter was never raised again and I stayed on there until I qualified in 1948.

In addition to their academic studies, all students were required to do some form of military service. The University Air Squadron and its Naval equivalent were restricted to people who were working for commissions in those services and so most medical students were drafted into the Senior Training Corps (STC), which was incorporated into the Home Guard. We did military drill and exercises at least one half day a week, as well as weekend camps. Our instructors

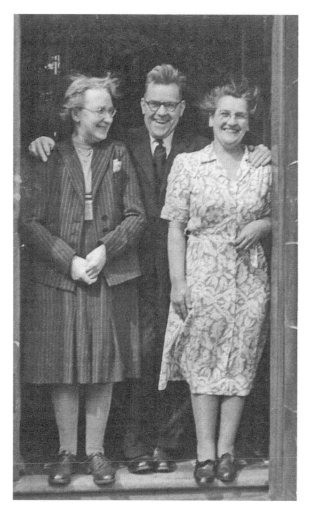

FIGURE 2.1 Left to right: Kit Harkess, John (Jock) Harkess and Mrs Williamson (my landlady), Edinburgh 1948.

were non-commissioned officers from the Highland Light Infantry and other Highland Regiments. Their favourite sport was to march us through roads thick with horse dung and to yell 'Under effective fire!', whereupon we were to lie down on the road instantly. Lord help the tardy or reticent. The 'sector' that we were to defend against the German Invasion was Dalkeith, about eight miles from the centre of Edinburgh. We marched there in full equipment, being passed by Scottish Motor Traction busses bearing the logo 'Take the bus it's more convenient'.

We were taught Physics by Dr Beevers, a scientist who was not used to boisterous medical students and who found it very difficult to deal with us. In return we took advantage of him and subjected him to flying paper darts, bottles rolling down the stepped lecture theatre floors, and other pranks. When he entered the lecture theatre on D-day he was faced with a sea of newspapers. The First Professional Examination in Physics was scheduled for a few days later, but members of the STC were ordered by the military authorities to report to the Waverley Station to unload wounded soldiers from the ambulance trains arriving there at the same time as the examination. The vast majority of the male students went to the station – the women, unfit males, and a few other males sat the examination. The paper was absurdly simple.

Dr Beevers could do nothing but set a separate examination later for the STC members. The paper that he set was extremely difficult, and a large number of the male students, including many of his tormentors, failed it. Their summer holidays were spent preparing for the 're-sits'. They were in a potentially disastrous situation because any student who failed an examination twice was sent down. They then lost their exemption from conscription and were 'called up' almost immediately.

On 8 May 1945 the war in Europe ended and I remember particularly the bright daylight when I fell asleep in Princes Street Gardens wrapped in an old Union Jack at about midnight. One evening during the summer vacation I went to the Royal Dance Hall in Tottenham. My school friend, John King, was there on leave from the Navy and he told us that an atom bomb had been dropped on Hiroshima. We did not recognise the significance that night, but I have always been deeply aware that I, and many of my contemporaries, survived to have careers and families because of it.

My first clinical firm was in the ward of Dr A Rae Gilchrist, an eminent cardiologist with a peculiar vocal presentation, and a reputation for being a martinet. A few days after starting on the ward we were shown a patient whose complaint was that he had become breathless when being chased by an elephant – quite true, he was a big game hunter. I was told to take his pulse, which was very slow and completely irregular. I reported this and was then ordered to listen to his heart. Deeply confused by now, I said, 'I can hear two sounds, Sir, and a third'. Dr Gilchrist screamed at me, 'Who told you that?' I had no idea what he was talking about but replied, 'No one'. Apparently this patient had a split first sound, a presystolic murmur and was in atrial fibrillation – all gobbledygook to me! I became the blue-eyed boy, was offered the opportunity to work in Rae Gilchrist's ward during the coming summer holidays, and to be considered for his house job on qualification. However, when I went back to the ward in the vacation it was full of returning ex-service doctors being re-trained. I was rapidly forgotten.

Ray Gilchrist's ward was the centre for an experiment with the new wonder drug called penicillin. All cases of a fatal heart disease called subacute bacterial endocarditis from the whole of the east of Scotland were brought to our unit so that they could be given penicillin by injection every three hours, night and day. We were expected to monitor their progress. At the other end of the clinical scale university medical students were required to do 'dispensary practice' in which we acted, under remote control, as unqualified general practitioners in the slums of Edinburgh.

As a result of this diversity of training I qualified as a doctor having seen thirteen cases of subacute endocarditis and one of measles! Also, while we were doing dispensary practice we were taught to vaccinate against smallpox and I was issued with a certificate stating that I was recognised as 'a public vaccinator'. Without that piece of paper I could not register as a medical practitioner.

Our medical education was at a very high academic level, but we needed more experience in clinical medicine outside the university in order to be competent doctors. During our six weeks summer holiday we were required to find some sort of clinical work near to our homes. In my first summer break I went to Shrodells Hospital in Watford and the following year I was accepted at St Leonard's Hospital in Shoreditch, a large London County Council (LCC) ex-workhouse full of very sick, mainly elderly, patients. The medical superintendent was Dr Bernstein, a brilliant clinician and a wonderful teacher. I learned more about examining and treating patents in six weeks there than I did in three years on the wards in Edinburgh, where the superb teaching was diluted by the numbers of students in each ward.

During my fourth year I held an undergraduate house job at the Western Infirmary in Edinburgh. We took bloods, clerked patients and made ourselves as useful as possible acting as 'housemen' to the housemen. In return we were given free board and lodging and practical experience. In that year my career prospects also changed. Sidney Smith did not take the course on Forensic Medicine. The lecturer we had was very boring and that, combined with my lifelong ability to sleep immediately after lunch, meant that I missed the entire course. I passed the Professional Examination, but knew that I had no future in that department. I decided instead that I would be an obstetrician and gynaecologist.

In my final year I was attached to the surgical clinic of Professor Sir James Learmonth, who I found to be particularly unpleasant. Each student was expected to 'clerk' a number of patients and on our first ward round we stopped at one of my patients who was enclosed in a weird contraption of metal rods, wires, strings and pulleys. The professor asked me what the device was for. I said it was to stop the patient bending his knee, whereupon Sir James pulled on one of the bits of string and miraculously the knee bent. He yelled at me,

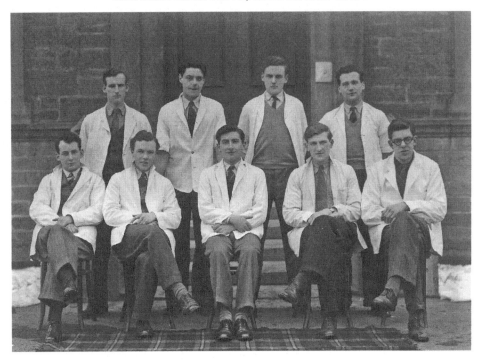

FIGURE 2.2 Undergraduate, and one graduate, housemen, Western Infirmary, Edinburgh, 1947.

'You'll never make a doctor!' To be told that by the Professor of Surgery did not suggest that my future was to be a bright one, and so you can imagine how we both felt when he had to give me a first class merit certificate in surgery at the end of the term.

Obstetrics and Gynaecology were also part of the final year studies and we were required to conduct at least twelve normal deliveries. There was a long tradition of Edinburgh students going to Dublin to do their midwifery, which persisted during the war and after it. Everyone wanted to go to the Rotunda Hospital but by the time I came to book it was full and so I, and most of my close friends, went to the Coombe Hospital, deep in the slums of Dublin. Because I could not get a direct boat from Glasgow to Dublin I went via Belfast and I remember being astonished to see British police carrying guns. In the train from Belfast to Dublin there was a large notice listing all the items banned in the south and the harsh penalties that could be imposed. Contraceptives headed the list, but like most medical students my pockets were stuffed with them because they were easily sold in the Free State and were a useful form of currency.

We arrived at the Coombe to find that it had been double booked, but they assured us that they would find sufficient cases for us and they told us we were to go out in pairs. That winter was one of the most severe in living memory, the whole of the British Isles being frozen. The fuel situation in the [Irish] Free State was even worse because coal could not be imported from the United States, and so, although there was ample food in the shops, including things that we had not seen for years like beef steaks, there was only gas for two hours a day and cooking was very difficult. After a few days my suit got stained and I took it to the cleaners. As we left the shop Jimmy and I realised that our entire stock of contraceptives was in the pockets. When we collected the suit a few days later the pockets were empty.

Students went out in pairs. The homes we went to work in were hovels deep in the Dublin slums and in disused old British army barracks. To describe the poverty as 'grinding' was an understatement – it was almost unbelievable and unbearable. On one occasion Jimmy Harkess and I went to a residence in the disused Curragh barracks. There was an absolute rule that once you went to a house you could not leave until the baby was delivered and this woman's labour went on for many hours. All three of us were frozen until I produced the best piece of obstetric equipment that we had, my British Army greatcoat. We covered her up. Hours later, when none of us could keep their eyes open, I uttered words that were to become famous in my year 'Move over woman', and crept in beside her fully clothed and went to sleep.[2] Fortunately she finally delivered a healthy baby.

I found the poverty and the squalor of Dublin very distressing and when my last case was delivered I headed for the boat. I swore I would never return to Ireland again. However, years later I had to visit the country representing the British Medical Association (BMA) and after my daughter married an Irishman we became regular visitors. It was wonderful watching the country progress to an unbelievable level of prosperity as a result of its membership of the European Economic Community.

The Final Professional Examination took place over several weeks in June 1948. It was a harrowing experience with many written examinations, oral examinations, and worst of all clinical cases. So much depended on who the Examiner was and how he felt, and also of course whether or not you knew your stuff. Like most of the other students I was convinced that I had failed, although I had never failed an exam in my life. The few days that we spent waiting for the results seemed like an eternity and even alcohol could not ease our misery.

Monday 5 July 1948 was the day that the National Health Service Act of 1946 came into effect, or to put it more dramatically, that day the NHS started. On the radio the reader of the early morning news said, 'Today is a great day for British medicine'. It was, because at six o'clock that evening the results of our final degree examination were to be posted on the wall of the university. When the results went up I had passed, but sadly several of my friends had not. Rosemary Davey, the genius of our year said to me, 'I suppose you're going to get drunk', to which I replied 'Too bloody true', and I did.

In those days, doctors registered with the General Medical Council (GMC) for life by paying a single fee of two guineas. I registered on the 14 July 1948 at the GMC office in Edinburgh and became a Registered Medical Practitioner. At that time, there was no legal restriction on a doctor's practice following registration and the concept of pre-registration and organised vocational training was years away.

I went back to London and visited St Leonard's Hospital just to tell Dr Bernstein and his colleagues that, thanks to them, I was now qualified. I was asked if I would like a job as a locum while I looked for a permanent position. I accepted and asked when the job started, to which they replied, 'Now'. That was how my clinical career started – as an unsupervised locum casualty officer.

That night a 90-year-old man with acute retention of urine was admitted. I arranged for a surgeon to come in and asked where I could find an anaesthetist. I was told, 'It's you'. I gave the chap an injection of Pentothal,[3] he went to sleep, and stopped breathing. I vaguely remembered seeing someone somewhere putting a tube down the throat of an anaesthetised patient, and so I closed my eyes and shoved the tube somewhere – luckily it went into his trachea and he resumed breathing. He survived, but I'm sure that if he had died no one would have been blamed for allowing a barely qualified young doctor to administer the anaesthetic. That is what medicine was like in the 'good old days'.

I saw a job advertised at Wembley Hospital, which, the advertisement claimed, was to become part of Charing Cross Hospital, a prestigious London teaching hospital. Wembley Hospital had been a general practitioner hospital with visiting consultants and was run by a board of governors who were all local GPs. General practitioners still had the right to admit their own patients and treat them with or without consultant advice. My duties during my first six months' appointment included being the casualty officer, the paediatric houseman, the ears, nose and throat houseman, and an occasional anaesthetist. During my second six months' appointment I looked after the surgical, gynaecological and orthopaedic cases. The hospital had about a hundred beds with a staff of three – me, one other houseman and one resident surgical officer, who was alone in being allowed to use the single primitive electrocardiogram machine!

We had a large collection of eminent and not so eminent London consultants who were very keen to come to Wembley because they acquired a considerable number of private patients through their contacts with the local doctors. I had three ear, nose and throat surgeons to look after, but my main function was to be

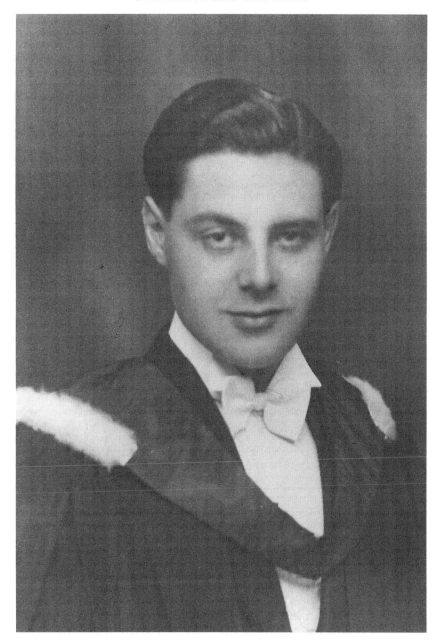

FIGURE 2.3 My graduation photograph, July 1948.

the casualty officer. On my second night on duty two young men were brought in after a motorcycle accident, having been carried into Alperton bus garage on the front of a bus. One of them died in minutes, but I managed to resuscitate the other man. I believe the first one had the better deal because when I left the hospital almost a year later the other one was still lying there semiconscious, with multiple fractures to his limbs.

One day I admitted a man with a very high temperature. The story was that he had had intermittent attacks of fever, and his general practitioner had been giving him sulphonamide drugs for months on end. He obviously had septicaemia, from which he died in a couple of days. When I wrote 'septicaemia' on the death certificate the other doctors told me that if I did that there would be an inquest, and that I should give a different cause of death. I declined to do so because I believed there was a distinct possibility that his death was related to a well-known complication of sulphonamide drugs – they could damage bone marrow. The condition is called agranulocytosis. Such patients can no longer fight infection and before antibiotics they invariably died. The registrar notified the coroner's officer and a post-mortem was arranged. An eminent pathologist from London was appointed to do the post-mortem examination, which I attended. He did a very cursory examination and decided that the man had died naturally from a form of leukaemia. Unlike that eminent gentleman, I removed a piece of bone marrow and sent it away for analysis, though of course the result came back long after the inquest had been forgotten.

I went to the inquest at Whetstone in a panic because I was certain the first question would be, 'How long have you been qualified Dr Marks?' I met the general practitioner who had been treating the man. He had qualified in Ireland many years before, had a huge list of patients all of whom thought that the sun shone from him, and was in high spirits but rather angry that his golf was delayed. A verdict of natural causes was given and everyone was happy but me. Months later I received the results of the bone marrow examination. They proved that the man had died of a condition called aleukaemic leukaemia, a great rarity and completely irrelevant to the doctor's actions. So, both the eminent pathologist and the cocky houseman were completely wrong. More importantly, I learned that in those days some people in the profession were quite happy to cover up other people's mistakes – even to lie in order to do so – and that they were prepared to put pressure on others to do the same.

Another interesting case involved a patient who was brought in with very severe burns affecting most of his body. We gave him the usual analgesic injections and put up a saline drip. Only then did I ask him what had happened. It was an incredible story. He worked at the British Oxygen Company (BOC) at Wembley and had been smoking while he was pouring out liquid oxygen.

His cigarette fell through the grill over the well where the waste liquid oxygen fell, and he removed the grill and went into the well to rescue it. The poor man died from his injuries.

I now had to attend my second inquest. The coroner asked me if the man had told me what had happened and I said, truthfully, 'Not at the time'. Before I could say another word I was dismissed, but I remained at the back of the court. I was recalled to the witness box and asked by an angry coroner if I had been told later what had caused the accident. When I told the court what the patient had told me all hell broke loose – one after the other lawyers stood up claiming to represent the man's family, his trade union, his employer, their insurers and goodness knows who else. I learned another lesson at that moment – medicine does not exist in a vacuum.

The paediatric unit at Wembley had about a dozen beds and the visiting consultant from London was a pompous, self-important man. As far as he was concerned the main duties of the houseman consisted of meeting him at the door of the hospital when he arrived and carrying his bag. Teaching was non-existent. No visitors were allowed until a child had been in hospital for at least six weeks, and in those days when we had cases of rheumatic fever and osteomyelitis in the ward that was not rare.

Tuberculous meningitis was invariably fatal. A new drug called streptomycin was being used experimentally to treat it and when we had a case admitted it was included in the trial. Every day I had to inject the drug into the child's spinal canal, an unpleasant exhausting experience for both of us. I also had to complete numerous forms in quadruplicate. Miraculously, the child survived but sadly its mental state was incompatible with a normal life.

I earned the princely salary of £250 a year. When I had finished my first six months appointment I was automatically appointed to the other job in the hospital and I had to be replaced. My position was advertised and there were countless applications for it, as there was for every other medical vacancy in the country. A friend of mine, George Goodman (now a retired radiologist in Vancouver, British Columbia) was one of the applicants. When the members of the selection committee had finished playing poker with the housemen and winning most of their meagre salaries from them,[4] they discussed the applicants. The decision was made to interview all of them and then to appoint 'John Marks' friend'. That was the norm for those days and no one gave it a second thought.

Each houseman was allowed one afternoon off a week and one weekend of each month. Even then we were expected to be available on telephone. We were of course exploited, but were happy to be part of the great new experiment in health care – the National Health Service (NHS). My paediatric consultant, who also did general medical outpatients, was inundated with requests for wigs. The public did not accept that going bald was a natural phenomenon – it was an illness that the NHS was expected to treat. Fortunately, after a while both clinicians and the state refused to go along with that. However, it was wonderful to watch my chief's face each time someone asked for a wig, because he was as bald as a coot.

The other physician at the hospital was a young man who had recently been appointed at St Thomas's Hospital as well as Wembley. His name was Dr John Richardson MVO. He had gained that medal for treating King George VI for a chest infection in North Africa. In contrast to some of his colleagues, John Richardson treated housemen kindly and as professionals and spent time teaching them.[5] Years later he was knighted, and I had many contacts with him when he was president of both the GMC and the BMA. His wife was a well-known artist Sylvia Trist. I still have a small pencil study that she did of me at a meeting of the Guild of St Luke held at the RSA on 25 March 1976 where I was a speaker and her husband was a guest of honour.

The surgeons who I worked for were all very different people. One, Mr Grant Batchelor, was the typical upright West End surgeon, complete with black jacket and striped trousers. He was meticulous and fastidious. He insisted on keeping his hernia cases flat on their backs for two weeks and claimed that he had never had a recurrent hernia – it never dawned on him that they might have gone somewhere else. My other chief was John Shirley Callcut, who had been a general practitioner surgeon on the staff of the hospital for many years and who was highly respected by all the local general practitioners and their grateful patients. The new NHS bureaucracy decreed that John Callcut could not be a consultant because he did not have the magic letters FRCS after his name. He had sat the Fellowship once, but when the examiners failed him he refused to meet them again. The managers graded him as senior hospital medical officer, but as far as everyone else was concerned he was a full-blown consultant and had the largest private practice for miles around.

There were three perks for housemen: cremation fees, private certificates, and presents from the chiefs for assisting at their private operations. The fee for the statutory certificates required for cremation was one guinea (one pound one shilling, now £1.05). The doctor kept the pound and the shilling went to the hospital porter. Private certificates were very rare – they were a perk of the general practitioner. Occasionally one of the consultants did a private operation at Wembley and most of them gave a cash donation to the housemen who assisted them.

I enjoyed my year at Wembley, and I learned a lot of medicine. However, looking back I wonder how much damage unsupervised partly trained doctors like me did to patients. Many years later when I was involved in medical training and in medical discipline I realised that training alone did not make good doctors and that supervision did not weed out the poor ones.

Towards the end of my second house job I received notification of my impending call-up into the Army. I reported at the Royal Army Medical Corps (RAMC) depot at Crookham on the scheduled day in October 1949. The British Army commissioned qualified doctors as full lieutenants with two pips. It was necessary to convert educated, unenthusiastic 23-year-olds into officers within six weeks and so the course was intensive. We started with square bashing and, as in the STC, we were trained by Scottish Regimental sergeant majors who had no great love for middle-class university graduates. However, we were officers and they were not, so we could only be abused in terms such as 'Pick your bloody feet up, Sir' and 'Get your bloody hair cut, Sir'. We also received intensive training in military law and how to behave as an officer and a gentleman.

We then moved to Mychett, where the RAMC had its Public Health Training School. After that we were granted two weeks embarkation leave, but before going home we were given injections against typhoid and paratyphoid fevers. Nobody reminded us about the effects of alcohol after these injections and by the time I got to the platform at Ash Vale station I felt ghastly – by the time I got home I had a high fever and spent the next few days in bed.

Before being sent on leave we had been given a 'choice' of destination. I made it clear I did not want to go to the Middle East. A far as I was concerned it was the second worst posting available, West Africa being the worst because there was a war going on there. I was duly posted to the Middle East and embarked on the *Empire Windrush*[6] for my journey to Port Said. As an officer I travelled first class, which meant I had a small cabin to myself and ate in a dining room. Other ranks travelled on 'troop decks' where they were packed in like sardines and slept in hammocks.

On arrival at Port Said we were moved to General Headquarters Middle East, which was at Fayid, on the Suez Canal, south of Ismalia. Once again we were asked to choose our postings and I requested anywhere but Egypt and so I was promptly sent to Moascar, headquarters of British Troops Egypt alongside the town of Ismalia. There, for the third time, I was asked to choose my destination and again I requested that I be sent to any part in Egypt but the Canal Zone. I was dispatched to the headquarters of the Canal Zone where I met Colonel Malveney, the Assistant Director of Medical Services (ADMS). I don't know what he was like as a doctor but as a disciplinarian he was an absolute Tartar. As there was no obvious posting for me at the time I remained in his office for a week or two as Deputy Assistant Director of Medical Services (DADMS) where I learned a great deal about medical administration in the Army.

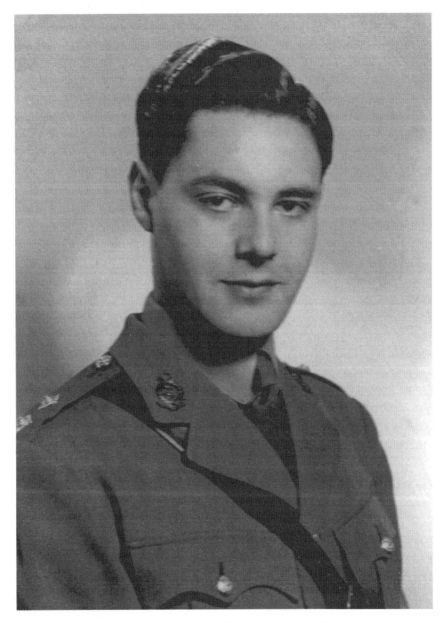

FIGURE 2.4 Lt Marks RAMC 405940, October 1949. On embarkation leave.

I was then finally posted to the Supply Reserve Depot at El-Kirsh, a few miles west of the Canal and about seven miles north of Ismalia. That unit was unique. It comprised a large number of aircraft hangars full of food and other supplies sufficient to maintain an army in the field for months and was commanded by a lieutenant-colonel in the RASC. Apart from me, one or two other specialist officers and a War Office civilian scientist, all the officers were from the RASC.

Life was very pleasant at El-Kirsh, where I lived in the officers' mess and became part of their community. I was the general practitioner and hygiene specialist for the officers and men of the garrison and the few families who lived there. Soon after my arrival I was consulted by the colonel, who had a monumental hangover. I concocted a simple mixture for him and it worked like a charm. My professional status was enhanced forever.

Among the troops in the garrison was a company of Mauritian 'guards' which was employed and deployed solely to guard the garrison perimeter. I found it difficult to reconcile the medical documents of these men, which showed them to be perfect human specimens, with the weedy individuals who stood in front of me. I was then let in on a great secret. When the sugar crop failed in Mauritius there was very little work around, but the British Army had a recruiting centre that was actively seeking men. My puny individuals signed on and were then asked to attend for a medical examination to see if they were fit to serve. Before the medical examination, substitutions occurred with a fit, strapping specimen presenting himself using a recruit's name. The substitute got his payment, the weed got into the Army, and the recruiting office got its recruits. Everyone was happy.

I had a subsidiary job at El-Kirsh. Once a week I was driven into Ismalia to inspect civilian premises to see whether they were fit for British Service families to rent because there was insufficient accommodation for the large number of wives and children who accompanied the regular Army personnel in the Moascar garrison. The thing that mattered above all was the state of the kitchen, which was shared by the householder and the British wife. Ismalia was a mixed community of Arabs, Greeks, and the occasional French family, each with very different standards of hygiene. My job did not make me popular with locals because if I turned down their kitchen I turned down their income. In the end I had to be accompanied by an armed guard.

Our civilian scientist was posted home and the War Department did not provide a replacement. One day the colonel sent for me and told me they were having a special board and that I was to replace the non-existent analyst. We went into one of the hangars where there were literally hundreds of thousands of tins of condensed milk with expiry dates that had been passed by many years.

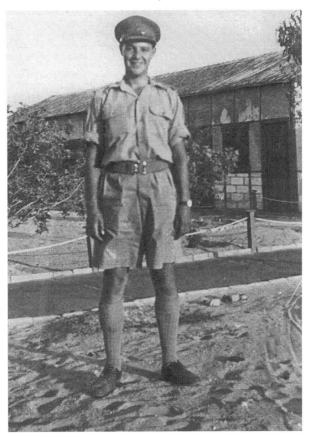

FIGURE 2.5 At Supply Reserve Depot, El-Kirsh, Egypt, 1950.

The officers looked at one or two tins, prodded them, and pronounced that they could have their expiry date extended by another year or two. Someone then produced a piece of paper and asked me to sign it. I looked at it carefully and noted that I was giving a professional opinion supporting the extension of the 'use-by date' of the milk. I explained carefully that there was no way that I was going to sign that piece of paper as I had no training or experience in food science and if my opinion was challenged I would, quite rightly, have looked to be an idiot. The colonel was very unhappy but I was adamant and so the entire consignment was condemned as unfit for human consumption. A hole was dug in the desert and the tins were buried deep in the sand, but the next day they were freely available in the markets in Ismalia at a knockdown price.

I was very happy at El-Kirsh, but after about nine months I was moved to the garrison at Moascar, where I was the officer commanding the Medical

Reception Station (MRS). This was a small medical unit with about 20 beds for soldiers with minor illnesses who, in civilian life, would have been treated by a few days in bed at home. I had a corporal and about nine other ranks. The unit was within the curtilage of the Military Families Hospital commanded by a lieutenant-colonel who was a trained gynaecologist, although in reality most of the gynaecology and obstetrics was performed by a National Service lieutenant from Leeds called Henry Shapiro, who had been qualified for two or three years. To make matters more complicated, as the commanding officer of the MRS I was responsible for the discipline of the 'other ranks' on the hospital staff.

Like every other commanding officer in the British Army I held a morning 'orderly room' where I dished out minor punishments such as 'confined to barracks' (CB), with more serious cases being referred to headquarters in Moascar. I lived in the garrison mess, which was dominated by officers of the Signal Corps, many of whom had been involved in the troubles in Palestine and taken part in the arrest and internment in Cyprus of Jews fleeing from Europe to Palestine in the closing year of the mandate. That was the one and only time that I met open anti-Semitism in the Army. On the other hand, the Army provided regular transport for Jewish officers and men to attend religious services on Friday nights, which could be held in Ismalia, Port Said, Suez, or even Tel-el-Kabir. The Jewish chaplain Captain Alec Ginsberg, for whom I had the greatest admiration, conducted them. He was followed everywhere by the Egyptian secret police, but to us he was a hero. I remember the supreme irony of having a Passover service, which commemorates the exodus of the Israelites from slavery in Egypt, at which we were served by very unhappy Egyptian servants.

The Korean War broke out on the 25 June 1950. Shortly afterwards an order was issued that all officers and other ranks were to assemble in their units to hear a broadcast by the Prime Minister Clement Attlee. He told us that conscription was to be extended from eighteen months to two years. I had to deal with the anger and disappointment of my own troops as well as those of the hospital, but to their surprise my anger, my misuse of the English language, and my capacity to swear, far surpassed theirs.

The thieving of medical stores in Egypt was a highly developed and sophisti-cated skill. The storeroom of my Medical Reception Station had a skylight that was less than two feet square, but one night local thieves got in through it and removed all my stores. I was arraigned before a disciplinary board, but all the officers serving as members of the board were my patients and they decided that I had not been negligent. Instead, they said it was disgraceful that a young national service medical officer should be exposed in the way that I was. I then had a wonderful lesson in military ingenuity. Headquarters sent me a lieutenant quartermaster RAMC who had been in the Army before I was born. My 'second-in-command' convened another board, comprising only National Service medical officers. He produced a piece of cloth that he tore into small pieces. He then said to the other officers, 'Fifty sheets written off', and they were. He did the same with all sorts of pieces of junk that had acquired the status of 'valuable medical equipment' and at the end of the day all the equipment had been written off, the Army was off the hook, and I was still a commanding officer.

I was by now a bit of an embarrassment to the Army. Someone had a brilliant idea of sending me to Tel-el-Kabir as senior medical officer, a post that carried a major's pay but not the rank. Tel-el-Kabir was one of the worst postings in Egypt. It was an isolated garrison, halfway to Cairo, with enormous stores of military hardware, subject to periodic armed raiding by bandits and guerrillas who objected to our being there and who had a ready market for their stolen goods.

I entered the officers' mess dining room and sat down next another medical officer who asked me what I was doing in Tel-el-Kabir. I told him I was a new senior medical officer. He looked at me and said, 'Rubbish. I am the new senior medical officer.' He then asked who had sent me to Tel-el-Kabir. When I replied, 'GHQ British Troops Egypt', he smirked and said, 'I was sent here by GHQ Middle East'. GHQ Middle East was the senior headquarters and so after lunch I was driven back to Moascar.

I solved the Army's problem of my being an embarrassment to them by being taken ill with a high fever that required admission to the British Military Hospital at Fayid. Investigations were started and some genius decided that I had malaria. I was started on quinine by mouth and as I got worse they gave me intravenous quinine. The next day I was deeply jaundiced because I, and half the officers of the unit I'd been with, had infective hepatitis. I was in Fayid hospital six weeks and enjoyed three weeks convalescence following that.[7]

To make amends for my fruitless journey to Tel-el-Kabir they gave me the best posting in the Canal Zone for a non-specialist medical officer, looking after Army families in Ismalia and in the huge transit camp alongside the town. The medical inspection room, which I shared with another RAMC officer, Captain Campbell, was in the transit camp and the job we did was exactly the same as general practice in the United Kingdom. Needless to say it was not without incident.

I was consulted by a large, aggressive German woman, the wife of one of the senior warrant officers of the garrison. She had a trivial skin condition that I decided I could treat, but she took the view that I had to send her to a dermatologist and I insisted that she did not need specialist care. Her husband complained to his commanding officer and once more I was dragged up in front of a senior officer for chastisement. The warrant officer came in, saluted smartly, and gave his story. I was asked for my views and I said that in my clinical opinion she did not require specialist advice and furthermore I intended to consult my Medical Defence Organisation in London. A hushed silence descended and the warrant officer and I were both asked to leave the room. I was asked to return and I was followed by the warrant officer who saluted smartly, withdrew his complaint, and immediately retired. I would love to have been a fly on the wall and to have known what happened during my absence. In retrospect, medical officers who were not regulars were a complete pain to the Army because they desperately needed us but we did not respond to the normal pressures that exist in any hierarchy.

That posting also demonstrated the different attitudes that the Royal Air Force Medical Service and the Royal Army Medical Corps had towards its officers. By coincidence my close friend, David Atkinson, was doing exactly the same job in Ismalia. I was by now a captain – he was a squadron leader, equivalent to a major in the Army. As a matter of interest, years later Dave became Air Vice-Marshall Sir David Atkinson, head of the Medical Services of the Royal Air Force. Another of my contemporaries, Sir Alan Rae, became Lieutenant-General Alan Rae, Director-General of the Army Medical Services, two weeks after Dave's promotion

It was strictly forbidden to go on leave outside the theatre of operations but several Jewish officers managed to go on holiday to the new State of Israel. The ploy was to go on leave to Cyprus, to change into civilian clothing there, pick up your passport which a parent had sent to you post restant, and then go to Israel as a civilian. I'm sure it never dawned on any one of them to desert, nor to act as a spy for Israel. Finally it was the turn of a doctor from Glasgow, who I will call Bernard, to go. For some reason or other the Army decided to recall him from leave but no lieutenant of his name could be found in Cyprus, although there was a record at the airport of a civilian of that name having flown to Israel.

When Bernard came back to Cyprus he was arrested and returned to Egypt where he was interrogated by the commander-in-chief's minions. He pleaded innocence of the orders but the general said that, although he would accept Bernard's excuse, no one else would be able to use it again, and it was reiterated in general orders that to leave the theatre – the 'British' Middle East – was a serious offence. I went to Cyprus on leave and I looked for two weeks at a signpost that said 'Jerusalem 200 miles'.

One day in the spring of 1951 I was examining a child with sores all over his face and in his mouth. During the examination the child coughed and I was aware of something going into my left eye. A few days later my left eye began to water and became red and painful. I saw the consultant ophthalmologist and was admitted to the Military Hospital at Fayid with the diagnosis of herpetic corneal ulceration. I was treated very simply – I had atropine drops to dilate my pupil and rest my eye and nothing else. I made a full recovery and returned to duty within a week. I will deal later with this problem, which recurred for the first time when I was working as an assistant in Chingford in 1954 and which ultimately led to my becoming blind in my left eye.

My term in Egypt having came to an end, I came home and was demobilised. I thought my military career had finished, but in October 1953 I was called up again as part of the 'Z reserve' and was instructed to report to Thetford in Suffolk for two weeks' military service. We set up a field ambulance to deal with the expected [mock] casualties that might be sustained by the troops taking part in a night exercise. It turned out to be an absolute waste of time and the only real casualty, a chap with a broken leg, received medical care at an abysmal level.

FOOTNOTES AND REFERENCES

1   Jamieson EB. *Illustrations of Regional Anatomy*. 7th ed. London: E & S Livingstone; 1947.

2   Tyler R. The cheeky chappie. *You Magazine*. 1988 Jun 12.

3   Sodium thiopental, better known as Pentothal (a trademark of Abbott Laboratories) is a short-acting barbiturate drug used as an intravenous anaesthetic.

4   This is not fantasy – it is the absolute truth. Working life in small cottage hospitals was very different from that in prestigious teaching hospitals or in the hierarchical, municipal ones.

5   Richardson, John Samuel, later Lord Richardson of Lee in the County of Devon (1910–2004). Kt 1960; LVO 1943; MRCS 1935; Hon FRCS 1980; MB BCh Cambridge 1936; MD 1940; MRCP 1937; FRCP 1948; Hon FRPharms 1974; FRCP Edinburgh 1975; Hon FRCP Ireland 1975; Hon FFCM 1977; Hon FRCPsych 1979; Hon FRCPSG 1980.

6   The ship originally called the *Monte Rosa* had been built in Germany. During the Second World War it was used as a troop ship and then a hospital ship. Seized at Kiel, it was refitted as a British troop carrier and renamed *Empire Windrush* in 1947. Its most celebrated journey took place the following year when it brought the first batch of immigrants from Jamaica to the UK. The full story can be found at: www. icons.org.uk/theicons/collection/ss-windrush/biography.

7   My period of hospitalisation coincided with a crisis in Iran when the Government of Muhammad Mossadeq was threatening to nationalise Anglo-Iranian Oil. There were suggestions that the British Army in Egypt would be used in the Persian Gulf, and the officers who visited me had on at least one occasion been actively prepared for such action.

CHAPTER 3 From lorry driver to
principal in general practice

I RETURNED TO A UNITED KINGDOM WITH A GLUT OF DOCTORS. WHEN the short-term locum post that I secured at the North Middlesex Hospital in Edmonton came to an end there was nothing else in sight, so for three weeks I earned my living working for my cousin, driving a lorry full of dresses up and down the Great North Road.

At that time I wanted to be a gynaecologist and I was looking for an appropriate house job. I applied for many but never got as far as an interview. My friend Jimmy Harkess was finishing a surgical house job at St Martin's Hospital in Bath and an obstetric job there became vacant. I was not keen to apply for it because it was not recognised for the Diploma in Obstetrics or for training for any other higher qualification. However there was no other job on the horizon and Jimmy's influence there secured my appointment in the same way that my influence at Wembley had helped George Goodman.

St Martin's was an old municipal hospital with a large obstetric unit staffed by three consultants, two housemen, and a Resident Surgical Officer. It had a vague link with the prestigious, ex-voluntary hospital, the Royal United. All three chiefs worked at both hospitals and the St Martin's housemen attended the odd gynaecological outpatient there as part of their training.

On my first night on duty a woman was admitted with her fourth illegitimate pregnancy. I examined her and decided that she had a breach presentation; the other, more experienced house surgeon also examined her and decided that she had a normal, so-called cephalic presentation. During the night the pair of us delivered twins! I managed to persuade the three obstetricians and the hospital administrators to change their arrangements so that I could apply to have the post recognised for the Diploma in Obstetrics and I then persuaded The Royal College of Obstetricians and Gynaecologists to accept it as fulfilling the requirements for training.

During one operating session a nurse came in a state of extreme agitation and told us that the King had died and that we now had a Queen. At another session the chief, Mr Leach Wilkinson, looked at me over his horn rimmed spectacles and asked me 'Marks, how many thumbs do you think you have?' I answered, 'Two Sir'. And he replied, 'I can count at least ten. Might it not be a good idea if you rethought your career prospects?' He was telling me what are already knew, that my poor manual dexterity would guarantee that I would fail as a surgeon and therefore could never be a gynaecologist.

Before I started work at Bath I met a girl who lived in Brighton called Sylvia Stroh and in time I fell desperately in love with her. Occasionally we met in London and one of those meetings took place on the day of King George VI's funeral. London was almost deserted. I had arranged to take Sylvia to Quo Vadis, a fashionable restaurant in Soho. When we arrived there I found to my horror that I had left most of my money back in Bath. I then had a piece of extraordinary luck. Sitting at another table was the owner of the garage in Tottenham where I took my car for servicing. He was sitting with a woman who I knew was not his wife. I strolled over and asked him if he could lend me some money for a short period and the speed with which he gave it to me was almost indecent.

When my six-month job at Bath came to an end I again joined the ranks of the unemployed. In those days doctors did not draw unemployment pay, they scrounged from their parents. I ultimately landed a job as a trainee assistant with Dr Harold Bloom of Teddington. The trainee assistantship scheme was dreamt up allegedly to improve the standard of general practice, but I believe the real motive was to give employment to a group of very discontented doctors. At least a third of my contemporaries had emigrated. Of my own close friends, Jimmy Harkess was in Louisville, Kentucky, Bill Graham was in South Africa, and George Goodman was in Canada.

Harold Bloom was a keen, caring, single-handed general practitioner whose surgery was attached to his house. He had very progressive ideas about the effects of emotional conflicts on the body and he taught me to look out for them. Domestic arrangements for trainees varied, but this one lived with the family and was constantly available. The first few weeks I sat with Dr Bloom whilst he did his surgery, accompanied him on visits, and drove his children to school. Gradually I saw patients on my own in the surgery and in their homes. As far as off-duty was concerned I had one half-day a week and every other weekend after Saturday surgery. The rest of the time I was on duty.

That winter we had a great smog and doing visits became a nightmare – I well remember driving along a pavement thinking I was on the road. Even in the early days of the service complaints of 'failure to visit' were extremely common and were dealt with harshly by the NHS authorities. Bad weather was not a valid excuse! Even then patients knew what they considered to be 'their rights', which in reality bore no relationship to what was actually possible.

During my traineeship I went with my brother Vincent to a dance at the Bonnington Hotel in Bloomsbury, which was organised by the London Jewish Graduates Association. There I met a young woman from Leeds called Phyllis, but nothing came of that relationship. I then went to a weekend party in Brighton arranged by the Graduates, where I first saw Shirley Nathan, a pretty girl in a green dress. We started going out together. When I finished my year at Teddington Dr Bloom wanted another trainee assistant and so I suggested to Shirley that she should apply for the job. She was appointed but for some inexplicable reason Harold Bloom did not like her. On the other hand his wife Bella, who loathed me, thought she was wonderful.

After my traineeship finished I found a job in Chingford with Dr Henry Blair, a first-class general practitioner. It was a straightforward assistantship with no 'view to partnership'. Henry and I got on well together and he taught me a great deal. In addition to his National Health Service practice he had a thriving private practice. I knew that there was enormous pressure from the Essex Executive Council for him to take a partner because he had a huge list of patients who needed two doctors to look after them and the NHS authorities wanted principals to provide that care, not transient assistants.

Shirley's parents were both born in the East End of London. Her father, Alec Nathan, entered the Civil Service at the age of 14 and progressed up the ladder, a large part of his life being spent in the Inland Revenue, where he became responsible for staffing. When I met him he had reached the rank of Principal in the Ministry of Supply, and when he retired he was awarded the OBE. He was a typical English gentleman and had acquired the classical clipped accent. Shirley's mother Esther had been head girl of her school, but following her marriage gave up work and became a doting mother who was also deeply involved in many charitable organisations. She too acquired an accent that could only be classed as 'received pronunciation', and was not particularly enamoured with their daughter's boyfriend's Cockney speech.

Our courtship survived its ups and downs and in November 1953 Shirley and I became engaged. When I told Harold Bloom he told me that I was mad – Bella expressed similar views to Shirley. They were both wrong.

Over the years my father-in-law and I became very close. He had part of his lung removed for cancer at the age of 75, gave up smoking, and enjoyed life for another 16 years. In spite of our early differences, in time I became quite fond of my mother-in-law, who also lived to the ripe old age of 89.

At the time of our engagement both of us were sitting the examination for the Diploma in Obstetrics of the Royal College of Obstetricians and Gynaecologists. In fact we became officially engaged between the written paper and the oral parts of the examination. Ironically, our euphoria made our interviews seem easy and we both passed. The great value of the qualification D (Obst) RCOG – now defunct – was that the NHS authorities were compelled to accept its holders on the 'Obstetric List', which meant that the doctor could look after pregnant women and deliver them in their homes and be paid at a higher rate for the job than those who were not on the list.

The wedding was set for the following June, after which we were going on honeymoon to Lake Como in Italy. We were well aware that many of our contemporaries were doing very well abroad but we both had fairly strong family ties and were not keen to break them. We decided that, if within three months of marriage we had not found the sort of practice we wanted, we would either 'go to Wigan' or 'catch the boat'. At that stage I still had delusions that Henry Blair might offer me a partnership.

We scanned the advertisements in the *British Medical Journal* (*BMJ*) every week looking for a practice advertised by an Executive Council in London or the Home Counties, or a partnership in the same area. In January 1954 we spotted an advertisement for an assistantship with view in Borehamwood, Hertfordshire. The practice had been started three years earlier by Philip Sattin. It was located on a huge housing estate that was being built by the old London County Council (LCC.) Sattin came from a wealthy family whose money came from the fashion industry. A couple of years later he took as a partner the young Glaswegian Carl Hodes, always known professionally as Charles Hodes, and they opened a branch surgery on a second estate being built to the north of Borehamwood Village. The surgeries became known as the Manor Way and the Theobald Street surgeries respectively. It was obvious to me that this was going to be a very progressive, forward-looking practice; a 'group practice', based on the ideas of Dr [later Lord] Stephen Taylor, which were being implemented in Harlow, New Town.[1] Unlike the publicly owned premises in Harlow, those in Borehamwood belonged to private landlords.

They had 120 applicants for their job. I was selected for interview. The interviews took place at the home of Philip Sattin, about six weeks before Shirley and I were due to be married. I received a formal offer of a partnership subject to a short assistantship to find out if we could work together. I was to receive a small share of the practice profits, the minimum third that the Government required, and I would progress to parity with the other partners over a seven-year period. It was illegal to buy and sell goodwill; however, there were other ways whereby new partners could subsidise existing ones. In my case the two premises used by the practice were leased from the landlords on a 30-year lease at a rate of £750 per year. As both buildings could have been bought quite easily for well under £5,000 each, the return on the capital was enormous. The landlords of the surgeries were the two partners' wives.

When I was offered the partnership in Borehamwood I went to see Henry and reminded him that he would have to take a partner sooner or later and that he and I worked very well together. One of the problems was his private practice, which, as far as the Executive Council was concerned, had to be included in the 'practice earnings' of which any partner must have a one third share. I got one of his famous smiles and he said 'I'm getting married at the weekend John.' He married a woman doctor, gave her half his list, solved his problem, and left me with no option but to accept the offer of a partnership in Borehamwood.

I was very keen to go to the Borehamwood practice and money had never been a very important factor in my life, but when I discussed the problem with our families they told me not to accept. However, I ignored that advice and told Philip and Carl that I was prepared to accept their terms and then reminded them that I was due to be married in June and that I had a honeymoon booked. They look horrified and told me quite simply that if I wanted to join their practice I could forget about a two-week honeymoon, but as a concession I could have a long weekend off. In those days I was too naive to argue with them and did not realise the strength of my position. I went back to Shirley's home to discuss the matter with her. She could see how keen I was to join the practice, but was very disappointed with the idea of giving up her honeymoon. In the end we agreed to do so, but she never forgave the partners.

We were married at Hendon Synagogue on Thursday June 17 1954. The local minister, Reverend Leslie Hardman who was the first British Army chaplain to enter Belsen, married us. Our reception was held at the Brent Bridge Hotel and the following morning we went to Northolt airport to catch a plane to Jersey for our weekend honeymoon. There was brilliant sunshine at Northolt and thick fog in Jersey and so we did not take off until the early afternoon. We stayed at the L'Horizon Hotel, a luxury that we would not be able to afford again for many years to come. On Sunday we returned to our new home, the upper half of a semi-detached house in Edgware, four miles from the practice, which we rented furnished while house hunting in Borehamwood.

I started work on the following Monday morning, 19 April 1954. Each doctor did a morning and evening surgery at both buildings, which were two miles apart, and anything up to 20 home visits a day. The Theobald Street estate was one huge building site with no street names or lighting – we had mobile

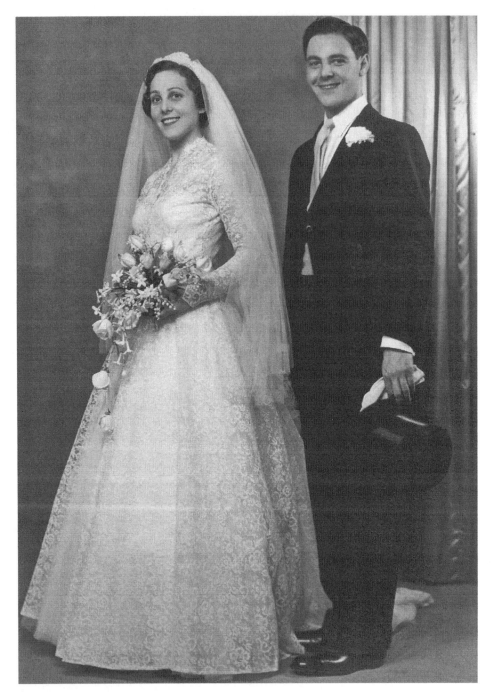

FIGURE 3.1 Wedding photograph with Shirley Nathan, 17 June 1954.

searchlights fitted to our cars. At the Manor Way surgery the main competitor was Dr Bowman, a very nice man who had been in practice in Kensington and had been appointed by the Executive Council to the vacancy in Borehamwood. He was a fish out of water. On the other hand I could empathise with the working class people who were being moved into the area from London or from the older LCC estates because they had priority points for council housing. Many of them had tuberculosis, asthma, a large number of children, or psychiatric illnesses, often with one or more permutations in the same patient.

As soon as they were properly housed the women became pregnant, often for the third, fourth, or more times. At one stage I was taking on up to a hundred new patients a week and in my first year I was involved in over a hundred home deliveries. NHS bureaucracy decreed that our obstetric facilities should be based at Edgware General Hospital but that the women would be delivered at Bushey Maternity Hospital, a converted cottage hospital miles away, while our other hospital facilities, including gynaecology and the treatment of miscarriages, were based at Barnet.

There was such a shortage of beds that we had to deliver women at home who should have been delivered in hospital. There was an obstetric flying squad based at Edgware which fortunately I only had to use once. More by luck than judgement we never lost a mother, although sadly another practice in Borehamwood did – a Jehovah's Witness who strenuously refused a blood transfusion.

Our workload was so high that colleagues refused to believe us when we told them how many patients we saw during the day, or the number of visits we did at night. It was rare to be on duty without being out of bed at least once – my record was four times in one night.

On the other hand we were fortunate in having Dr Geoffrey Knight, a very progressive County Medical Officer, who believed in promoting general practice. In no time at all we had a nurse attached to us; then a midwife; and finally we acquired a health visitor. We became a group practice, although the term was not yet in common use. Carl became interested in computer science and the county granted him access to their computer, which filled the whole room. As a result, the immunisation programme of our practice was computerised and we had the highest uptake of immunisation for miles around, which to a slight extent boosted our relatively low earnings.

Shirley and I needed accommodation near to the practice but nothing that we could afford ever appeared. One day, the estate agent's assistant asked us if we were interested in an unfurnished flat in Hollywood Court, a block of flats backing on to Elstree station which was built in the 1930s when Borehamwood was striving to become the 'Hollywood of Britain'. We jumped at it.

Within a year it became obvious that the practice needed another doctor. Unfortunately we had work enough for at least four doctors but not enough income to support four families. Shirley had been working intermittently as a casualty officer and as a clinical officer in family planning clinics. It was obvious that she would be of great benefit to the practice, but my partners insisted that we advertise a vacancy because Carl objected to women doctors. However, no one was interested in joining our practice with its low income and abnormally high workload and so we had to negotiate terms of entry for Shirley.

It was finally agreed that she should be a full-time salaried partner, her salary being £500 a year. She would do the same amount of work as the three male partners, including her share of weekend and night work, but should she become pregnant she would have maternity leave and then return to the practice working part-time for the same salary. She became a partner in June 1955 and our son Richard was born a month prematurely in March 1956. Because he weighed 6 lbs. 2 oz. we were teased that we could not calculate dates properly, but he acted like a premature baby and within days became deeply jaundiced. Dr George Newnes, the consultant paediatrician, told me that he needed an exchange transfusion. When I asked what would happen if he did not have it, Newnes replied 'He'll be dead by the morning'. The exchange took place and Richard recovered, but for the first two years of his life we were worried that the jaundice might have damaged his brain.

Finding a decent house that we could afford with our combined income was difficult – the most we could borrow was £3600. That was a considerable sum in those days but Elstree was a very desirable area and the house prices were correspondingly high. A private developer offered a corner plot for £4500. We could just about raise the necessary deposit and we reserved it. While it was still undeveloped we were invited out to dinner one evening at some friends of the Sattins – Teddy and Margot Goldman. Another guest there was Mr Wilkinson, a director of Boots the Chemist. He was being moved to Nottingham and was selling his house in Elstree. The house, Cotswold, was a large semi-detached Edwardian building on three floors on the south side of Barnet Lane, which runs along the ridge forming part of the rim of the London basin.

Although our house agent had the house on its books he had not sent details of it to us, and we were therefore free to negotiate directly with Mr Wilkinson. We offered him our maximum, the princely sum of £4500, which he accepted. At the time the nation was in the middle of one of its recurrent credit squeezes and raising money was very difficult indeed, but the Scottish Equitable Insurance Society offered me an endowment mortgage. It was to be a policy without profits and the interest was fixed at 3.5 per cent, payable for 30 years. We accepted, although we were told that we were stupid. Years later, as a result of inflation and high interest rates, we would still be paying £350 a year on our mortgage – a pittance – while others were paying more than that monthly for much smaller houses.

While working for Henry Blair I had the first recurrence of herpes in my left eye. Henry recommended that I consult an ophthalmologist by the name of Joseph Minton. I was given steroid eye drops with disastrous effects. I will not go into details, but over the years I suffered constant recurrent pain in my eye and for a long periods I wore a patch, looking just like a pirate. I was sent by Mr Minton for second opinions to a host of eminent specialists, including the doyen of British ophthalmologists, Sir Stewart Duke Elder. The way that I was handled by most of them was disgraceful. They took one look at me, told me to come off steroids, and sent me back to Mr Minton. I had x-ray therapy at the Middlesex hospital and subsequently I was referred to another radio-therapist who refused to allow my wife into the examination because he did not approve of women doctors. Vaccine therapy also failed. Finally, Mr Minton did a tarrsoraphy operation which involved stitching my eyelids together. He botched that too.

I met a house surgeon from Moorefield's Eye Hospital socially and he arranged for me to see his chief, Mr Stephen Millar. When I met him I felt for the first time that somebody really cared about me. I had a series of corneal graft operations that transformed a useless painful eye into a useless painless eye. Stephen Millar became ophthalmologist to the Queen and was subsequently knighted, but he continued to treat ordinary patients like me with great courtesy and great kindness until he retired.

Many years later when I was on holiday in Florida my eye broke down again and, by telephone, my partner Laurence Buckman arranged for me to see yet another ophthalmologist, Mr Paul Hunter from Kings College Hospital.[2] Once again I was lucky in my choice of specialists, and I have been treated by him ever since.

My friends knew that my eye condition was a direct result of my military service and suggested I apply for a pension. I took the view that that being a pensioner might be an encumbrance but as I got older I changed my mind and in January 1971 I wrote a letter to the Ministry of Social Security informing them that I believed that I was entitled to a pension[3] because my loss of vision was a long-term result of the illness for which I had been admitted to the military hospital in Fayid. A few weeks later I submitted a formal request[4] and informed Stephen Millar of my decision.[5] He wrote a report confirming that I was blind in my left eye as a result of corneal herpes and surprisingly the records of my stay in Fayid were found and confirmed the history. I was seen by a medical board and granted a 30 per cent disability pension which, after several reviews, was extended for life. It was a relatively small sum, but it is exempt from assessment for income tax.[6]

Our practice grew steadily and the partners developed outside interests. Philip Sattin had been involved in the making of medical films before I joined, and any money that he made from that enterprise was excluded from the practice income. Carl Hodes was interested in practice organisation and also in the use of computers in medicine. The philosophy of the practice now permitted each of the doctors to involve themselves in other activities apart from medicine while their colleagues supported them. Shirley involved herself in the magistracy. I unwittingly became interested in medical politics.

FOOTNOTES AND REFERENCES

1 Taylor S. *Good General Practice: a report of a survey*. London: Nuffield Provincial Hospitals Trust/Oxford University Press; 1954.
2 Paul Hunter later became President of the Royal College of Ophthalmologists.
3 Letter dated 7 January 1971 to Ministry of Social Security.
4 Pension for disablement. Reference O/M2/57709. 7 April 1971.
5 Letter to Stephen Miller dated 7 April 1971.
6 Department of Health and Social Security (War Pensions). Form MPB 19, Reference 0/M2/57709. 26 July 1971.

CHAPTER 4

My involvement in abortion law reform

WHEN I STARTED IN MEDICINE ABORTION HAD BEEN ILLEGAL IN THE United Kingdom since the passing of the Offences Against the Persons Act of 1861, the only exception being to 'preserve the life of the mother'.[1] In 1938 an eminent gynaecologist Alec Bourne terminated the pregnancy of a girl under the age of fifteen at St Mary's Hospital in London. She had been gang-raped by a group of guardsmen. He and a series of expert witnesses argued in court that continuation of the pregnancy would leave the girl a mental wreck. He was acquitted[2] and 'The Bourne Case' introduced a certain degree of flexibility, but every doctor involved in an abortion placed themselves in jeopardy before both the criminal courts and the Professional Conduct Committee of the General Medical Council.

In early 1968 I was consulted by Betty H, a young woman patient who had a gynaecological problem. I referred her to a local gynaecologist for her opinion, but while waiting for the consultation Betty became pregnant for the fourth time. The consultant gave Betty a letter for me which she opened at home. It said that there were no grounds for terminating the pregnancy – a subject that I certainly had not raised. In spite of Betty's begging me to do something, after that letter I had no possibility of securing a 'legal' termination in the NHS and she could not afford a 'medical' termination in the private sector.

Betty left the consulting room, went to the local chemist, bought a Higginson's syringe, used for giving enemas and douches, and attempted a self-induced abortion. She dropped dead on the bathroom floor of her mother-in-law's home, where she and her family lived in one room. I was called from my surgery and I can still see that young woman lying dead on the bathroom floor with the syringe in her hand and her clothes raised up around her waist. Her distraught husband was widowed and three young children were left without a mother.

That incident made me a convinced supporter of abortion law reform. I had seen countless poor women damage themselves in futile attempts to remove an unwanted foetus. So called 'septic abortion', with its terrible consequences of death, chronic ill-health and infertility, was almost always the result of illegal interference with an unwanted pregnancy by the patient, a 'friend', or a rogue doctor or midwife acting as a professional 'back street abortionist'.

In 1966 David Steel introduced a Parliamentary Bill to liberalise the rules of abortion and it went on to become The Abortion Act of 1967. Unfortunately the Act did not become effective until 28 April 1968,[3] just too late for Betty. A few weeks after her death any two doctors could have had the pregnancy legally terminated. Although the 1967 Act allowed termination only on 'medical grounds', it was permitted when there was 'a risk of injury to the physical or mental health of any existing children'. That was one of the so-called 'social clauses'. The elderly reactionary leadership of the BMA decided that although such abortions were legal they were unethical. They presented that policy to the Annual Representative Meeting (ARM) at Eastbourne in July 1968. The meeting was held in a theatre with a huge notice outside advertising its programme – 'The follies of 1968'. The irony was lost to the BMA hierarchy!

I took part in a debate on a motion asking the BMA to reconsider its opposition to the 'social clauses'. I told the representatives the story of Betty and how she had unsuccessfully begged and pleaded with me. I reminded the meeting that so called 'social abortion' was nothing new but that unfortunately the so-called medical grounds are more readily accepted for a woman if she has £100 cash in her handbag. I was booed. I continued by saying, 'We are a responsible and humane profession. The borderline between illness and environment is so poorly defined [that] we are encouraging the opening of Chairs in Social Medicine. I submit it would be barbaric, hypocritical and not Hippocratical to oppose this motion'. I was booed off the platform.

The next supporting speaker was Mr Stanley Simons, a young consultant gynaecologist from Windsor and Slough, who said that the Abortion Act was on the statute book, reflecting society's changed attitudes and that he had recently done an abortion solely in the interests of the other children. His level of booing exceeded that of mine, and the motion was rejected by a huge majority. (In 1990 Sir Stanley Simons became President of the Royal College of Obstetricians and Gynaecologists!) Our two speeches and Betty's story received wide coverage in the national and local press. On the other hand there was at least a theoretical possibility that Mr Simmons or a like-minded doctor could be expelled from the Association by the Ethical Committee for unethical conduct. The General Medical Council took the saner view that if a doctor acted within the law they were not interested in disciplinary proceedings.[4,5,6,7]

The first serious assault on the Abortion Act in Parliament was the James White Bill of 1975. When I opposed it at the Conference of Local Medical Committees I said, 'The introduction of words like 'grave' and 'serious' to limit the criteria in the Abortion Bill would put things back a decade'. The Conference overwhelmingly supported the motion opposing the Bill, reflecting general practitioners' acceptance of the improvements which had taken place.[8] I reported to the Select Committee of MPs examining the White Bill the BMA's view that a mere change in the Regulations would be sufficient to curb the abuses which undoubtedly existed, and therefore a new Act was unnecessary. The Royal College of Psychiatrists, the Royal College of Pathologists and the Association of Anaesthetists all gave similar evidence.[9] A Professor of Gynaecology from the London Hospital, situated in one of the poorest parts of the city, told the Committee that he could not find a case of 'septic abortion' to show his students, but before David Steel's Act he would have had dozens.

At the next annual Representative Body (RB) meeting representatives heard that those speaking for the BMA at the Standing Committee had demolished the Bill 'clause by clause'. One of the speakers supporting the Association's stand in the debate was Dr Shirley Nathan, representing the Barnet Division. There was the usual abusive opposition by the 'pro-life' brigade, headed by Prof Myer Sim, a psychiatrist from Birmingham. He accused the BMA of becoming too liberal by associating with Marxists, Trotskyites and lesbians, while David Steel's Act was merely a 'money-making racket'. The meeting overwhelmingly supported the BMA's actions over the Bill.[10] I subsequently made several television broadcasts on the subject and was paid for some of them – a new experience.[11]

In January 1977 William Benyon introduced yet another Bill to amend the Abortion Act. The ARM was told that although the Bill had failed to gain parliamentary time, there was still a risk that it could be reintroduced later that year and so a debate took place. It took the usual form – I opposed the Bill, the pro-lifers supported it, and they lost the vote.[12] Before the next ARM I decided to take the offensive and at that meeting I put forward a motion: 'This meeting deplores the persistent attacks on the 1967 Abortion Act, and reaffirms its belief that it is a practical and humane piece of legislation'. It was debated and passed by a huge majority. The following year the former Secretary of State for Health David Ennals, speaking against yet another Abortion Act Amendment Bill sponsored by John Corrie, quoted the ARM resolution, which he, Mr Ennals, supported.[13]

In January 1980 Shirley and I wrote to the Jewish Chronicle because we were amazed and appalled to see in it 'emotive but misleading advertisements by the self-styled Society for the Protection of Unborn Children (SPUC) asking for support for Corrie's Bill'. We noted that: 'there are many readers of the Jewish Chronicle who have themselves had a safe termination of pregnancy; others' wives, sisters or daughters have had one. If the Corrie Bill had been passed they might not have been so fortunate'.[14]

This provoked a response from 'a practicing Jew'[15] who was 'amazed and appalled' at the way Drs. Marks and Nathan had so arrogantly flaunted their contemptuous ignorance of Jewish law and sensibility and that it was audacious that such people should go over the heads of those who should be the leaders in these matters – our rabbis, not our doctors. He then went on to say that the argument that 'decent women will once more be driven to backstreet abortionists' just would not wash, and then made the amazing allegation that such [Jewish] women may be 'ordinary' but they were certainly not 'decent'. That letter showed the typical attitude of anti-abortionists to the real problems facing women in the latter part of the Twentieth Century.

A few weeks later I joined David Steel on the platform at a National Rally in Westminster where, according to the *Daily Express*, some 12 000 people were present while thousands more queued in Parliament Square to lobby their MPs. Mr Steel asked, 'Do the anti-abortion campaigners really want a return to the dark days of butchery, death and desperately costly abortion? . . . A vociferous minority opposed to abortion is trying to dictate to the majority in the country what the law should be'.[16] I pointed out that medical opinion had completely changed with regard to abortion over the past 13 years and that that change of mind had come about because the profession had seen the benefits which have flowed from the Act.[17]

THE GILLICK CASE

Victoria Gillick appeared at the High Court in July 1983 seeking a declaration that none of her five daughters – aged 1 to 13 – could be prescribed drugs or be advised on birth control until they were 16. Counsel for Mrs Gillick had argued that the act of giving contraceptive advice or treatment was 'very close' to the criminal offence of aiding and abetting unlawful sexual intercourse. Mr Justice Woolf, who later became the Lord Chief Justice, ruled against her application and also rejected her attempt to prevent the Department of Health and Social Security (DHSS) distributing circulars advising doctors that they could give contraception to under-16 year olds without parental consent. He told the court: 'I would regard the pill prescribed to the woman as not so much the instrument for a crime or anything essential to its commission, but a palliative against the consequences of the crime'. According to the BBC when she heard the verdict Mrs Gillick burst into tears and collapsed into her husband's arms shouting, 'God Almighty, that's ridiculous'.[18]

She appealed against the decision, lost again, and went to the House of Lords in 1985, where she also lost. In his judgment there Lord Fraser said that the degree of parental control varied according to the child's understanding and intelligence, and Lord Scarman said that parental rights only existed so long as they were needed to protect the property and person of the child. He concluded: 'As a matter of law the parental right to determine whether or not their minor child below the age of 16 will have medical treatment terminates if and when the child achieves sufficient understanding and intelligence to enable him to understand fully what is proposed'.[19] The subsequent development of case law of what became known as 'Gillick competence' showed that confidentiality related to the particular child and the particular treatment, and there have been cases where a 17-year-old has been found insufficiently competent to refuse medical treatment, while in other cases much younger children have been deemed sufficiently competent.[20]

A serious difference of opinion developed between the GMC and the BMA over the issue of confidentiality relating to the prescribing of contraceptives to girls under the age of 16. Professor Ian Kennedy advised the GMC they could no longer tell doctors they must observe secrecy; and were free to inform parents if they judge the girl too immature to enter into a 'contract of confidence'. Nicholas Timmins in an analysis of the confusing situation pointed out that the BMA was adamant that its legal advice was that there was still nothing to stop the GMC insisting that the normal rules of secrecy applied. The BMA Council had urged the GMC to reconsider its advice and revert to the previous situation whereby a doctor who breached the girl's confidence would have to justify his action.[21]

THE ANTIABORTIONISTS PERSIST IN THEIR ATTACKS

In 1987 there was yet another attack on the Abortion Act, this time promoted by David Alton. His Bill would have lowered the upper limit of abortion to 18 weeks. Six leading medical organisations publicly joined forces against the new Bill, warning that it could lead to about 500 handicapped babies being born each year and that a new era of backstreet abortion would also open up.[22] Another Bill by Sir Russell Braine MP, a well-known pro-lifer, scarcely made a ripple.

A RABBINICAL INTERVENTION

I received a letter dated 21 January 1988 from the Chief Rabbi of the United Synagogue, Rabbi Sir Immanuel Jacobovitch, which had been sent to a large number of doctors who had been identified by his office as being 'Jewish'. I knew that some non-Jewish doctors had received it and that they were highly amused. The letter stated that 96% of all abortions were for social reasons and pleaded that nothing whatsoever be done to assist in the perpetuation of what constitutes 'a grave offence'.

I was angry and I replied as follows:

> I received your letter of the 21st January 1988, and I wish to pick up your phrase 'a grave offence'. I happen to believe that to alter the Abortion Act, which in my view is a piece of humane legislation, is a grave offence. People's memories are short. I am sufficiently long qualified to remember the terrible things that happened before David Steel's Bill became law. I have personally witnessed the death of more than one young mother from a self-induced abortion because she was desperate. I also remember when hospital wards were full of septic abortions which left the women crippled and often sterile.
>
> The law of this country does not recognise 'social abortion'. It requires two doctors to certify in good faith that the patient satisfies one of the four criteria in the Act but, thank goodness, we can take account of the patient's total environment.
>
> I am particularly proud of being Jewish, but I totally reject the idea that religious views should influence the way that I care for patients. I will do everything possible to ensure that the only change that will flow from the disastrous Alton Bill will be a reduction of the age of viability to 24 weeks.
>
> I hold human life as valuable as anyone else. However I believe that the life and health of mothers has been ignored for too long by those who label themselves 'pro-life'.

I sent a copy of my letter to the *Jewish Chronicle*. Under the heading 'Doctors clash with Chief' one of their reporters quoted me as saying that if Sir Immanuel's beliefs were carried out Jewish women would be amongst those seeking back-street abortions. Dr Lionel Kopelowitz, President of the Board of Deputies of British Jews and also a member of the BMA Council, expressed his concern as to how the names and addresses of Jewish doctors had been obtained. The *Jewish Chronicle* told him how – the extremely orthodox Lubavitch Foundation had 'guessed' its way through the Medical Directory and then involved the chief Rabbinate which sent out the letters.[23] Fortunately the Alton Bill joined the increasing pile of rejected abortion amendment bills.

In 1990 the Human Fertilisation and Embryology Act[24] changed parts of the 1967 Abortion Act by imposing a time limit of abortion at 24 weeks for most cases, in line with the majority of medical opinion. That was the first occasion when Government time had ever been provided for a discussion on abortion, which was always considered a matter of conscience and not political orientation. However, by that time I was out of medical politics.

FOOTNOTES AND REFERENCES

1 Offences Against the Person Act, 1861 24 & 25 Vict. c 100, s.58.
2 *The King v. Bourne* [1938] CCC. July 18, 19.
3 Abortion Act, 1967 15 & 16 Eliz. 2, c. 87.27.
4 Women who take pills like sweets. *Evening Argus*. 1968 Jun 27.
5 Prince J. Warning on unethical abortions. *Daily Telegraph*. 1968 Jun 28.
6 Shearer A. *Guardian*. 1968 Jun 28.
7 Barnet doctor in abortion debate. *Barnet Press*. 1968 Jul 5.
8 Bill will put abortion back ten years – Doctor. *Evening Echo*. 1975 Jun 12.
9 Doctors join to fight abortion change. *Guardian*. 1975 Jun 24.
10 Parry M. Abortion law 'unworkable'. *Yorkshire Post*. 1975 Jul 11.
11 *Calendar*. Yorkshire Television. 1975 Jul 14.
12 Herbert H. Doctors back present law on abortion. *Guardian*. 1977 Jul 22.
13 Hansard. House of Commons. 1979 Jul 13: 906.
14 Marks J, Nathan S. Abortion bill. *Jewish Chronicle*. 1980 Jan.
15 Garfield A. The abortion debate. *Jewish Chronicle*. 1980 Feb 8.
16 Dover C. Doctors – scrap this baby bill. *Daily Express*. 1980 Feb 6.
17 Ferriman A. Minority dictating on abortion, MPs say. *The Times*. 1980 Feb 6.
18 *BBC News*. 1983 Jul 26.
19 *Law Reports* [1985] ALL ER 402.
20 In 2002 Mrs Gillick, by now the mother of 10 children, lost a libel case that she brought against the Brook Advisory Centre, a long-standing highly reputable family planning organisation. The judge in the case was Mr Justice Gray.
21 Timmins N. Pill: the doctors dilemma. *The Times*. 1986 Mar 8.
22 Dover C. Doctors slam bid to limit abortions. *Daily Express*. 1987 Dec 3.
23 Levitt L. Doctors clash with Chief. *Jewish Chronicle*. 1988 Feb 5.
24 The Human Fertilisation and Embryology Act 1990 s.37.

CHAPTER 5

I get further involved
in medical politics

The most senior doctor in the Borehamwood and Elstree area was Dr Wynn Everett, the daughter of Sir Percy Everett, a woman who had qualified in medicine 4 years after I was born. One day in 1960 I was summoned to her surgery at Schopwick House – almost literally. Wynn said, 'Marks (first names were not used to inferiors), I have been doing the Local Medical Committee, the BMA, and the St John Ambulance Brigade for years and it is time for me to give up. You will do them.'

The St John's Ambulance Brigade was easy – Dr Everett just told the local superintendent that I was the new Divisional Surgeon. My duties included the teaching of volunteers, holding first aid classes for the general population and attending public events with the Brigade. I was elected unopposed to the Hertfordshire Local Medical Committee (LMC) by the local GPs and I continued to attend the Barnet Division of the BMA as an ordinary member.

There were fairly radical changes in the practice too. Philip Sattin gave up medicine to concentrate on making medical films. At that time Britain had a shortage of doctors but we managed to persuade Godfrey Ripley to return to the United Kingdom from Jamaica by giving him a disproportionately large share of the practice income. Once more the Marks family was at the wrong end of the stick.

At that time general practitioners were paid solely by capitation fees through a fixed 'pool' of money known as the 'global sum'. It was distributed to general practitioners on a per capita basis. This method of payment, which had existed in the National Insurance since 1913, was accepted by the profession when it joined the health service in 1948 and was the basis of The Spens Report of

1946 which fixed GPs' pay and perpetuated it.[1] Spens's findings were based on the Inland Revenue figures, which in turn relied on GPs' returns. Many patients paid their general practitioners in cash, which some doctors failed to declare. I believe the low rates of pay for general practitioners in the United Kingdom compared with other countries stemmed from the artificially low baseline that reflected those activities.

Each capitation fee included an element representing practice expenses, which bore no relationship to the actual expenses that the practice had incurred.

In 1951 Mr Justice Danckwerts was appointed to arbitrate on a pay claim by GPs and his report published on 24 March 1952 gave them a massive increase. Even *The Times* admitted that the award showed that the family doctor has been underpaid by the State ever since the health service was launched.[2] This did not please the consultants, who were excluded from the exercise, nor the Government, which responded in March 1957 by appointing a Royal Commission on Doctors and Dentists Remuneration. It reported three years later.[3] The most important part of the report was the appointment of an Independent Review Body whose first chairman was Lord Kindersley.

By 1964 general practitioners were completely disenchanted. The third, fourth and fifth reports of the Review Body[4] recommended that the pool should be increased by 5.5 million pounds, most of which would go to the introduction of a proposed scheme for the partial direct reimbursement of the cost of ancillary help and maintaining practice premises. Illogically the Review Body, while recognising that the number of general practitioners was falling, refused to increase GPs' pay as an aid to recruitment, and refused to recognise the increase in general practitioners' workload due to the increasing age of the population. Furthermore, it ignored evidence of practitioner emigration, although this was well known, a third of my cohort having left for the United States, Australia, New Zealand, South Africa and other places where they were much better paid.

The direct reimbursement scheme would benefit those doctors whose expenses were very high because they had invested in decent premises or employed ancillary staff. Such doctors, including our practice, were being grossly underpaid by the pool system, while those who had inadequate premises and negligible staff were being heavily subsidised.

The profession's leaders reacted strongly to the reports and Dr Stevenson, the Secretary of the BMA, wrote to every doctor telling them that both the BMA's Council and the General Medical Services Committee (GMSC) would be discussing what action to take. The GMSC sent a copy of the Review Body reports to every general practitioner along with a copy of a pamphlet, *GMS Voice*.[5] At that time the political representation of doctors was inefficient and unbelievably complex. The profession as a whole was represented by the British Medical Association and its Council. However, general practitioners also had a separate and parallel system based on Local Medical Committees (LMCs), which met in a Conference that in effect made policy for the GMSC. (A fuller explanation of these anomalies appears in Chapter 9 below.)

Dr James Cameron, the Chairman of the GMSC, said that the award seriously raised in general practitioners' minds the question of whether it was in the best interests of patients for the profession to continue to offer professional services within the NHS [sic]. Realising that the major issue facing general practitioners was not money but their terms and conditions of service, the GMSC appointed a small subcommittee whose report was published as *A Charter for the Family Doctor Service.*[6] The committee asked general practitioners to submit their undated resignation from the NHS to BMA House to be used if necessary. Within a fortnight 14 000 were received, including those of our partnership, and a Special Conference of LMCs was convened for the 25 June 1965.

I have often been asked why doctors like me – deeply committed to the service – were prepared to risk damaging it by submitting our resignations. We did so because we believed that without a properly organised and properly paid workforce the NHS would, ultimately, collapse. The general practitioner contract, based on Parliamentary Regulations, left us with no alternative but resignation in the face of Government intransigence.

By now I had become Vice-Chairman of the Hertfordshire LMC. The proposed indirect reimbursement scheme would be a great boost for the relatively young doctors of Hertfordshire and our decision to support a motion at the Special Conference requesting that that part of the 'new deal' should be implemented 'forthwith'. Our usual representative disagreed with our decision and declined to speak to the motion, and so I was appointed to go to BMA House in his stead. I did not realise it but that was the moment when my career in medical politics at the national level began.

At the Conference Dr Cameron proposed that the direct reimbursement scheme should be implemented from 1 October 1965, whereupon one of the old guard introduced a wrecking amendment insisting that nothing should happen until all the charter had been implemented. I learnt rapidly – I had to speak against the amendment, but needless to say the elderly, well-heeled, established doctors in the hall supported the amendment and nothing further was done.[7]

As a result of decisions whose origins were lost in time the Representative Body of the BMA and the Conference of Local Medical Committees each debated the same issues separately, sometimes coming to conflicting decisions. The Council of the Association called a Special Representative Meeting (SRM) at which the Barnet Division of the BMA was entitled to have one representative.

This had always been an old man, Dr Melvyn Scott, known as 'Beardy Scott', who was also entitled to attend the meeting as a member of the Council. Although he had moved to Devonshire he announced his intention of attending the meeting as Barnet's representative, his motivation being to prevent my progressing up the medico-political ladder because he disliked me intensely. He had extreme right-wing views and was absolutely convinced that I was a Communist because I strongly supported the National Health Service and the philosophy behind it.

The members of the Barnet Division did not take kindly to this and at a meeting called on the 18 June I was appointed to deputise for Dr Scott at the SRM.[8] When I arrived at BMA House my credentials were challenged by Dr Scott, with the support of Dr Derek Stevenson, the influential and smooth Secretary of the Association. He looked like the famous actor Rex Harrison, but was known to the general public as 'Docker Stephenson', because he was associated in their minds only with doctors' pay claims. I was not easily browbeaten and threatened to make a scene, which convinced Derek that I should be allowed to take my seat.

That spring I contested my first election for the BMA Council in the local constituency. I was bottom of the poll by a mile.[9]

I began getting local recognition. When I spoke at the dinner dance of the local division of the St John's Ambulance Brigade I was quoted at length in both the *Borehamwood Post* and the *Herts Advertiser*.[10,11] Both articles were accompanied by photographs of me and my wife Shirley. I pasted them on the first page of my new scrapbook. The Elstree Rural Council's General Purposes Committee nominated me for two NHS authorities and objected when I wasn't appointed to either.[12] As the Vice-Chairman of the LMC I received a (routine) invitation to a reception to meet Kenneth Robinson, the Minister of Health, while at the other end of the scale I was invited by the editor of the *Borehamwood Post* to attend the Borehamwood and Elstree civic festival queen competition.

By now I realised that if I were to influence the future of general practice, to move it and the BMA in what I believed to be the right direction, I needed to be on both the General Medical Services Committee and the Council of the Association. I carefully considered whether, as a member of a Faculty Board, I should participate more fully in the activities of the Royal College instead – to stand for election to its Council, rather than the BMA's. I concluded that the Association was the more important organisation and I have never regretted that decision nor changed my opinion.

I knew that if I were to progress I would need to make speeches and as my oratorical skills were nonexistent I registered for an evening course in public speaking at Hendon College – now part of the University of Middlesex. I learned

The District Post. Thursday, April 15, 1965

PUFFING AWAY

IT'S still "twenty, please" at Boreham Wood.

Cigarette sales have only been slightly affected by the Budget. Sixpence on cigarettes.

Mr. G. Jones, the manager of "Candies," said "The sales are usually affected the first couple of days, but never for long."

Mrs. E. Ives, the manageress of "Rolands," who put their prices up on Friday, said: They did drop off at first, but now they are beginning to rise

First aid knowledge can be so valuable, says surgeon

DIVISIONAL surgeon Dr. J. Marks stressed how valuable a knowledge of first aid was when he spoke at the fourth annual dinner and dance of Elstree and Boreham Wood Division of the St. John Ambulance Brigade at the Plough public house, Elstree, on Saturday.

Dr. Marks also stated how pleased he was that the St. John Ambulance Brigade had such an enthusiastic following in the district.

About 58 members and friends attended the event.

Mr. J. Borman, chairman of the social committee, mentioned the many successful outings and events that had been organised by the committee in 1964, and gave details of forth-coming events.

He thanked the committee and members for their help at the children's Christmas party and said how successful this event, the first of its kind to be organised by the committee, had been.

A Christmas party for children would continue to be held every year, he added.

Mr. C. Sansom, superintendent of the ambulance division, spoke on the full programme of duties carried out by the brigade in the district and appealed for help in the brigade's annual flag day collections to be held from May 17-22.

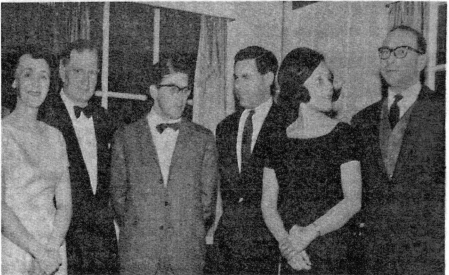

POST PICTURE—72261

Here are some of the principal guests: Mrs. M. Borman, Mr. C. Sansom, Dr. I. Campbell, Dr. J. Marks, Dr. S. Nathan and Dr. D. Goddard.

FIGURE 5.1 My first press cutting. Speaking at the St John Ambulance Brigade dinner in Elstree. *Borehamwood Post*, 15 April 1965. © Times Series Newspapers.

how to project my voice and how to fix, and hopefully hold, an audience. That training served me in good stead

AN ATTEMPT TO BAN AMPHETAMINES IN HERTFORDSHIRE
Although the BMA is regarded by many people solely as the doctor's negotiating body it also played a large part in maintaining medical standards and educating the public on health matters. I was always totally convinced of the importance of this aspect of the Association's work although many doctors thought it was a waste of the Association's time and their money. On many occasions in the future I was proved right as our commitment to maintaining the public health, in its widest sense, improved our image amongst the general public. This helped enormously during the major political crises of the 1980s.

In the late 1960s drug abuse, and particularly the misuse of stimulants in the amphetamine group, became an increasingly serious problem. At the Annual Representative Meeting of 1970 Dr Frank Wells, at that time a general practitioner in Ipswich, proposed that doctors should operate a voluntary ban on the prescribing of amphetamines and similar substances. He described how such a ban had been introduced in his area with the full co-operation of the general practitioners and the local pharmacists. The motion was passed, thereby becoming BMA policy.[13] Shortly afterwards Frank joined the staff of the BMA and ultimately became responsible for the ethical and scientific divisions of the Association and editor of the British National Formulary, a joint venture between the BMA and the Royal Pharmaceutical Society. Later he left the Association's staff to become Medical Director of the Association of the British Pharmaceutical Industry (ABPI). His views and opinions were respected both nationally and internationally, particularly in maters related to fraudulent medical research.[14]

In Hertfordshire there was a huge problem of amphetamine abuse. The drugs were made at Welwyn and were readily obtainable on a lucrative black market. Following the BMA's recommendations the Hertfordshire Local Medical Committee agreed to a voluntary ban on prescribing amphetamines in March 1971. The Local Pharmaceutical Committee agreed that chemists would not keep the drugs on their premises after their existing stocks had run out, although they would be obtainable on prescription with 48 hours notice. We had already established good relationships with the local press during the Review Body crisis the previous year, and as a result we had a very good attendance at a press conference, which I convened jointly with the Chairman of the Local Pharmaceutical Committee. Headlines like 'Doctors in new war on drugs'[15] and 'Doctors ban hits out at drug pushers'[16] appeared in local newspapers, but in spite of all the publicity, and a real effort on the part of the professions, we made very little impression on 'recreational drug-taking' in the county.

FOOTNOTES AND REFERENCES

1 Parliament. *Report of the Inter-departmental Committee on Remuneration of General Practitioners.* (Cm. 6810.). London: HMSO; 1946.

2 *The Times.* 1952 Mar 26: p. 5.

3 Royal Commission on Doctors and Dentists Remuneration, 1957–1960. *Report.* (Cm. 939.). London: HMSO; 1960.

4 Review Body of Doctors and Dentists Remuneration: *Reports.* (Cm. 2595). London: HMSO; 1965.

5 *GMS Voice* 1965 Feb 4; **4.**

6 British Medical Association. *A Charter for the Family Doctor Service.* 1965.

7 *BMJ.* 1965 Jun 26 (Suppl. 1): 287.

8 *Notice of Meeting.* Issued by Dr John Muende, Honorary Secretary, Barnet Division of the BMA.

9 *BMJ.* 1965 May 22 (Suppl.).

10 First aid can be valuable, says surgeon. *Borehamwood Post.* 1965 Apr 15.

11 *Herts Advertiser.* 1965 Apr 17.

12 A doctor is nominated. *Herts Advertiser.* 1965 Nov 5: 4.

13 Prince J. Doctors vote to ban pep pill prescriptions. *Daily Telegraph.* 1970 Jul 7.

14 Wells F. Fraud and misconduct in biomedical research. *Newsletter of the Chief Scientist Office.* 2003; **22.**

15 Currell R. Doctors in new war on drugs. *Watford Evening Echo.* 1971 Mar 24.

16 Doctors' ban hits out at drug pushers. *Borehamwood Post.* 1971 Mar 24.

CHAPTER 6

I get started in medical politics at the national level

ALTHOUGH I STOOD FOR ELECTION EACH YEAR IN THE LOCAL constituency of the BMA Council I knew that I had no hope of being elected because the incumbents were well respected and well liked individuals. In fact, I had to wait until one of them retired in 1973 before I could contest the local seat successfully. Years later I wrote, 'Had anyone suggested that one day I would chair the Council I would have recommended psychiatric treatment. Cockney, Jewish, Grammar School general practitioners were not 'the right material'.[1]

Elections at the Representative Body demonstrated democracy at its worst. Representatives from Birmingham and all points north paid allegiance to a 'northern block' controlled then by Dr George Cormack from Morpeth and they sent delegates to a semi-secret meeting held the night before the main conference where they produced a 'slate'. After appropriate horse trading it was duplicated and circulated amongst block members. Any doubts that I may have had about the block, whose existence was of course strenuously denied by its affiliates and the BMA establishment, vanished when somebody gave me my voting instructions because I was wearing an Edinburgh University tie! People like me, obvious southerners, had no chance of being elected by that route to either the BMA Council or the GMSC, and I am tolerably certain that similar arrangements existed at the Conference of Local Medical Committees (LMCs).

I stood unsuccessfully for the local seat on the GMSC in 1965, 1966 and 1967 – I had been elected to the chair of the Hertfordshire LMC in May 1967[2] and was beginning to feel that I had reached the pinnacle of my medico-political career. However, Hertfordshire LMC nominated me for election yet again in

1968. Our constituency, known as 'Group S', elected two members to the GMSC, our electorate being the members of five local medical committees: Hertfordshire, Bedfordshire, Southend-on-Sea, Essex and North East London. The votes were 'weighted' according to the number of GPs that the LMC represented. Each candidate was entitled to write an election address, which was distributed for them by the BMA Secretariat.

Until the reorganisation of London's Local Government in 1964, Essex and North-East London had been one constituency. Just before the local GMSC election I attended a meeting somewhere in Essex organised by the Royal College of General Practitioners (RCGP).

I went to the toilet and stood between two men who I did not know, but from their conversation I soon realised that they were Dr Weller from Essex, one of the Group S representatives, and Dr Arnold Elliott from North-East London, who held one of the seats on the GMSC reserved for the Medical Practitioners' Union (MPU). In 1968 he was standing in the group election for the first time. One of the men in the toilet suggested to the other that they should each support each other's candidates as they had always done in the past, and thus guarantee that they would secure both places on the Committee. I heard them out and then, to their embarrassment and consternation, I revealed my identity. I realised then that the only way I could possibly be elected would be to persuade all the other electors to use just one vote.

At my own expense I wrote a separate election address to the members of the other three LMCs, telling them about the mathematics of the election and explaining that if they used two votes I could never be elected. They resented the chicanery that I had exposed, they used one vote each, and to the surprise of everyone in Essex, Dr Weller and I, not Drs. Weller and Elliott, were elected.

When I attended my first meeting of the GMSC there were four other new members of the Committee elected at that time – Drs. Brian Whowell, John Ball, Benny Alexander and Gyels Riddle – all of whom in due course would hold high office within the BMA. During one of the more boring meetings John Ball, a talented cartoonist, produced several draft logos for the committee. The one finally adopted showed two cockerels with their necks entwined, demonstrating the committee's well-known ability to talk cock in two directions at once.

Going back a year or two, in 1966 I attended the joint Annual and Special Conference of Local Medical Committees in London as the representative of the Hertfordshire Local Medical Committee. I had noticed that the Agenda Committee prepared a list of speakers for the Chairman, and the names were placed in the order in which they were received, no attempt being made by the Committee or the Chairman to produce a balanced debate.

My first speech related to the phasing of the Review Body award. I told the meeting that although I personally was prepared to resign on that issue in line with BMA policy, the constituents who sent me to the meeting were not. More controversially, I suggested an amendment to the GMSC's constitution to increase the number of directly elected representatives and reduce those appointed by other bodies including the Conference itself and the Representative Meeting. As many of the more elderly members of the Committee were elected through these routes they, and their friends in the hall, made sure that the Hertfordshire motion was overwhelmingly defeated.[3]

A few weeks later I attended my first Annual Representative Meeting (ARM) which was held in the University of Exeter – in fact the University was being built around us. I discovered that the arrangements for debates and the selection speakers were the same as those that I had met at the Conference and that the Agenda Committee and its members had enormous power. They could, and did, put their own names higher on the list of speakers than others. Within a couple of years I had succeeded in getting elected to the Agenda Committee of both the Conference and the Representative Body.

One of the more asinine motions tabled for debate at Exeter proposed that 'the Council should not issue press statements until the opinion of the periphery has been determined'. Speaking against it I said, 'Imagine the situation if the Ministry of Health's statement on private practice [which had been released just before the meeting started] had been made next week instead of this one, and the BMA had told the press to go away and come back in six weeks after every division has met to consider it and given us [the BMA] their views'.[4] I won, and I learned.

Dr SJ Carne from West London proposed that the election to the BMA Council of one special woman representative, which the Council wanted to stop, should continue.[5] Having declared an interest because I was married to a woman doctor I opposed Stuart's idea because I wanted to see women sitting on the Council 'in droves' but they should be there in competition with doctors of both sexes, because they considered themselves the best candidates available.

I went shopping in Exeter for a present for Shirley and in one shop I met two other new representatives doing the same thing – Benny Alexander from Manchester and Gyels Riddle from Gateshead. In time the three of us became close personal friends. I bought Shirley a vanity case which the three of us agreed was a brilliant gift, but when I gave it to her she burst out crying because she thought it was an abomination. I was forbidden to buy her any more presents; instead, each time I went away from home I bought a board game for the children and the well-used collection is still in my daughter Laura's attic.

A few weeks later I wrote my first letter to the medical press as 'a relatively young member of both the Conference of LMCs and the Representative Body'.

Dr John Maxwell from Liverpool had written to *Pulse*, a free newspaper paid for by drug advertisements, claiming that the Conference of LMCs and the ARM were undemocratic and hinting that the proposed extra payments for special experience were a bribe which would line the pockets of medical politicians. I did my best to educate him and the other readers of the newspaper and finished my letter:

> Finally for Dr Maxwell to suggest that high office in the BMA or the GMSC should automatically exclude one from payments for special experience (a subject which was causing considerable friction within the profession at the time) is sheer impertinence. He may like his leaders to be chosen only from the mediocre and inexperienced – I do not.[6]

A year later I became president-elect of the Hertfordshire branch of the BMA[7] and was given the honour of proposing a vote of thanks to the chairman of the Conference, Dr Ben Ridge of Enfield. Six years later he and I would stand against each other for the chairmanship of the GMSC.

REFORM OF THE GMC

In the middle of the Nineteenth Century the British Medical Association played the leading role in getting parliamentary approval for a system of regulating the medical profession, so that the public could choose between properly qualified practitioners and quacks. In spite of enormous opposition from vested interests after 18 unsuccessful attempts a Medical Act was passed in 1858, establishing a General Medical Council for Medical Education and Registration, always known as the GMC, which would be responsible for keeping a Medical Register available for public consultation.[8] As I noted earlier, the registration fee of two guineas when I registered in 1948 was paid at the time of qualification and lasted for life. Until the introduction of the pre-registration year in 1953 there was no legal requirement for doctors to undertake any form of postgraduate education.

On 4 April 1968 the report of the Royal Commission on Medical Education (*The Todd Report*) was published.[9] It proposed that the professional training of British doctors should consist of an intern year, three years general professional training, and a period of further training leading to the normal responsibilities of a professional career. On 4 July 4 the Secretary of State announced the government's acceptance of the Royal Commission's recommendations and of its intention to introduce legislation to ensure that the GMC could carry them out. A few months later the Chief Medical Officer Sir George Godber wrote to the BMA proposing that multiple fees should be payable by the profession to meet the 'substantive administrative costs [which] will be incurred'.[10]

The Medical Act of 1969 implementing those changes and the Council of the BMA agreed to a retention fee of two pounds per year, without consulting the profession. That angered doctors throughout the country. Matters became so bad that a Special Representative Meeting (SRM) was convened by the Council. It met on the 12 February 1970. Although I did not know it at the time, that Special Representative Meeting would be another of the turning points in my medico-political career.

A large number of Divisions of the BMA sent in resolutions opposing the charges and also demanding changes in the Constitution of the GMC so that a majority of its members would be doctors who had been directly elected by their colleagues. Before the SRM opened a meeting was held in one of the committee rooms of BMA House to draft a composite motion on the GMC's constitution for consideration by the SRM. There were about 70 representatives present and they chose Dr Morgan Williams, an articulate general practitioner who practised in the West Midlands, to move the motion on their behalf. Dr Ray Outwin, a maverick member of the Agenda Committee, whose job was to take the message back to the chairman took a different view and, on his own initiative, reported to the chairman and the Agenda Committee that the meeting had chosen me, the representative of the Barnet Division, to move the composite motion.[11]

By now I had become a fairly seasoned debater and I knew that what mattered above all else was the reply to the debate before the vote was taken. I was allowed to make an opening speech of three minutes, and then I did the unthinkable – I left the platform and sat in the front row of the hall making notes. The Treasurer of the Association, Dr Jack Miller, a general practitioner from Glasgow who was well liked, gave the representatives a lecture on acting 'responsibly'. The debate went on for well over an hour, but the rules gave me just three minutes to reply. I told the chairman of the Representative Body, Dr John Noble, that I could not possibly reply to such a debate in such a short time, and I was allowed to speak for much longer. I dealt in turn with the points made by the Chairman of Council and others and then I came to Jack Miller. I told the Representative Body that I, like Jack Miller, was a registered medical practitioner and that I too was responsible. I was responsible to the profession and in exercising that responsibility I urged them to support the Barnet motion. They did, by a majority of 214 to 85, well above the two-thirds majority needed to change the Association's policy. I was the hero of the hour.

Another motion was passed saying that in the event of the retention fee being imposed against the profession's wishes the Association would advise members to withhold payment. Pandemonium broke out, the meeting adjourned, and the Council held an emergency meeting during the adjournment. There was talk of resignation, and in my view and that of many other representatives the Chairman of the Council, if not the whole Council, should have resigned. When the meeting resumed it quietly passed another resolution recommending that doctors should make a single payment to the GMC of two pounds 'without prejudice'.

The *Guardian* published a reasoned article written by Anne Shearer, its welfare correspondent, under the heading 'Doctors tie strings to £2 levy'. It explained the significance of the decisions and pointed out that they were in no way illegal.[12] *The Times* relied on a staff reporter and its report appeared under the title, 'Victory for militants in BMA vote'.[13] I think that was the first time I was called a militant in public – it certainly was not the last.

1970 A VISIT TO TORQUAY AND THE ANNUAL CONFERENCE

For some unaccountable reason I was invited to attend the Annual Conference of the South West Region of the Institute of Hospital Administrators in Torquay, one of the other speakers being the then Under Secretary of State for Health Dr John Dunwoody MP. At that time I was advocating group practice as a means of dealing with the shortage of doctors and also as a means of improving the services provided to patients. Considerable prominence was given to my then heretical views that patients should be transported to doctors' surgeries rather than doctors visiting patients in their homes.[14,15,16] I was also asked to make the obligatory after-dinner speech proposing the toast 'The Institute of Hospital Administrators'. Of itself that visit to Torquay was of no great importance, but it showed that I was already being recognised by others as a competent public speaker.

GMC REFORM CLASHES WITH A REVIEW BODY CRISIS

The Regulations imposing the annual retention fee were introduced in March 1970 and in the same month a working party was set up under the chairman-ship of Sir Brynmor Jones to review the composition of the GMC. It included members from the BMA, the GMC, and the Royal Colleges and Universities. The BMA establishment had its revenge on me – they made me one of the BMA's representatives. By chance, that appointment also accelerated my medico-political progress, because one of the meetings of the Brynmor Jones Committee was held on the Friday before the Spring Bank Holiday.

In the taxi on the way back to BMA House Dr Stevenson told the very senior members of the BMA present, including the Chairman of Council, that he had been notified that a letter from the Prime Minister was waiting for them at BMA House. It told them that the Government had decided that it would 'not be right' to consider the current Review Body Report, its 12th, in the middle of a general election. The medical politicians immediately started discussing the problem and what to do about it. Suddenly, they realised a complete outsider was present, but by then it was too late to do anything about it. I was trusted to maintain secrecy and was privy to the plans that were drawn up to force the Government to publish the Report. The letter was also released to the press.[17] Even then governments published unwelcome news or took unpopular actions when there was a distinct possibility that the public would be too busy to notice at times such as bank holidays. They hoped that when the country returned to normal the issue would have been forgotten. Fortunately, Dr Stevenson had arranged for a small skeleton staff to stay on in BMA House and action started immediately with the issuing of a press statement.[18]

On 28 May the leaders of the BMA and the British Dental Association met Prime Minister Harold Wilson and Secretary of State Richard Crossman. After the meeting Downing Street issued a statement that said, 'in view of the strength of feeling within the profession the government would publish the Report on the fourth of June' – seven weeks after they had received it. The Report was amazingly simple – it recommended a 30% increase across the board for all doctors and dentists.[19] That rise was linked to the high level of inflation, something the Government was keen to conceal and which explained the delay in publication. The Prime Minister, on behalf of the Government, accepted the Report as far as junior doctors were concerned, but referred the rest of it to its own National Board for Prices and Incomes. The professions found this intolerable, but far more importantly the entire Review Body resigned. That night I appeared on the BBC *Money Programme* to explain the profession's point of view, for which I received the princely sum of 20 guineas.[20] That night I learned a lesson – it is very important to get any interviewer on your side if you possibly can, especially on radio or television.

The Association, through its front organisations, the British Medical Guild (*see* Chapter 9 on the Chambers Report and the Industrial Relations Act) advised all doctors to stop collaboration with the NHS Authorities and requested general practitioners to stop signing certificates of incapacity for work. As doctors hated doing that anyway, and it did not harm patients, it was a very popular form of industrial action.[21]

I called a meeting of Hertfordshire doctors for the evening of Monday 8 June to discuss the Review Body crisis. Doctors shun meetings on Mondays like the plague because it is the busiest day of the week, but of the 360 doctors in the county 170 turned up – every practice in the county was represented because they all wanted to know what was going on and what they needed to do. I also knew that a national newspaper strike was extremely likely and that a strike was threatened throughout Fleet Street. I had arranged for a press conference to be held immediately after the meeting to which all the Hertfordshire newspapers were invited. They all turned up.

The following day the *Watford Evening Echo*, a daily evening paper with a wide circulation, had banner headlines over two major stories.[22] The first, 'Fleet Street: Wilson in last ditch bid' reported that a complete shut down of Britain's national newspapers was just a few hours away, and the next day national newspapers disappeared from the streets, although both local and regional newspapers continued to be produced and sold. The second headline, 'Herts. Doctors: "We won't sign"', reported our decision to follow the BMA line. It also published the extensive list of under-doctored areas in Hertfordshire that I had given at the press conference, so that the public could be reminded of how fragile their health service was. The following Friday the story appeared in all the weekly local newspapers circulating in the county. [23,24,25,26,27]

The Labour Government was defeated in the election and the new Secretary of State, Sir Keith Joseph, invited the leaders of the BMA to meet him. They left the Annual Meeting in Harrogate in order to do so. I too left the meeting in Harrogate because my eye had broken down yet again and Stephen Miller did my second tarrsoraphy, which at least put me out of pain. Needless to say the new Government did not pay the whole balance of the Review Body award but made sufficient concessions so that the profession could go back to normal work without loss of dignity.

BACK TO BRYNMOR JONES

The Brynmor Jones Working Party on the Constitution of the GMC reported in March 1971. It was a compromise because there was no absolute majority of directly elected members on the proposed council, but it did recommend that such members should always exceed by one the number of representatives of the academic institutions. That was described as 'political double-think' by Dr Michael O'Donnell, who had been a prime motivator in the campaign to reform the General Medical Council.[28] Later that year in his article on the Annual Representative Meeting he graciously described me as a promising up-and-comer in BMA politics and reported how I helped to get Brynmor Jones accepted by the BMA by persuading the representatives to accept a compromise.[29] In the crisis over the proposed reforms of the NHS in 1989/90 the government and its supporters claimed that I was unable to compromise. Brynmor Jones showed I could and did.

Subsequently the government announced its intention to introduce a Bill to reconstitute the GMC. At the same time about 5000 doctors refused to pay the annual levy and the GMC retaliated by announcing its intention to strike those doctors off the register. To avert the massive crisis in the NHS which would have followed such a stupid action by the unreformed GMC, Sir Keith announced a public inquiry into the structure and function of the GMC to be headed by Dr Alec Merrison. The BMA's evidence prepared by a committee chaired jointly by John Happel and me was approved by the ARM in 1973.

The Merrison Committee reported in April 1975. It recommended that the profession should be self-regulated by an independent body, the GMC, with ten more elected members than all the other members combined. A massive victory for the BMA, but nothing happened. Only after constant badgering by the BMA for two years did David Ennals announce in July 1977 that a Medical Bill would be introduced which would deal solely with the constitution of the GMC and the establishment of a Health Committee which would consider if a doctor was unfit to practise by reason of poor health.

The Bill, introduced to the House of Lords on 10 November 1977, was described, accurately, as feeble and a depressing blow to all those who had campaigned for reform.[30] I attended many of the sittings in House of Lords and briefed speakers, particularly Lord Hunt, one of the founders of the Royal College of General Practitioners. He introduced a whole series of amendments. One of them, the so-called Hunt Clause 5, said that 'the powers of the General Council shall include that of providing, in such a manner as the Council thinks fit, guidance for members of the medical profession on standards of professional conduct or on medical ethics'. Part of the problem with the GMC was that it could not give such guidance to doctors trying to avoid acting unprofessionally. The government did not like the Hunt amendment and when the Bill came to the House of Commons in a bid to save debating time it proposed that the report stage of the Bill should be taken in a Commons committee. The Tories vetoed that move, described by Dr Gerry Vaughan, one of their spokesmen on health, as 'unprecedented'. In the end the amendment was accepted in its original form.

John Hunt successfully changed the Bill to such an extent that the government spokesman, Lord Wess-Pessel, said that 'so far as I personally am concerned, there has been no other occasion since I have been a member of your Lordship's House, so far as I can remember, when the opposition has got everything they asked for. It is the very first time'. The Bill passed all its stages in the House of Commons quite rapidly, and received the Royal Assent as the Medical Act 1978 on the 5 May.[31] In an article I wrote for *Pulse* a few weeks later under the heading 'The mouse that roared as a lion' I set out the entire history going back to 1970 and reminded the readers that they should appreciate that no organisation but the BMA had the resources required to deal with such a major project.[32]

John Hunt's role in the reorganisation of the GMC was emphasised in the excellent account of the crisis which appeared in the *History of the British Medical Association Volume II*.[33] No mention was made of my part in this major achievement for the Association, although others were more generous.[34,35] Dr Elston Grey-Turner, one of the authors of *History* became Secretary of the Association in 1976 – he was a perfect gentleman of the old school, a wonderful example of the old medical establishment, but he was never really happy in the new medico-political climate. Three years later he left office, being replaced by Dr John Havard, a very different man. John was a former Cambridge blue, had worked his way up the BMA staff ladder, and had demonstrated both his toughness and his intellectual powers over the years.

In life and in politics things do not happen in isolation. In June 1978, just before the ARM, the medical press started speculating as to who would be the next Deputy Chairman of the Representative Body of the BMA.[36] Much earlier in the year I had informed my friend Benny Alexander that if he wished to stand for the office I would not oppose him. When I told Tony Keable-Elliott and Keith Davidson what I had done they were very angry and told me that I had no right to make such a proposition because they thought I would do the job well and that I had a duty to stand for election. I accepted what they had said and then had a difficult task of explaining to Benny that I was opposing him. He accepted the new situation philosophically.

Although I had a very good chance of being elected anyway, my chances improved after I had spent most of a session at the RB leading the debate on the General Medical Council, described in the *BMJ* as 'A Major Triumph for the BMA'.[37] There were three candidates for the deputy chairmanship – Dr Ralph Lawrence, chairman of the Organisation Committee, Benny Alexander, who had been a very successful Chairman of the Conference of LMCs and who was also extremely popular amongst members of the RB, and me. When the votes were counted I had more votes than the other two candidates put together. In a leading article the medical magazine *General Practitioner* said 'The election which we record with the greatest pleasure is that of Dr John Marks as deputy chairman of the RB', pointing out that the post carried a place on the Executive of the BMA Council and almost invariably lead to the chairmanship of the RB, which it described as 'an important and influential post'.[38]

I have already described how Benny Alexander, Gyels Riddle and I had become friends way back in 1966. In no time at all the three of us got ourselves elected to the Agenda Committee of the RB. We were determined to change the way the business was conducted. The list of speakers presented to the Chairman, usually through the Deputy Chairman, had born no relation to the substance of the motions – the first 10 members wishing to speak might all be in favour, whilst the only one who objected appeared in the 11th place. As a result, many of the so-called 'debates' were completely one-sided, were statements of the obvious, and became unbelievably boring. They continued until the Chairman thought that the representatives had had enough.

Gently we began to produce two lists for the Chairman – those for and those against the motion. By the time I became Deputy Chairman I was able to cut non-controversial discussions to one or two speakers on each side and to leave ample time for real debates. That was part of my long-term wish to see the BMA transformed from an old man's talking shop into an effective medico-political machine. As a bonus, the press, radio, and television became more interested and gave more and more publicity to the Association's activities.

A FINANCIAL INTERLUDE – I BECOME CHAIRMAN OF A PUBLIC COMPANY

Even when I was deeply involved in medico-political matters I found time to do other things. In the autumn of 1971 my brother-in-law Stanley discovered a company called Biting Rubber Estates, a defunct plantation company whose sole asset was a claim for £17 000 compensation against the Indonesian government. Stanley, his solicitor, his accountant, his broker and I all bought a few shares. It was run by three elderly disinterested gentlemen, rather like the BMA. We wrote to some large shareholders and asked them for their proxies and we notified the press that an extraordinary general meeting had been called and that we had the support of 30 to 40 per cent of the votes.[39,40] At the EGM I became Chairman of the Board.[41] A year later it was reported that over 50 companies had approached Biting with a view to 'reverse take over'.[42] However, nothing came of all these approaches, we lost interest and another speculator took over the company. He had no more success than we did.

In later life I took great pleasure in reminding people that I had been the chairman of a public company quoted on the stock exchange, and that therefore my knowledge of business was not negligible! They, like me, thought the whole thing a great joke.

FOOTNOTES AND REFERENCES

1 McPherson G, editor. *Our NHS: a celebration of fifty years.* Oxford: Wiley-Blackwell; 1998.
2 Hertfordshire Local Medical Committee. Minutes. 10 May 1967.
3 *BMJ.* 1966 Jun 18 (Suppl.): 257.

4 *BMJ*. 1966 Jul 16 (Suppl.): 17.

5 Stuart Carne, who with his wife Yolanda became our close friends, was President of the Royal College of General Practitioners in the 1980s. He was also Chairman of the Standing Medical Advisory Committee.

6 Marks J. Committee. *Pulse*. 1966 Jul 30.

7 Anonymous. *Hertfordshire Branch News*. 1968 Dec 20.

8 *BMJ*. 1858 Aug 7.

9 Royal Commission on Medical Education, 1965–68. *Report* (Cm. 3569.). London: HMSO; 1968.

10 *BMJ*. 1969 (Suppl.): 4, 5.

11 The composite motion said 'The Representative Body is not opposed to the introduction of an annual retention fee of £2 . . . provided that . . . the GMC shall contain a majority of members who have been directly elected by the profession . . . [and the representative body] shall agree with the GMC and the Government on the functions and composition of the GMC following an immediate review thereof . . .'

12 Shearer A. Doctors tie strings to £2 levy. *Guardian*. 1970 Feb 13.

13 Victory for militants in BMA vote. *The Times*. 1970 Feb 13.

14 Group practice 'answer to GP shortage'. *Daily Telegraph*. 1970 Apr 11.

15 Minister discounts fears over NHS. [*Torbay*] *Herald Express*. 1970 Apr 10.

16 *Western Morning News*. 1970 Apr 11.

17 *The Times*. 1970 May 23.

18 *The Times*. 1970 May 25.

19 Review Body on Doctors and Dentists Remuneration. *12th Report*. (Cm. 4352). London: HMSO; 1970.

20 BBC contract dated 15 June 1970 [*sic*] and letter from BBC Lime Grove Studios dated 8 June 1970.

21 British Medical Guild. *Review Body Report: Message 4*. British Medical Association; 1970 Jun 6.

22 Jackson G. *Watford Evening Echo*. 1970 Jun 9: 1.

23 Doctors in Herts join pay war. *Borehamwood Post*. 1970 Jun 12: 8.

24 Herts doctors are 'very upset'over broken pay deal. *Barnet Press Series*. 1970 Jun.

25 Under-doctored Hertfordshire. *Watford Observer*. 1970 Jun 12: 3.

26 County's doctors vote to join ban. *Hitchin Gazette*. 1970 Jun 12.

27 Doctors could resign warning. *Herts Observer*. 1970 Jun 19.

28 O'Donnell M. The mountain gives birth. *World Medicine*. 1971 Mar 24: 9.

29 O'Donnell M. *World Medicine*. 1971 Aug 25: 31.

30 Editorial in *World Medicine* (presumably written by Michael O'Donnell). 22 Feb 1978.

31 Parliament. *The Times*. 1978 May 6.

32 Marks J. The mouse that roared as a lion. *Pulse*. 1978 May 20.

33 Grey-Turner E, Sutherland FM. *History of the British Medical Association (Vol II)*. London: British Medical Association; 1982.

34 Ministers seek change in Medical Bill's Hunt clause. *Pulse*. 1978 Apr 15.

35 Lord Hunt wrote an article, 'The Medical Act 1978: Passage through Parliament' in the *BMJ* in September 1978 which he based on the speech he had given at the GMC dinner on 24 May 1978. He mentioned particularly the help given to him by Elston Grey-Turner, Dr John Happel, Doreen Warner and me.

36 The contenders. *Pulse*. 1973 Jun 17.
37 General Medical Council: major triumph for BMA. *BMJ*. 1978 Jul 29: 366.
38 A new chairman takes his seat. *General Practitioner*. 1978 Jul 21.
39 Biting hard. *Evening Standard*. 1972 Jan 24.
40 Biting Rubber. *Financial Times*. 1972 Jan 25.
41 *Financial Times*. 1972 Feb 11.
42 Biting Shell Suitor Settled in the Summer? *Evening Standard*. 1972 Mar 29.

CHAPTER 7   A Royal College, an academic approach and a doctorate

IN 1950 AN AUSTRALIAN DOCTOR, DR JOSEPH COLLINS, WROTE A REPORT 'General Practice in England Today – a Reconnaissance', extracts of which were published in *The Lancet*.[1] He described a poor service staffed by overworked, exhausted and demoralised doctors, who provided a very poor standard of care. That report received enormous attention and could not be ignored by the Government or the profession.

In 1951, Dr Fraser Rose of Preston, who was deeply involved in the BMA General Practice Committee, and Dr John Hunt from London, who had served on a Royal College of Physicians' Working Party on General Practice and had important connections in the elite of London medicine, wrote a letter to the *British Medical Journal* setting out the need for a College of General Practitioners.[2] Subsequently, they met with Dr Geoffrey Barber of Dunmow, Dr Talbot Rogers and others and set up a 'Steering Committee' to plan for such a College. Dr Hunt managed the committee and arranged for Sir Henry Willink, Master of Magdalene College, Cambridge, and a past Minister of Health, to chair it. There was considerable opposition to the idea of a new College, particularly among the consultants involved in the existing Royal Colleges, but in spite of this, in November 1952, less than nine months after its first meeting, a College of General Practitioners was legally constituted and a Foundation Council was formed. In January 1953 'Foundation Membership' was offered to established GPs who satisfied criteria and within six weeks almost 1700 doctors had joined.[3]

I believed passionately that we needed a College because general practice was looked upon as the dustbin of medicine, mainly because it had no academic base and no criteria for entry. Even as late as 1958 Lord Moran, then President of the Royal College of Physicians, would describe general practitioners as 'people who fall off the ladder' when giving evidence to a Royal Commission.[4] Like many other ex-trainees and assistants, Shirley Nathan and I were not eligible for Founder Membership because we had not been in practice for five years. To encourage doctors like us to join a new category of 'Associate Members' was created and we became two of a very small band of 'Foundation Associates'. A few years later we, along with our two partners, applied to become members. While the other three were granted membership without any quibble I, a Founder Associate, had to attend for an interview in London. Dr Annis Gillis, a prominent member of the College, chaired it and she was extremely aggressive towards me, but I was accepted and could put the letters MCGP after my name. The College became incorporated in 1962, and in 1972 HRH the Duke of Edinburgh became the first president of the Royal College of General Practitioners.

I became a Fellow of the College in 1976. In April 1981 Shirley was awarded the Fellowship and the ceremony took place in Glasgow. Like everyone else she wore the Fellowship gown. Two medical journalists noticed that I was at the meeting and one took a photograph of Shirley and me together wearing the same gowns.[5] The other was more perceptive and asked me why I was not wearing the scarlet MD gown that I normally wore at College gatherings. I admitted that, although I considered the MD more prestigious than the Fellowship, I was wearing the black gown to identify myself with my wife and her being honoured.[6] In time Shirley became Chairman of the North West London Faculty and was a member of the College Council for a while. I was elected to the board of the Northern Home Counties faculty and to its successor the board of the North West London Faculty.

I developed a love-hate relationship with the College. I passionately believed we needed it to improve our status. On the other hand I believed its meddling in medical politics was damaging to the representative machinery of general practitioners. This feeling towards the college influenced many decisions I made later in life.

MY EARLY PUBLICATIONS

On 10 April 1965 I saw a patient in the surgery with acute bronchitis who also had Addison's disease. She told me that she had no history of drug sensitivity and so I started her on ampicillin, the new wonder drug derived from penicillin, which was marketed under its brand name of Penbritten. Within 10 minutes of taking her first dose she felt very ill with itching of her hands and feet, immediately followed by irritation of her throat and a feeling that she was 'swelling up inside'. She phoned me from a local phone box and collapsed. I reached her within a few minutes, by which time she was unconscious. She was admitted to Barnet General Hospital and after appropriate treatment she made a full recovery. Subsequent inquiries from the hospital where she was being treated for her Addison's disease revealed that she was known to be sensitive to penicillin. This episode taught me to be very careful in the future about relying on a patient's statements concerning drug sensitivity. My patient was the first known case of true anaphylaxis resulting from oral administration of ampicillin, but attempts to get the case published met a great deal of opposition. However, it finally appeared in the July 1966 edition of *Practitioner*, my first venture into academia.[7]

My interest in dermatology stemmed from my own experience as a teenager when I had severe acne. All the doctors I consulted, both in Tottenham and Edinburgh, treated me with indifference, completely ignoring the severe effect that the facial disfigurement had on my psyche. Barnet General Hospital had a scheme whereby general practitioners could work as unpaid clinical assistants to some of their consultants and luckily I was appointed as assistant to Dr Peter Borrie, an eminent dermatologist from Barts. Under his guidance I acquired a considerable knowledge of the subject and my colleagues in the practice referred all their cases to me.

Later I was appointed as a paid clinical assistant at both Mount Vernon and Watford General Hospitals. At Watford I learnt just how devious NHS management could be. The dermatologist there 'had a problem' and was often away from work for short periods. Finally he had to give up and had to be replaced. But the appointment procedures for new consultants were complex and took a long time. I was the sole dermatologist for the area and, quite rightly, I could not be allowed to work other than under consultant supervision, even if that supervision had been, at best, purely nominal. The administrators found a solution – I was appointed as a locum consultant with the appropriate terms of service because that could be done without reference to any committee! It suited me, it suited them, but it was a disgrace. The arrangement lasted for several weeks and years later I could tease my consultant colleagues at the BMA by telling them that at one time I had been one of their constituents. They were not amused.

One clinical condition that fascinated me was otitis externa – dermatitis affecting the external auditory meatus. It was known then that mild acid applications, especially a solution of aluminium acetate, relieved the symptoms. A new group of drugs known as corticosteroids were being used in the treatment of dermatitis, and it dawned on me that they might be useful in treating otitis externa, particularly if they had a low pH, meaning that they were 'acid'. Betnovate ointment, a fairly powerful steroid, was made by Glaxo. I wrote asking them for information about the ointment and explained why I needed to know its pH. I was invited to meet Dr Ray Garrett, who headed their Clinical Investigation Unit, and he helped me in this investigation and in subsequent ones.

Over a 12-month period I collected 29 cases of the disease, 20 of which had been treated previously and 9 new ones. The practice nurse and I treated them by packing their ears with gauze saturated in a cream sold as Betnovate C, which contained Betnovate and a mild antiseptic called chloraquine. Its pH was five. An unpleasant side effect was that until the packs were removed patients who had the problem in both ears were rendered deaf by the treatment. The results appeared to be good – certainly as good as those from other treatments and possibly better. My results were published in the *British Journal of Clinical Practice* in March 1968.[8]

My next project was a joint study into the use of the new antibiotic cephalexin in general practice, once more arranged by Ray Garrett. The trials were conducted by 12 doctors in 10 separate practices working under normal NHS conditions. Unfortunately, bacteriological control was not always available because it depended on the goodwill of the local bacteriologist, or more likely the lack of it. Our results suggested that the multi-centre trial had shown cephalexin was effective in most of the infections seen in general practice. I was invited to speak on the subject at an international conference in Brighton arranged by the Fellowship of Postgraduate Medicine in May 1970, the results being published as a supplement to the *Postgraduate Medical Journal*.[9]

In 1973 the Journal of the Royal College of General Practitioners published another of our papers comparing the use of topical corticosteroids in the treatment of eczema and psoriasis in general practice.[10] We explained that the trial was conducted under the everyday conditions of general practice and that the results showed that betamethasone-17-valerate (Betnovate) was more consistently and more rapidly effective than the product of a competitor. The standards required of clinical trials are now, quite rightly, far higher than they were 30 years ago, and I am sure that those that we did would be completely unacceptable now. Nevertheless, by the standards of the time they were a genuine attempt to do serious research work in an ordinary group practice.

A VERY SIGNIFICANT AFTER-DINNER SPEECH

On the 27 May 1970 I gave a speech that, unbeknown to me, was to change my whole life. I proposed the toast 'The Conference of Local Medical Committees' at the Annual Conference dinner, held at the Dorchester Hotel in London.[11]

When I received the invitation I had asked within BMA House for information about the origins of the Conference and the GMSC and found that no one had any idea at all about them. I started researching in the archives of the BMA and in the *British Medical Journal* and found that Local Medical Committees had been set up following Lloyd George's National Insurance Bill of 1911 and had been given statutory recognition in the National Insurance Act. Two years later the first conference of Local Medical Committees was held at Brighton on 24 July 1913 in the middle of the Annual Representative Meeting. The first motion considered was 'that as far as possible there be fusion between Local Medical Committees and divisions of the British Medical Association'. It was not passed – but when the word 'co-operation' was substituted for 'fusion' it was. The rest of the agenda, which was a single typewritten page produced on one of the old-fashioned 'jelly' duplicators, included matters which are still debated at conferences: certification, representation and fees.

My speech was very well received. Dr Jimmy Ross of Welwyn Garden City suggested that it could be the basis of a MD thesis, which it was not, but I agreed that it needed to be published. The Society for the Social History of Medicine promised that if I read a paper on the subject at one of their meetings they would publish it. I honoured my part of the agreement but they did not honour theirs. I then approached the Trustees of the General Medical Services Defence Trust, who agreed to fund a booklet. Later in the year *The Conference of Local Medical Committees and its Executive: a review of 60 years* appeared and 7000 copies were sent to Local Medical Committees for onward distribution to their members. In 1979 a second edition[12] was published, which included an account of the constitutional crisis within the BMA that followed a report by Sir Paul Chambers. I will deal with that later (*see* Chapter 9).

By now I had become completely immersed in the subject and was determined to write a doctorate thesis. The University of Edinburgh told me that I was eligible to submit a thesis under old regulations which were about to expire – to be acceptable a thesis had to lie within the scope of any subject taught for the MB degree, and the university authorities accepted that my work was part of the discipline of Social Medicine. Over the next two years I researched the subject at the National Newspaper Library at Colindale, as well as at BMA House. I was still working full-time in the practice and was also a national negotiator at the General Medical Services Committee (GMSC). Mrs Cynthia Harwen, who had been my practice secretary, typed and re-typed over 110 000 words and over a thousand references – in those days computers and word processors were in their infancy and I did not have one.

I submitted my thesis in early spring 1974 and heard nothing further. Barely a week before the graduation ceremony I received a message that my thesis

THE CONFERENCE OF LOCAL MEDICAL COMMITTEES AND ITS EXECUTIVE:

An Historical Review

by
John Marks
M.D.(Edin), F.R.C.G.P., D(Obst) R.C.O.G.

1979
Published by the Trustees of the
General Medical Services Defence Trust

FIGURE 7.1 Pamphlet, *The History of the LMC Conference and its Executive*, 1979. © British Medical Association.

had been accepted and would I please present myself at the McEwen Hall at 10.00 a.m. on the appropriate day. Hasty arrangements were made for Shirley and my mother to travel with me to Edinburgh. I also had to get an MD gown. I went to the appointed university outfitters where I was given the choice of hiring one or buying a second-hand one for the equivalent of three hirings. I chose the second alternative, and it turned out to be a wonderful bargain as I have worn that gown at least once a year for nearly forty years.

The degree ceremony opened with a procession of the graduates. The first degree awarded was an Honorary Degree of Doctor of Science to a famous international scientist, Dr Marthe Louise Vogt. The next in order of precedence was the degree of Doctor of Medicine awarded to me for my thesis *The History and Development of Local Medical Committees, Their Conference and Its Executive.*[13] I walked up to the Vice-Chancellor in my scarlet splendour, was capped, received a certificate and a few words of congratulation, and returned to my seat. My mother was very proud of me. For my part I had succeeded in making the study of the politics of medicine a respectable academic discipline.

The following March I gave the Pfizer Lecture at the North and West London Faculty of the Royal College of General Practitioners and an article based on it appeared in the *British Medical Journal* under the title 'General practitioners and the state – an unequal struggle?'[14] I also gave the prestigious Annual Oration on Medical Politics at Medical Society of London, choosing as my subject 'Medical politics – the myths and realities'.[15] I started by remarking that 'medical politics' were two dirty words to many doctors and then gave an account of the relationships between the medical profession and the English State from the passing of the Sanitary Act of 1388 until the time of the lecture.

FOOTNOTES AND REFERENCES

1 *Lancet.* 1950; **1**: 555–8.
2 *BMJ.* 1951; **II**: 908.
3 Tait I. *The History of the College.* Royal College of General Practitioners. Available from: www.rcgp.org.uk/history
4 Lord Moran. Evidence to the Royal Commission on Doctors and Dentists Remuneration. *BMJ.* 1958; **27** (Suppl.)
5 *General Pratitioner.* 1981 Apr 17.
6 *Pulse.* 1981 May 2.
7 Marks J, Williams DE. Anaphylactoid shock introduced by oral ampicillin in a woman with Addison's Disease. *Practitioner.* 1966; **197**: 85–7.
8 Marks J. A study of otitis externa in general practice. *Br J Clin Pract.* 1968; **22**.
9 Marks J, Garrett RT. Cephalexin in general practice. *Postgrad Med J Suppl.* 1970 Oct.

10 Marks JH, Garrett RT. Topical corticosteroids: a comparison in the treatment of eczema and psoriasis in general practice. *J R Coll Gen Pract* 1973; **23**: 225–7.

11 Menu of the Conference of Local Medical Committee's dinner, April 1970.

12 Marks J. *The Conference of Local Medical Committees and its Executive: an historical review*. Trustees of the General Medical Services Defence Trust; 1979.

13 Programme of Graduation Ceremonial, McEwen Hall, University of Edinburgh, 26 June 1974.

14 Marks J. General practitioners and the state: an unequal struggle. *BMJ*. 1975; **2**: 97–9.

15 Marks J. *Transactions of the Medical Society of London*. 1987: 81–90.

CHAPTER 8

Early attempts at NHS reform and heart transplants

THE NATIONAL HEALTH SERVICE IN BRITAIN WAS SET UP ON A TRIPARTITE system – the Hospital Services; the Executive Council Services, which dealt with general medical practitioners, dentists, pharmacists, and opticians; and the Public Health Services provided by local authorities. There was no provision for co-ordinating decision-making or the delivery of services. The first moves for integration came from the profession – in 1962 the BMA and the Royal Colleges set up a committee under the chairmanship of Sir Arthur Porritt which concluded that the tripartite division of the health service was harmful to its proper development and that it should be replaced by unified administrative units to be called Area Health Boards.[1] That principle was supported by the Conference of LMCs and the GMSC in 1965.[2]

In November 1967 the Minister of Health, Mr Kenneth Robinson, announced that he was making a careful examination of the administrative structure of the service, and on 23 June 1968 a Green Paper outlining his proposals was issued for discussion and consultation.[3] That was the first time the Green Paper was used as a tool whereby a Government proposal could be discussed publicly before the issue of a formal White Paper. The BMA set up a working party which came up with the sensible suggestion there should be a pilot scheme to evaluate the effectiveness of any changes before they were implemented nationally. The Government did not agree with that sensible idea, setting a pattern from which no government of any political persuasion has ever departed.

The GMSC, on behalf of general practitioners, insisted that the existing structure should be retained until a suitable agreed alternative had been accepted by the profession, and put that point of view to a Special Conference. The young progressive doctors of Hertfordshire were not happy with that and their Local Medical Committee tabled a proposal that 'a unified administration of the National Health Service is desirable'. Making one of my first speeches as a member of the General Medical Services Committee I loyally accepted the Committee's policy but insisted that the Hertfordshire motion was not in conflict with it. Hertfordshire lost by a surprisingly narrow majority of 72 votes to 98.[4]

TRANSPLANT POLICY

In clinical medicine renal transplants had become commonplace in the United Kingdom in the 1960s and Professor Christiaan Barnard had carried out the first heart transplant in South Africa in 1967. This aroused enormous interest worldwide in both the medical profession and the general public, and the subject was scheduled to be considered at the BMA meeting in Aberdeen in 1969, which I would be attending. I decided to oppose the whole idea on the grounds of cost effectiveness – the cost of one heart transplant, about £15 000, being equivalent to the cost of treating five or six other surgical patients needing routine operations. I wrote a speech to that effect and tried it out on my children over Sunday lunch. My son Richard, then 13, listened carefully and said, 'Daddy you are stupid. Of course the transplant must go on. When I am your age the one case will be a brain transplant and the others five heart transplants'. I realised at once that he was talking sense and rewrote my speech, quoting Richard directly. The speech was widely reported in the national press, being quoted verbatim in some of the more serious papers.[5] The Association decided to support the continuation of heart transplant surgery within the NHS and the Government ultimately agreed to fund such a programme. At the time of my writing this Richard is older than I was when I made that speech. We have not yet seen a brain transplant, but we have seen a face transplant and heart surgery is now routine, so at least part of his prophecy has been fulfilled.

AN ATTEMPT AT INTEGRATION

Following the Conservative election victory in 1970, Sir Keith Joseph became Secretary of State. By now there was a strong feeling that the tripartite system set up by Aneurin Bevin was not working properly, that it was inefficient and costly, and that there should be some integration of the three parts.[6] An expert study was set up, headed by a team from McKinsey and Co. Inc., a large American management consultant group. A steering group to assist the study group was formed and two members of the GMSC were appointed to it by Sir Keith. One was a very reputable senior member, Dr Chris Wells from Sheffield, and the other one was me. I firmly believed that an integrated service was necessary and my experience in general practice turned out to be very useful. The Government had laid down certain criteria for the reorganisation, one of which was that the boundaries of the new NHS would be 'coterminous' with the reorganised local authority boundaries which would take effect on 1 April 1974. That turned out to be far from easy.

One evening the team took me to the top of the DHSS building at the Elephant and Castle along with a map of Borehamwood and the surrounding area. They asked me to show them where my surgeries were and I pointed out our two sites in Borehamwood, Hertfordshire. They then asked where I sent my hospital cases and I pointed to Barnet General Hospital in the London Borough of Barnet, and to Edgware General Hospital also in the London Borough of Barnet where our maternity cases went for their outpatient care. Those women were subsequently delivered in Bushey Maternity in Hertfordshire. When I told them that I sent a large proportion of my surgical cases to the Westminster Hospital in Central London they became even more confused, until I explained that the Westminster Hospital had a very short waiting list, that I knew the Professor of Surgery very well, and that my cases would be dealt with by a senior consultant and operated on before they would have been seen at Barnet General Hospital.

I then revealed that I was a clinical assistant in dermatology at two hospitals, Mount Vernon in the London Borough of Harrow, and Watford General in Hertfordshire. When it came to explaining the public health services that covered Borehamwood and Elstree things became even more complicated. The vast majority of our patients lived in Borehamwood and were the responsibility of the Hertfordshire County Council, but about four hundred patients whose addresses were in Borehamwood were actually in the London Borough of Barnet, and another hundred or so in Harrow. I told the team about a case of suspected typhoid that occurred in a hotel known then as the Thatched Barn. The boundary between Hertfordshire and the London Borough of Barnet actually ran through the hotel and I had great difficulty in persuading the Medical Officer of Health(MOH) in Barnet that he, and not the chap in St Albans, was responsible for dealing with this infectious case. Real coterminosity between local authorities and their health equivalents was a good concept but almost impossible to implement fully. All sorts of compromises were necessary. I met Sir Keith during the time that the review was taking place in my capacity as Chairman of the Hertfordshire Executive Council when he opened a Health Centre in Hoddesden.[7] I am sure that protocol and good manners would have prevented my discussing anything remotely concerning the proposed reorganisation on that occasion.

The original intention of the Government had been that the lowest tier of health service management would be the Area Health Authority (AHA), but the steering committee persuaded the study group that a lower tier was necessary. We were to some extent constrained by the Government's insistence on coterminosity and McKinsey's attachment to the concept of consensus management, but we ultimately came up with the idea of a District Management Team (DMT), which would have two separate components. Three of the members – a general practitioner, a hospital consultant and a nurse – would be elected by their peers. The other three, a community physician, the administrator and the treasurer would be appointed by the NHS authorities. These teams would have no chairman and no formal voting. They would reach decisions by consensus.

The report of the study was published in a document which became known as the 'Grey Book'.[8] Its cover was grey, its presentation was grey, and it was so poorly produced that it fell apart with a minimum of handling – rather like the changes in the health service that it proposed. The *Sunday Times*, under the headline 'Doctors win again', complained that Sir Keith Joseph had produced a sane and logical administrative structure for the NHS, but that left consultants as king.[9] The official historians of the BMA[10] recorded truthfully that in due course the BMA welcomed the decision to create the district management teams, one of the most successful of the 1974 innovations. The reality was somewhat different – Chris Wells and I pushed it through the Conference and the ARM against considerable opposition and outright hostility.

At a reception given by Sir Keith Joseph to honour the former members of the study group[11] he told me that he feared that we had 'created a charter for bad doctoring', a view which I tried to correct. Members of the group begged him to try out the system before imposing it on the whole country, but he declined, citing the need to have it up and running by 1 April 1974. That was the first time untried 'reforms' were imposed on the Service without any form of pilot study. In fact I cannot think of any 'reform' of the health service by any government of any political persuasion that has been subjected to proper scientific testing before being introduced on a national scale. Although most of the district management teams worked very well, in some places they were a complete failure – in one north-eastern port the members of the team refused to sit in the same room because of some minor conflict between two of the members. The whole concept of consensus management also fell into disrepute within a few years, both in the health service and elsewhere.

FOOTNOTES AND REFERENCES

1 British Medical Association. Annual Representative Meeting: minutes. 1963.

2 British Medical Association. Conference of Local Medical Committees: minutes. 1965.

3 Ministry of Health, National Health Service. *Administrative Structure of Medical and Related Services in England and Wales*. London: HMSO; 1968.

4 *BMJ*. 1969 Jun 1.

5 Prince J. Doctor clash over cost of transplants. *Daily Telegraph*. 1969 Jul 4.

6 National Health Service. *Reorganisation Consultative Document*. London: HMSO; 1971.

7 Secretary of State visits East Herts. *Mercury*. 1971 Sep 17.

8 *Management Arrangements for the Reorganised NHS (The Grey Book)*. London: HMSO; 1972.

9 Doctors win again. *Sunday Times*. 1972 Aug 6.

10 Grey-Turner E, Sutherland FM. *History of the British Medical Association (Vol II)*. London: British Medical Association; 1982: 127

11 Invitation from the Government Hospitality Secretary addressed to 'Mr [*sic*] JH Marks' to attend a reception on 6 September 1972 'in honour of the members of the former NHS Reorganisation Management Study and DHSS Review Study'.

CHAPTER 9   # An outdated constitution and
Sir Paul Chambers' report

I AM VERY AWARE THAT THE CONSTITUTION OF THE BMA IS NOT OF much interest to most readers, but I do have to explain how the BMA came to be recognised as the only body that could speak on behalf of all doctors, whether they were members or not. Ill-conceived attempts to change the Constitution led to the so-called 'Chambers crisis', which almost destroyed the Association in the early 1970s. I played a major part in defusing that crisis, which helped to advance my medico-political career.

On 19 July 1832 Dr Charles Hastings and about 50 other doctors met in the boardroom of the Worcester Infirmary and set up the Provincial Medical and Surgical Association, which became the British Medical Association. In 1874 the Association became a limited company with Articles and Bylaws, one of which forbade it from becoming or acting as a trade union. The general [company] meeting of the Association delegated most of its powers to the Representative Body, elected by all the members. Alongside that there was a Council elected by the Representative Body itself.[1]

The treatment of the sick poor in England was a considerable problem. Doctors were paid either directly by the patient or by local sickness clubs, often 'Friendly Societies', which collected contributions from subscribers and contracted a local general practitioner to provide services for them. That system was known as Contract Medical Practice, or, more colloquially, as 'the club'. The clubs paid their doctors on a per capita basis.

A large number of the sick poor were not members of clubs and certainly could not afford fees and they were treated on a charitable basis, if at all. In February 1910 the BMA issued a report that criticised the existing methods and laid down three principles which were to play an important part in all its future relationships with the state. These were:

1 The medical services rendered on behalf of the state should be paid for by the state.
2 That the payments should be adequate and in accordance with the professional services required.
3 That there should be adequate medical representation of all committees formed to control the medical assistance.[2]

In May 1911 the then Chancellor of the Exchequer David Lloyd George introduced a National Insurance Bill to Parliament. One of its objectives was to provide general practitioner and pharmaceutical services to low-paid workers, using Friendly Societies as the state's agents.

Two months later a Special Representative Meeting (SRM) of the BMA considered the Bill and established six cardinal points, its basic conditions for co-operating in the establishment of any state-funded service. One of the points was that there should be statutory recognition of a local medical committee (LMC) in the district of each Health Committee, and later such committees were set up under the Act.[3] The Association established a State Sickness Insurance Committee, and that committee recognised that there was a need for a Conference of LMCs. It proposed that such a conference should be held during the Brighton Annual Representative Meeting.

THE FIRST CONFERENCE OF LOCAL MEDICAL COMMITTEES

Unbelievably, the politically naive Council of the Association declined to pay for the Conference and it went ahead only when the local Brighton Division agreed to fund it. It met in the Brighton Pavilion on 24 July 24 1913. The BMA changed the name of its State Sickness Insurance Committee to the Insurance Act Committee, and the Conference asked that Committee to be its Executive. When the Insurance Act Committee met on 8 July in 1948, three days after the start of the National Health Service, it changed its name to the General Medical Services Committee (GMSC).[4]

That system of representation, which became known as the LMC/Conference/ GMSC axis, served general practitioners well, although many considered the arrangements to be an anomaly. Within the hospital services a similar arrangement developed whereby all consultants, whether BMA members or not, were represented by a BMA committee, the Central Committee for Hospital Medical Services (CCHMS), but only in their dealings with the NHS bodies that employed them. In professional matters they were represented by the Joint

Consultants Committee (JCC), which included representatives of the Royal Colleges.

THE BRITISH MEDICAL GUILD

The dispute with the Labour Government in the 1940s exposed the weakness of the BMA as a negotiating body. There were increasing demands for it to become a trade union but doctors, who are by nature individualists, were not enthusiastic about the idea. In February 1949, lawyers advised the Council that conversion of the Association into a trade union was not practicable because it was already a limited company, and in any case doctors did not fall within the definition of 'workmen' in existing Trade Union Acts. The lawyers recommended that the BMA could acquire many of the powers it needed by setting up a Medical Guild, which would be independent of the BMA. The trustees of the Guild would be the members of the Council of the BMA, and those trustees could lawfully invite doctors to take collective action in any dispute with their employers! Furthermore they could make payments to any doctor who suffered financial hardship as a result of loyalty to the collective policy. This clever idea was accepted at a SRM a few weeks later.[5]

TRADE UNION AND THE INDUSTRIAL RELATIONS ACT 1971

On 5 October 1970 the newly elected Conservative Government issued a consultative document relating to a proposed Industrial Relations Bill.[6] The Department of Employment made it clear that the Bill was intended to cover the medical profession and that because the only form of registration under the Bill would be as a trade union, the BMA, being a limited company, was ineligible. High-powered meetings, including some with the Sir Keith Joseph, produced no solution and an Industrial Relations Bill was introduced to Parliament in December.

The GMSC considered the possibility of the autonomous committees registering separately under the proposals of the Bill, but that was found to be incompatible with the Act.[7] Dr Elston Grey-Turner, the then Deputy Secretary of the Association, suggested to the Department that a provision should be inserted in the Bill recognising the professional negotiating bodies with their status and constitutions as they existed on the 5 October 1970, the date of the Government's proposal. His idea was accepted – they were registered as 'staff organisations' in a special section of the register of trade unions in the Industrial Relations Act. The BMA, the British Dental Association and the Royal College of Nursing all signed up. The Council of the Association, not the Representative

Body, was recognised under the act as the Executive of the Union, and from then onwards all voting members of the Council had to be directly elected by the membership.

The 1971 Act was repealed by the Labour Government in 1974,[8] but the protected position of bodies on the Special Register was preserved. Since that date the BMA has had a distinctive status – in law it is both a limited company and a trade union, as well as being recognised universally as representing the majority view of the medical profession.

CHAIRMAN OF AN NHS BODY

Meanwhile, at a local level I had been appointed by the LMC to the Hertfordshire Executive Council, which was responsible for providing general practitioner, general dental, pharmaceutical and ophthalmic services to approximately one million people. In 1971 I became its Chairman and served in that capacity for three years. I learned a great deal about the administration of the health service and the problems within it, especially as the rapid growth of the population in Hertfordshire led to shortages of practitioners, hospitals and all sorts of specialist services.

THE CHAMBERS' REPORT

In 1970 the Representative Body decided that an independent body should examine and report on a revised constitution for the Association.[9] Sir Paul Chambers, Chairman of the Royal Insurance Group, accepted an invitation to do the job. He was asked specifically to consult the Association's chief officers, committee chairman and others, and to take account of the expected White Paper on National Health Service Reorganisation. The consultation process was, to put it mildly, perfunctory. Among those he failed to consult was Dr Alistair Clarke, the Chairman of the Conference of LMCs, who resented what he considered a deliberate snub.

Sir Paul's report was published in March 1972.[10] It recommended that there should be only one democratically elected central body, The Representative Body, which would determine policy. Subordinate to that would be a small central executive. Then came the dynamite. The autonomous committees would disappear, being replaced by four new committees. Two would deal with the terms of service of general practitioners and hospital doctors, while the other two would deal with pay and conditions. Each committee would have an equal number of senior and junior members. Sir Paul emphasised that only members of the Association could hold office of those committees and that there was 'no obligation on the BMA to provide central co-ordination for the work of Local Medical Committees as such'.

The national press paid considerable attention to the report, rightly described as radical by the *Glasgow Herald*,[11] while *The Times* welcomed the report on the grounds that it would increase the involvement of junior doctors in the Association and more importantly it could lead to the destruction of the two autonomous committees.[12] The newspaper questioned the will of the leaders and the members [of the BMA] to make the big adjustments necessary to look at the Association and to meet the needs of today or tomorrow. The BMJ commented favourably on the report but recognised the risk that it might lead to the Association being run by a professional committee supported by the secretariat.[13] However, medical journalists writing in medical newspapers recognised that the proposals to destroy the Association's autonomous committees would reduce the effectiveness of the leadership.[14,15]

Sir Paul addressed both the Council and the GMSC. The GMSC advised the Council not to endorse the report and in its draft report to the SRM convened for November the Council set out the problems that would flow from the implementation of Sir Paul's proposals. Sir Paul addressed the SRM for 40 minutes. As a member of the GMSC, and in effect speaking on its behalf, I was expected to try and hold the party line in the debate that followed. I was doing quite well until I came to dealing with Sir Paul's statement that only BMA local committees would be recognised within the new reorganised NHS. I said, correctly, that I knew more about the new NHS than anyone else in the room as I had helped to draft it. What a blunder! I could see and feel the audience slipping away from me and in the vote that followed Chambers in its entirety was accepted by 153 votes to 149. Fortunately, that was far less than the two-thirds majority required to change the Association's policy, but in an atmosphere described by Lawrence Dobson, a highly respected medical journalist, as 'resembling a revivalist meeting'[16] a proposal that the Chamber's Report be accepted in principle was carried by 217 votes to 82.

Countless meetings took place over the next few months. However, there were two small meetings that I have to mention specifically because they were important in my own medico-political career. The great advocate of Chambers was Dr Clifford Lutton, a general practitioner from Musselburgh, who was Chairman of the Organisation Committee at the time and happened to be an ex-championship boxer. He and I arranged a tour of the country at which we would debate the issue. The first was on my own home territory in Hertfordshire. I had a very high fever and was feeling awful. I made a long rambling speech with masses of details and Cliff won the vote by a landslide. On the way home Shirley gave me a lecture, pointing out that I had been too complicated in my arguments and too verbose and to stick to simple words. The next trip was to Torquay, a hotbed of pro-Chambers sympathy. I was expected to be the meat in the sandwich between Cliff Lutton and the local secretary, but using Shirley's technique I explained the problem to the ordinary members and won the debate by a huge majority. That was the pattern of all the meetings that followed on our tour and I learned yet another valuable lesson.

In 1973 a whole day was allocated at the ARM in Folkestone for the debate on Chambers because 126 motions on the matter had been received from divisions. The night before the meeting, Gyels Riddle and I hosted what was publicly described as a 'birthday party'. It was attended by the Chairman of the Consultants Committee and senior members of all the other negotiating committees within the Association. We planned our tactics carefully for the following days.

According to the official history of the Association, the meeting's acceptance of the Chairman of Council's proposal that each part of the Council's recommendations on Chambers be considered separately effectively disposed of 'Chambers in principle'. The following morning I moved the resolution tackling the issue of autonomy head on.[17] After a long intense debate, during which the Junior Hospital Staff Committee acquired autonomy for the first time, and following a roll call of the representatives, the first in living memory, it was passed by 246 votes to 86.[18] Chambers was dead and buried. I was seen as a great supporter of the craft committees, yet my loyalty to the BMA was never in question. That combination was to stand me in good stead later.

FOOTNOTES AND REFERENCES

1 Muirehead Little E. *History of the British Medical Association*. London: British Medical Association; 1932: 24.

2 *BMJ*. 1910; **1** (Suppl.): 41.

3 *BMJ*. 1911; **1** (Suppl.): 406.

4 Marks J. *The History and Development of Local Medical Committees, Their Conference and Its Executive* 2nd ed. Trustees of the General Medical Services Defence Trust; 1978: 10.

5 Grey-Turner E, Sutherland EM. *History of the British Medical Association (Vol II)*. London: British Medical Association; 1982: 295.

6 Department of Employment and Productivity. *Industrial Relations Bill: consultative document*. London: D.E.P; 1970.

7 British Medical Association. *Minutes of Special Meeting of General Medical Services Committee 24 July 1971*. London: British Medical Association; 1971.

8 *Trade Union and Labour Relations Act 1974*. C52.

9 *BMJ*. 1970; 3(Suppl.): p. 41.

10 British Medical Association. *Report of an Inquiry into the Association's Constitution and Organisation* (Chairman: Sir Paul Chambers; the 'Chambers Report'). London: British Medical Association; 1972.
11 *Glasgow Herald.* 1972 May 5: 6.
12 *The Times.* 1972 May: 4.
13 *BMJ.* 1952; **2**: 305.
14 *Medical News Tribune.* 1972 May 15: 11.
15 *World Medicine.* 1972 Jul 26: 5.
16 *Pulse.* 1972 Nov 25: 1.
17 'That no reorganisation of the BMA can be effective which does not take into consideration the LMC/Conference/GMSC structure and the parallel machinery of regional committees for hospital medical staff/Hospital Medical Staff's Conference/CCHMS, and which does not confer delegated authority upon the GMSC and CCHMS and any other committee of similar structure.'
18 British Medical Association. Annual Representative Meeting: minutes. 1973.

CHAPTER 10

I become involved in national negotiations

FOLLOWING MY ELECTION TO THE GMSC I PROGRESSED SLOWLY UP THE ladder. I was elected to some subcommittees and finally became one of the five 'negotiators' who acted on behalf of general practitioners in their dealings with the Government and other bodies. The other four members of the team were the chairman, Dr James Cameron, Dr Ben Ridge, Dr Tony Keable-Elliott and Dr Keith Davidson, who was Chairman of the Scottish GMSC. Dr Ridge had been involved in politics for many years and was the acknowledged authority on the Regulations that formed the basis of the general practitioners' contract. Ben was highly respected and well liked, and was the de facto Deputy Chairman of the Committee, but he was also known as 'Rigidity Ridge'.

Outside of the BMA I was becoming recognised as an expert on general practices in the NHS. In April 1972 I was invited to speak at the 79th Health Congress of the Royal Society of Health, in a session called 'The Family Practitioner Services – Future Possibilities'. I concluded that given sufficient goodwill, foresight and imagination and a willingness on the part of the community to accept the financial implications of progress, the future possibilities for the family practitioner services, and especially general medical services, were exciting and almost unlimited.[1] My hopes were never fully realised.

Nineteen seventy-three was a quiet year in medical politics for me. Apart from giving a talk on 'Reorganisation of the general practitioners' at the Postgraduate Medical Centre in Canterbury, there was only one major event – the BMA Council dinner. It was a white tie affair, held in the Great Hall in BMA House. The guest of honour was the Prime Minister Edward Heath. Unfortunately for Mr Heath, and us, the dinner took place in the middle of a coal strike when electricity was limited by Government diktats to three days a week. The hall was lit by candlelight and the microphones didn't work properly, and as a very new member of Council I sat with my wife at the bottom end of 'Table J', as close to the exit as it was possible to get.

By the following year it was recognised that Jim Cameron would be giving up the chair of the GMSC after the Annual Representative Meeting. Unfortunately, just before the Annual Conference, Jim was admitted to hospital with gastrointestinal bleeding and Ben Ridge became the Acting Chairman of the Committee and its spokesman at the Conference. Ben was seen to be unbending, and even worse, he wagged his finger at the members of the Conference while addressing them. Neither the members of the Conference nor the Committee were happy with his performance

The Conference took place a couple weeks after the announcement of my MD in the *BMA News*,[2] at a time when the profession was yet again in dispute with the Government over pay. Guided by the negotiators, the Conference rejected a plan for mass resignation from the NHS, but by a large majority decided to issue an ultimatum to the Government – from 1 January 1976 general practitioners would no longer issue national insurance certificates. It was also decided by a majority of two that from 1977 all general practitioner principals must have passed a vocational training course, and by a majority of three it rejected the concept of London weighting.[3]

It was well known that Ben Ridge and I would be candidates for the chairmanship, and we both had supporters and detractors, but quietly a head of steam was building up in support of Tony Keable-Elliott for the chair. I was eliminated in the first round of the ballot, and Ben in the second. Tony became the Chairman and turned out to be a superb one.[4] Ben was so wounded that he resigned from the committee. The GMSC had decided the previous year that it needed a Deputy Chairman, but was fearful that such a person would become the 'Chairman-elect', which happened routinely at the Representative Body. It therefore decided that its Chairman would appoint two Deputy Chairmen to eliminate the possibility of a 'Chairman-elect', rather than have an election for a Deputy Chairman. Tony appointed me and Keith Davidson as his deputies.[5]

In September I spoke at the Annual Postgraduate Meeting of the Association in Douglas, Isle of Man on the organisation of general practice. During the discussion my friend, Professor Harold Ellis from Westminster Hospital, claimed that the reliance of many GPs on deputising services was undermining the high standing of general practitioners. I expressed the view that without deputising services general practice in the centre of large conurbations would collapse. We needed to ensure there were high-quality and well-supervised services.[6]

Not for the first time general practitioners were unhappy with their contract and demanded a new one as a panacea for all their woes. Tony gave me the thankless task of chairing the New Contract Working Group, and we set about collecting evidence from LMCs and others. We very soon discovered that many of the proposals put forward were mutually incompatible, and by the middle of January 1975 I could accurately predict that the LMC Conference would 'tear the model contract to bits and send the Working Party back to the drawing board'.[7]

A CONSULTANT INTERLUDE

Although I was unaware of it at the time, a matter affecting another part of the profession played a considerable part in securing my election to the chairman-ship of the BMA Council years later. In September 1966 the Central Consultants and Specialists Committee (CCHMS) of the BMA took over from the Joint Consultants Committee (JCC) the right to negotiate for its constituents on pay and conditions of service with the Department of Health. Following long discussions between the Department and the profession a draft model contract for consultants was published in 1972. Thereafter negotiations made very little progress until 1974, when the new Secretary of State, Mrs Barbara Castle, set up a joint working party under the chairmanship of the Minister of State, Dr David Owen. In line with Labour Party policy its terms of reference included consideration of arrangements for phasing out pay beds from the NHS. At about the same time NUPE members at Charing Cross Hospital, led by their shop steward 'Granny' Brookstone, went on strike against working in the private wing and refused to feed the patients. The local Health Authority compromised with the stewards and the BMA took the matter up directly with the Secretary of State, making it an issue of principle and considering it as the thin end of the wedge to destroy private practice. Meanwhile, junior hospital doctors were also threatening to strike over their long working hours.[8]

The CCHMS recommended that consultants 'work to rule' by suspending all non-clinical activities. That situation continued until April 1975 when, following an all-night negotiating session, Mrs Castle 'clarified misunderstandings'. However, in August the Government published a Consultative Document on the separation of private practice from the NHS which the BMA described as 'perhaps the greatest threat to the independence of the medical profession since the controversy associated with the introduction of the NHS thirty years ago'. In September, the BMA and 15 other medical and dental organisations sent Mrs Castle a detailed critical commentary on the Government's plans. A month later, when the Prime Minister announced the appointment of a Royal Commission on the NHS, the CCHMS asked that this matter be referred to it. That request was flatly refused. The BMA then asked all senior hospital doctors to ban all NHS work except for emergencies. Junior doctors were already taking unofficial action in their dispute with the Government and that was 'made official'.[9]

There was a split in the Cabinet and Mr Wilson got cold feet. He asked his friend and solicitor Lord Goodman to chair a working party to look into the problem and I, whose private practice was negligible, was appointed by the GMSC to represent general practitioner interests. I had prolonged and close contact with consultant leaders and became friendly with David Bolt and Maurice Burrows, and especially with Tony Grabham,(later Sir Anthony Grabham) their Chairman. In her account of the negotiations Mrs Castle recorded in her diary of 5 December 1975, 'Grabham made all the running: he is by far the ablest negotiator they have got'.[10] I cannot think of anyone to date that has come anywhere near stealing that crown.

David Bolt christened as the 'Cullompton principle'[11] the profession's demand that private practice should be available to everyone in the United Kingdom. The group suggested a compromise that became known as the 'Goodman proposals', accepting the ultimate separation of private practice from NHS hospitals but insisting that the changes would be under the control of an independent board and not the Secretary of State. All concerned accepted that compromise.

COLLECTING UNDATED RESIGNATIONS

Within weeks of their election the new Chairman of the GMSC and his negotiating team were involved in a major political crisis. While gathering evidence for submission to the Review Body, the negotiators sought an assurance from Mrs Castle that the Government would honour any award that the Review Body might make. She said she could not give cast iron guarantees but insisted that the Government felt under 'a strong obligation' to honour any award. According to John Stevenson, a highly respected medical journalist writing in *Pulse*, 'any fluttering of a dove-like nature in Dr Keable-Elliott's conscience was wiped out by the intensity of the GMSC's scepticism'.[12]

As far as the negotiating team was concerned they did not trust Mrs Castle or any politician to publish a report that was likely to show that the country was in the grip of rampant inflation. They felt vulnerable to the accusation that they were inexperienced and weak and the situation was even more complicated because Tony Keable-Elliott and Barbara Castle were known to be next-door neighbours in Ibstone, a small Buckinghamshire village. The GMSC decided that the BMA should once more collect undated resignations from general practitioners to be used if the Government reneged on its commitments.

The Association wrote to every doctor explaining why it needed their undated resignations.[13] Dr John Fry, a leading light in the Royal College, wrote to the *British Medical Journal* criticising our 'over-militant postures' and accused us of 'over-emotional and crude leadership'. In my reply I reminded him, and the *British Medical Journal's* readership, of what appeasement had led to in the past.[14] This was one of the many occasions when leading members of the College attempted to undermine the authority of the BMA's negotiators when they were in dispute with Government, and exacerbated my love-hate relationship with the College.

Local Medical Committees all over the country held meetings and the Hertfordshire doctors were very supportive of the leaders. Headlines such as 'We'll quit threat by doctors'[14] and 'Herts. GPs may resign'[15] appeared in local papers, while the doctors in Finchley, Barnet and Edgware were equally militant.[16] About 60% of general practitioners in England submitted their resignations from the NHS to the Association, to be used if and when the GMSC decided to do so.

However, because of my past involvement in the Hertfordshire Family Practitioner Committee (FPC) I was aware from contacts with senior staff that more than a few doctors were phoning the office, warning the FPC that their resignations had been submitted, but insisting that if the crunch came they would withdraw the resignation. My studies of doctors' actions in such situations, going back to 1912, led me to believe that Hertfordshire was not unique.[17] The resignations were never submitted because the Government honoured the Review Body award in full, to the surprise of everyone, particularly the GMSC negotiators.

Whilst all this was going on I ventured once more into medical journalism writing a short history of the Medical Practitioners' Union (MPU), a recognised trade union representing at the most 5000 general practitioners, which was in favour of a full-time state-salaried general practitioner service. Aneuran Bevan had exerted enormous pressure on the GMSC to allow representatives of the Union to sit on the Committee and that wish was granted in 1950.[18] The Union had just two members in the Committee out of about 60, and although Arnold Elliot, who I have referred to previously, was well respected and influential the power of the Union faded over the years.

AN INTERESTING TWO YEARS

With a little help from me the 1975 Conference of LMCs overwhelmingly rejected the proposed new contract for general practitioners which my working group had produced. I warned the representatives that the closed contract which many of them were demanding would lead to their being employees rather than independent contractors with the advantages of self-employment. I also told them that 'with my own ears I have heard Mrs Castle saying that, deep down in her heart, she would like a full-time salaried service'.[19] By the time the next new contract for general practitioners was being drafted I had moved on.

The Association Secretary, Dr Derek Stevenson, was due to retire in early 1976 and the BMA Council had decided not to advertise the post on the assumption that precedents would be followed and that Dr Grey-Turner would quietly slip into it. Motions were submitted to the Representative Body demanding that the post be advertised A wild rumour that I was a candidate received a great deal of publicity and comment – the one that caused me the biggest problem was John Stevenson's statement that I 'refused to be drawn' on the subject.[20] I had no desire whatsoever to be the Secretary, which involved running committees and managing a staff of hundreds, for which I was completely untrained. The Secretary was in effect a medical civil servant. Admittedly, Derek Stevenson had enormous power because of his own personality and looks and because the elected officers at that time were unwilling and incapable of acting as the 'public face' of the Association and the profession. To his credit, John Stevenson later wrote that I had been genuinely surprised about the support building up on my behalf and did not see myself as the right man for the job.[21] It was only when I became Chairman of the Council 15 years later that the roles changed and I met the press and appeared on radio and television as the profession's spokesman. Elston was appointed as Secretary and served for three years, and when he retired the post was advertised.

In the autumn I was invited to speak at the Biomedical Section of the British Association for the Advancement of Science at their Annual Meeting, held that year at the University of Surrey. I believe that was the only occasion at which my brother Vincent and I spoke at the same meeting. Vincent was the Professor of Clinical Biochemistry in the University and his theme was 'NHS resources are wasted by useless clinical tests'.[22] My paper was an analysis of the benefits and risks of generic prescribing, which the Government was putting forward as a solution to the mounting cost of prescription drugs. I said, 'Government exhortations to prescribe generically should be weighed against the view that no amount of wishful thinking or administrative fiat could alter the fact that the bioavailability – the percentage of drug in unchanged form that reached the body's systemic circulation system – varied quite commonly'. Citing forty two drugs which were suspect I continued, 'There is evidence that GPs are willing and able to make value judgments between these opposing ideals'.[23] My speech was quoted almost verbatim by The Times.[24] The fact that I could speak scientifically to scientists would come in very handy a few years later when I met my first crisis as Chairman of Council in 1980. Then the Government decided that general practitioners would have to stick to a limited list of prescribable drugs, directly contradicting its own previous statements on the subject.

In December 1975 I received my first invitation to speak abroad. Boehringer Ingleheim, a French drug firm based in Rheims, invited me; Dr Donald Irvine, secretary of the Royal College of General Practitioners; Dr Jane Richards, a general practitioner from Exeter; Dr Paul Vickers, a very right-wing Accident and Emergency surgeon from Newcastle, and others, to speak about the British National Health Service. Peter Head, a long established medical journalist, expressed his amazement that over a hundred French doctors would attend a meeting on a Saturday evening, noting their intense interest in our system and their fear that a leftward trend in Europe would 'socialise' medicine in France.[25] Very early on it became obvious to me and the other Britons that our role was to

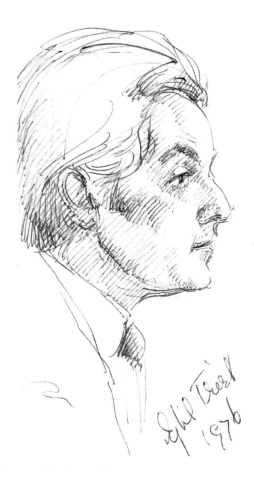

FIGURE 10.1 Sketch by Lady Richardson (Sybil Trist). Me speaking at Guild of St Luke Meeting, Royal Society of Medicine, 25 March 1976.

denigrate our nationalised health service, a role which we rejected. The French audience was astounded to find that we were very happy working in the NHS, although we had doubts about the way politicians manipulated it. A few years later Dr Vickers, who failed in his ambition to be a senior European medical politician, was jailed for the murder of his wife by poisoning her. His use of a rare 'prescription only' drug led to the rapid identification of the murderer!

The morning after the conference we visited a group practice in Rheims. Their whole concept of group practice was very different from ours. There were 17 doctors and two dentists in the group as well as a few general practitioners. To our astonishment we saw three gastroscopes hanging on the wall at a time when Barnet General Hospital had just one.

A few weeks later I received an invitation to speak at the third International Congress on Group Medicine to be held in Paris in June 1976. That meeting was opened by the French Minister of Health Simone Veil, who did nothing to allay the fears of French doctors about the steady erosion of their freedom to practice by Government interventions. I pointed out that the British public had the best 'value for money' in Europe but explained that one of the reasons for that was that we underpaid our doctors.[26]

In June I received a letter from William Rees-Mogg, then editor of *The Times*. He said, 'From time to time we hold lunches here and invite members of one particular profession for an off-the-record conversation. We are planning to hold such a lunch on July 14 for small group of distinguished members of the medical profession and I hope you will be able to join us'.[27]

When I received the guest list it included five medical knights, one being my ex-chief Sir John Richardson, and five members of *The Times* staff, including its medical correspondent. We had a very pleasant lunch and then a discussion started. I well recall feeling that my role was to be the whipping boy while the elders of my profession attacked the BMA in general, and me in particular, for supporting the junior doctors who were rebelling against the establishment by seeking changes in their training programmes and a reduction in their obscenely long working hours. To this day I do not know why a relatively junior member of the BMA leadership was picked out for this treatment but it certainly widened my horizons.

At the Council meeting that followed that year's Annual Representative Meeting Dr James Cameron, the former Chairman of the GMSC, defeated Mr Anthony Grabham in the election for the chairmanship. Dr Cameron was nominated by Dr Tony Keable-Elliott, who told the Council that if elected Dr Cameron 'would only serve for three years'.[28] Three years later those six words would become very significant, cause an upheaval within the Association, and lead to the break up of one of my long-standing friendships.

THE TIMES

Times Newspapers Limited, P.O. Box no. 7, New Printing House Square,
Gray's Inn Road, London WC1X 8EZ (registered office)
Telephone 01-837 1234 Telex 264971 Registered no. 894646 England

From the Editor   7th June, 1976

Dear Dr. Marks,

    From time to time we hold lunches
here and invite members of one particular
profession for an off-the-record
conversation. We are planning to hold
a lunch on July 14 for a small group of
distinguished members of the medical
profession and I hope that you would be
able to join us. It would be a great
pleasure if you can.

    We lunch at 12.45 for 1.00 p.m.

        Yours sincerely,

William Rees-Mogg

Dr. John Marks, MD, MBChB, RCOG, MRCGP,
121 Theobald Street,
Boreham Wood,
Herts.

FIGURE 10.2 Invitation to lunch with William Rees-Mogg, Editor of *The Times*.
Suddenly I am 'distinguished'. 7 June 1976.

MORE ABOUT PRIVATE PRACTICE

In 1976 a Health Service Bill was introduced to Parliament to implement the phasing out of private beds from NHS hospitals and the introduction of common waiting lists. The Bill also dealt with general practitioners and health centres, and the LMC Conference heard from myself and Tony Keable-Elliot that the Bill would dramatically alter the right to private practice in those centres that had only existed since 1967.[29] However, following pressure from the profession the Secretary of State put down amendments to the Bill which guaranteed the right of general practitioners to practise privately from health centres.[30] I received a letter from Patrick Jenkin, the Shadow Secretary of State, expressing his gratitude for the help and guidance I had given him and his colleagues during the Committee stage of the Bill in the House of Commons and saying how important it was that the opposition team in House of Lords receive the same backup.[31]

The Health Service Act 1976 set up a board to implement the changes. I was invited to attend a luncheon meeting of the Medical Journalists Association (MJA) to discuss 'Pay Beds and Related Issues' with Laurie Pavitt MP, the Chairman of the Labour Parliamentary Health Group. In his view two of the members of the board that would phase out pay beds would be 'hard line BMA types', adding that 'Dr Marks could be one of those'. To quote *Medical News*, 'the suggestion had the medical journalists falling about over their profiteroles . . . despite holding the record for putting down parliamentary questions on health matters Mr Pavitt was blithely unaware that in Tavistock Square at least Dr Marks is regarded as positively progressive in medical politics'.[32]

FOOTNOTES AND REFERENCES

1 Royal Society of Health. 79th Health Congress: General Medical Services. *Executive Council Journal of the Society of Clerks of National Health Service Executive Councils.* 1972 Jun; **23**: 109

2 History of LMCs. *BMA News.* 1974 Jun.

3 Milmo S, Turner C. At the Conference of Local Medical Committees. *Medical Week.* 1974; Jun 21.

4 With the benefit of hindsight I can see that the Committee made the correct choice. Tony was interested in general practice and understood money – I was interested in the wider issues of medicine and medical politics. Many years later Tony became one of the best treasurers the BMA ever had. We worked as well together then as we had when I was his deputy.

5 Heir is not apparent. *Pulse.* 1974 Sep 28.

6 Eagle R. Deputies 'undermining GPs high standing'. *General Practitioner.* 1974 Sep 27.

7   Griffiths H. New contract is the top target for GPs to aim at in 1975. *Pulse*. 1975 Jan 18.

8   Owen D. Politics and the NHS. In: MacPherson, G, editor. *Our NHS: a celebration of 50 years*. London: BMJ Books; 1998.

9   Grey-Turner E, Sutherland FM. *History of the British Medical Association (Vol II)*. London: British Medical Association; 1982.

10 Castle, B. *The Castle Diaries 1974–76*. London: Weidenfeld & Nicholson; 1980.

11 Cullompton is a small town in Devon, many miles from the nearest hospital private practice facilities.

12 Stevenson J. How the Hawks won. *Pulse*. 1975 Jan 18.

13 British Medical Association. *Why We Must Have Your Undated Resignation*. London: British Medical Association; 1975.

14 Marks J. Interim pay award [letter]. *BMJ*. 1975; Feb: 175.

15 National health pay award: Herts GPs may resign. *Borehamwood Post*. 1975 Mar 13.

16 Doctors set to resign. *Edgware Times*. 1975 Mar 14.

17 *Daily Telegraph*. 1913 Jan 1: 13.

18 Marks J. Past and present tensions of the MPU. *General Practitioner*. 1975 Mar 28: 18.

19 Langdon NR, Griffiths H. 'About face' euphoria at LMC Conference. *Pulse*. 1975 Jun 21: 2.

20 Stevenson J. Decision on top BMA post put off. *Pulse*. 1975 May 31.

21 The top BMA post may be fully advertised. *Pulse*. 1975 Jun 7.

22 NHS resources are wasted by useless clinical tests. *The Times*. 1975 Sep 2.

23 Generic prescribing is too risky, says BMA official. *Doctor*. 1975 Sep 4.

24 Ally against prescription criticism. *The Times*. 1975 Sep 3.

25 Head P. *Pulse*. 1975 Dec 20.

26 Head P. Concern at loss of freedom. *Pulse*. 1976 Jul 10.

27 Letter from William Rees-Mogg. 1976 Jun 7.

28 Handley S. Cameron the Conqueror. *Pulse*. 1976 Jul 24: 1.

29 Threat over health centres. *Doctor*. 1976 Jul 22.

30 GPs right to prescribe privately safeguarded? *Medical News*. 1976 Jul 22.

31 Letter from Patrick Jenkin MP. 1976 Aug.

32 First, find a chairman. *Medical News*. 1976 Dec 2.

CHAPTER 11   I appear before a disciplinary
body and I lose some friends

ALTHOUGH I HAD WRITTEN OCCASIONAL ARTICLES FOR THE PRESS
I had not been involved in serious 'professional' writing. However, my
extensive knowledge of the Regulations and the GPs' contract led to my being
commissioned to write a series of articles for the magazine *General Practitioner*
entitled 'Know the Terms of Service'.[1] The first one appeared in January 1977.
The publishers must have been happy with it because later that year I wrote an
article explaining the Obstetric List, what it was and how to get onto it[2] and a
whole series of other articles that attempted to make sense of NHS forms.[3]

While studying the origins of local medical committees I became increasingly
aware that ever since Lloyd George introduced his National Insurance Bill in
1911 the state had ruthlessly exploited doctor's vocational spirit. Civil servants
and politicians appreciated medico-political history and knew that doctors
were unwilling to take any action that would jeopardise their patients, and
that under pressure they would blame the BMA for their troubles and form
splinter groups. In my opinion these groups damaged the profession and helped
the Government or its proxies. I came across a whole host of them while
researching: the Association of Panel Committees, the National Medical Guild
and the National Association of Doctors in Practice, and others, all of which
had vanished without trace.

The General Practitioners Association, founded in 1963, was the best
example of a ginger group – in four years it acquired 7000 members, presented
a petition to Parliament, saw one of its leading members elected to the GMSC,
and then passed into obscurity. Having seen the damage done to the consultant
cause during the pay beds crisis by the mutual antipathy between the CCHMS

of the BMA and the Hospital Consultants and Specialists Association (HCSA), I wrote an article for *World Medicine* under their chosen heading 'My medico-political hobbyhorse – splinter groups'.[4] I started by explaining why I felt so strongly about them and then specifically referred to the break-up of the Owen Working Party and the way that Barbara Castle had treated the leaders of both the CCHMS and the HCSA. I compared that with the courteous way she had dealt with the GMSC negotiators at around the same time. This provoked a well-reasoned response from Dr Norman Simmons, a very senior member of the HCSA, defending their position.[5] The article stimulated a host of letters from senior officers of the BMA, HCSA,[6,7] and a long reply from me.[8] I also received a personal letter from Reginald Murley, President of the Royal College of Surgeons, who lived in Radlett. He held what I considered reactionary views and we had crossed swords at many medico-political meetings in Hertfordshire and elsewhere. This time he agreed with my views, emphasising that the consultants were 37 years behind the general practitioners in designing efficient negotiating machinery.[9]

One of the characteristics of the BMA is that its members often ignore its activities at the local divisional level. However, in parts of the country where the division has an active secretary, it can contribute a great deal to medical politics. In 1978 Rotherham was such a division, its Secretary, Dr Hamid Hussein, being a go-ahead general practitioner and an active member of the Representative Body. I was invited to speak at the Divisional Dinner in October 1978. I pointed out that politicians were encouraging patients to complain about doctors so that they could escape taking the blame for faults in the health service. I said that the profession should redirect the public anger and frustration to where it belonged – the politicians. I don't know how Hamid did it but to my amazement the story appeared the following morning in *The Times*,[10] the Manchester edition of *The Daily Telegraph*,[11] *The Yorkshire Post*,[12] *The Morning Telegraph*[13] and, less surprisingly, *The Rotherham Star*.[14] It was a wonderful example of the value of establishing strong contacts with the local media, rather like those I had in Hertfordshire.

Holidays have always played an important part in the life of the Marks family and in March 1978 Shirley and I went to Israel. During that visit I had a working lunch with Dr Elian, chairman of the Israeli Medical Overseas Fellowship. It dawned on me that if I wrote about it and the organisation of health care in Israel it might help to pay for the holiday. The article which I wrote for *General Practitioner* described a system in which most of the medical care was delivered through insurance schemes, the largest of which was Kaput Holim, the health insurance programme of the General Federation of Labour. I described a doctors' strike and the court case that followed when Kaput Holim was sued by a patient for failing to force its doctors to work, and how the head of the organisation finished up in jail having been convicted of fraud.[15]

In July 1978 I wrote to the Greek Embassy, enquiring about visiting the health facilities on the island of Corfu and a month later I received a reply inviting me to meet the chief of the Section of Hygiene of the island. The following May we went to Corfu and met Dr Tselik who told me how after the Second World War young doctors were required to spend part of their careers in the villages as rural doctors. During the military dictatorship the colonels enforced the law strictly but by 1979 things had become more lax. Greek doctors earned about the same as the British doctors but their standard of living was better because they worked for themselves and charged fees.

In November 1978 I had a most unusual experience – I chaired one of the sessions at a weekend course on Private Consultant Practice, arranged by the British United Provident Association Ltd (BUPA). I chaired the section on running a general practice. One of the other speakers at the weekend was Dr Jeremy Lee-Potter. Twelve years later he succeeded me as chairman of the BMA Council.

I APPEAR BEFORE A DISCIPLINARY PANEL

After 24 years in practice a complaint by a patient led to my appearing in front of a Service Committee. Had the whole incident, which exposed the sheer stupidity of the NHS disciplinary procedures not been so unpleasant, it would have made a script for an unsuccessful farce.[16]

In June 1978 Mr Blank came to see me by appointment having already arranged to have more physiotherapy for his backache at the local orthopaedic hospital, but they insisted on a letter from his GP. Mr Blank had received treatment from me, other GPs, and countless specialists over the past 20 years for his depression, hypochondrias, tinnitus and backache. Only two years earlier he had been diagnosed as having 'long-standing minor thoraco-lumbar kyphosis', for which physiotherapy had been given. I examined him thoroughly and then told him quietly that NHS resources were scarce, and that in any case further physiotherapy was unnecessary for his condition. At this he took great umbrage and became abusive, and so I told him to seek medical services elsewhere.

One month later I was invited by the Family Practioner Committee (FPC), which replaced the Executive Council after 1974, to take part in an informal hearing of Mr Blank's complaint. After consultations with my defence body, I declined. Soon afterwards, the formal complaint came, accusing me of a breach of my Terms of Service, which said 'a doctor shall render to his patients all necessary and appropriate medical services'.

Events then took a strange turn. The FPC wrote to say that although I had Mr Blank's very thick record envelope he had not been on my list or that of my partners since 1968 when, having entered a rehabilitation centre in another county, he had registered there. The word 'patient' acquired a new significance. There was no doubt in my mind that Mr Blank was a 'patient' in common sense and common law. But was he a 'patient' as defined in the Terms of Service?

Unbelievably, when the Executive Council reminded Mr Blank that he had not registered with a doctor when he returned to Hertfordshire he immediately tried to come back onto my list. My partners and I declined to accept him.

At the hearing in Hertford on 8 January 1979 I set out to show that legally I was not responsible for Mr Blank's care, and I succeeded. This annoyed the chairman more than somewhat. I then showed that even if I had been legally responsible I had provided adequate treatment in line with my clinical judgement, as I was entitled to do, and there was no case to answer. At the end of the hearing the committee had no option but to reject the complaint.

The ultimate lunacy was yet to come. Mr Blank complained to the FPC that my refusal to accept him on my list was victimisation! He refused to be removed from my list and, furthermore, he had such a high regard for my medical abilities that he was not prepared to register with any other doctor! The Deputy Administrator of the FRC put him right as gently as possible.

I am certain to this day that I was only prosecuted, almost persecuted, because I was the Deputy Chairman of the General Medical Services Committee and the chairman of the Service Committee wanted to make an example of me. He failed.

THE ARM IN LIVERPOOL AND A CHAIRMANSHIP ELECTION

Just before the Annual Representative Meeting Isabel Walker, a very experienced medical journalist, wrote an article under the heading 'Who will sit in Council chair?'[17] Although Jim Cameron had promised Tony Keable-Elliott that he would serve for only three years he began to have second thoughts, allegedly related to the premature retirement of Elston Grey-Turner. Isabel suggested that the Chief Officers (an informal group comprising the President, Chairman of Council, Chairman of the RB and Treasurer) and many Council members were trying to persuade Jim to stay on for at least another year. Nothing was farther from the truth as far as I was concerned. I believed that the BMA suffered because it was represented by two elderly men – one of whom had been known to fall asleep at important meetings. I believed that it needed a new image and a dynamic leader, and that it should be Tony Grabham, who was young, bright, and had a good personality and appearance. Miss Walker suggested that David

Bolt might be a candidate and that either John Noble or Jack Miller could be considered. Most of that was bordering on fantasy. She did say of me, 'RB deputy John Marks, who, some say, will make a very good Chairman of Council *after* he has chaired the RB, will definitely not stand'.[17]

It was a closely guarded secret amongst the Chief Officers and senior officials that the reputation and standing of the Association within the profession had plummeted so far that by then that only 49% of doctors were members. The resistance by the Chairman and the Treasurer to the demand by the Representative Body that ten more industrial relations officers and two more provincial medical secretaries be appointed was just one example of how out of touch the leadership was. Properly trained specialist members of staff were needed to give members the services, particularly trade union type services, for which they were paying.

The ARM was held in Liverpool and was certainly the most unpleasant BMA meeting that I had attended. Although I almost worshipped Jim Cameron, who had been my mentor since I had joined the GMSC, I knew that for the future of medicine and the Association he had to go. I therefore became the leading supporter, outside the consultant camp, of Tony Grabham. My close friend Gyels Riddle led the Cameron camp and publicly accused me of being a traitor! On the other hand, Benny Alexander shared my views, while many of the junior doctors did not trust Tony Grabham.

Before the Council meeting started Shirley and a couple of friends took Pam Grabham on a tour of Liverpool, through the Mersey tunnel and on to Wallasey, so that she could escape from the stress and unpleasantness. Tony was elected by a small majority and Gyels Riddle never spoke to me again except for essential business.

THE GMC ELECTION

The GMC elections had taken place during the summer, using the single transferable vote system. When the results were declared in the autumn there were a lot of surprises. Of the 50 successful candidates only 12 were general practitioners. Even more astonishingly, there was only one junior hospital doctor. To me this suggested that general practitioners and juniors did not vote for their own kind.[18] Isabel Walker commented that although 22 of the 50 candidates were sponsored by the BMA, this was not as good as it looked because BMA sponsored candidates had contested every seat.[19]

THE OVERSEAS MEETING IN HONG KONG

A joint meeting had been arranged with the Hong Kong branch, to be held in October 1979. Shirley and I had booked a pre-Congress tour of China arranged through the BMA. A few weeks before we were due to travel I noticed a black mark under the toenail on my right fourth toe. I was worried that it might be a melanoma, a very nasty malignancy. Unfortunately, Harold Ellis was on holiday and I saw his senior lecturer, who was concerned to such a degree that he phoned Harold on his canal boat. It was arranged that I would see his colleague Gerald Westbury, an authority on the treatment of malignancies, and my admission to the Westminster Hospital was arranged. Before I had my operation I phoned Tony Keable-Elliott and explained the situation and how I might well not be going to China. It was obvious that he was extremely distressed by my news.

Dr Stanley Feldman, a lifelong friend of my brother Vincent, anaesthetised me and when I came round I discovered that nothing had been found because during the preparation the black mark, which must have been a tiny speck of blood, had vanished. My wife Shirley maintains to this day that she knew I had stubbed my toe but she was unable to prevent the medical hysteria that took over my management. Furthermore, the removal of my toenail left me with a tiny spicule of nail that grows alongside the main toenail. This catches in my sock, and from time to time becomes inflamed and painful. Shirley says it is 'God's punishment'.

Arriving in Peking was like landing on the moon. The country was slowly recovering from the Cultural Revolution – everyone was in blue Mao jackets and there were hardly any cars on the streets, although there were thousands of bicycles. The hotels were very poor; but the food was acceptable. Although we had a printed itinerary we were warned that we were unlikely to stick to it, and we didn't. We spent a few days in Peking and then unexpectedly went to Nanking. Our next stop was Kwelin, where we boarded a boat for a cruise along the Yangtze. The mountains there looked exactly like those in Chinese prints – inverted ice cream cones sticking up towards the sky.

On several occasions we visited hospitals and other health facilities and when I returned home I wrote about them.[20,21] Our first medical contact at the Peking Institute of Cancer Research was its director Dr Wu, who had trained at the Marsden Hospital in London. Later that same day the first ever meeting took place between the Chinese and British Medical Associations. In Nanking we visited the hospital attached to the traditional medical school. Built in 1956, it had 350 beds. In addition to the usual departments such as surgery, paediatrics and gynaecology it had a special department for dealing with haemorrhoids, a very common condition in China, although we were told that cancer of the colon was a rarity.

At the Lungua No.1 Hospital in Shanghai we went into an operating theatre where a fully conscious patient was lying on the table. The anaesthetist inserted two acupuncture needles, one into the back of the right hand and one into the right forearm which was connected to a 9 Volt electric simulator. After 20 minutes induction, a surgeon appeared and removed an adenoma of the thyroid. One of our surgeons who had been completely sceptical told us that he was impressed beyond words. We also visited two communes where the medical facilities were extremely primitive, but we noted that the queues for Chinese traditional medicine were much longer than those for the Western scientific brand.

The meeting in Hong Kong was a great success. We saw its booming economy and its modern medical facilities. We also visited a modern block of flats, which was not on the official tour, and were quite horrified at the overcrowding. One tiny room was allocated to each family, but those families could consider themselves fortunate compared with many others. From there we returned home to the humdrum life of general practice and yet another Abortion Bill.

FOOTNOTES AND REFERENCES

1 Marks J. Know the Terms of Service. *General Practitioner.* 1977; Jan 7: 31.
2 Marks J. The obstetric list: getting your name down. *General Practitioner.* 1977; Sep 23: 33.
3 Marks J. Making sense of NHS forms. *General Practitioner.* 1977; Dec 9: 17–32.
4 Marks J. My medico-political hobby-horse: splinter groups. *World Medicine.* 1977; Oct 19: 42
5 Simmons N. Splinter, sharp reply. *World Medicine.* 1977; Nov 16: 15.
6 Goldman M. Letter. *World Medicine.* 1977; Nov 2: 14.
7 Shrank A. Letter. *World Medicine.* 1978; Jan 11: 16.
8 Marks J. Letter. *World Medicine.* 1978; Jan 11: 17.
9 Letter from Mr Reginald Murley. 1977 Oct 24.
10 Politicians 'trying to escape blame' for NHS faults. *The Times.* 1978 Oct 6.
11 Doctors NHS 'scapegoat', BMA told. *Daily Telegraph.* 1978 Oct 6.
12 Health service faults 'hidden by politician'. *Yorkshire Post.* 1978 Oct 6.
13 *Morning Telegraph.* 1978 Oct 6.
14 Lloyd T. Public 'conned' on NHS funds. *Rotherham Star.* 1978 Oct 6.
15 Marks J. A poor state of health. *General Pracitioner.* 1978; Nov 3.
16 This account is based on an anonymous article I wrote in *Pulse,* 19 May 1979 under their heading 'Rough justice'.
17 Walker I. Who will sit in Council chair? *General Practitioner.* 1979; Jun 30.
18 Landon N. GPs out-voted on reformed the GMC. *Pulse.* 1979 Aug 24.
19 Walker I. Representative GMC. *General Practitioner.* 1979; Aug 24.
20 Marks J. West meets East in Chinese medicine. *Pulse.* 1980 Feb 16: 17–18
21 Marks J. China's inventive and unorthodox medicine. *Pulse.* 1980 Feb 23: 17–18.

CHAPTER 12 I represent the profession
at home and abroad

BY NOW, AS DEPUTY CHAIRMAN OF THE REPRESENTATIVE BODY I HAD become almost part of the BMA establishment. After the publication of the second edition of my pamphlet on the LMCs, which included an account of the Chambers Report crisis, John Illman from *General Practitioner* interviewed me. We discussed the threat to the Association which followed that report, but fortunately he was unaware of the latest threat – the rapidly dwindling membership. I expressed the view that the space devoted to the Association's failures in the paramedical press was out of proportion to that given to its successes and that one day we would have no BMA – it would have been destroyed by the medical comics. We both agreed that outside the profession the BMA enjoyed the highest reputation and was considered by the public to represent British medicine. Only the members took it for granted.[1]

This elicited a rapid response from Cliff Lutton, the great proponent of the Chambers proposals. He wrote a letter that claimed Sir Paul Chambers was not a threat to the BMA – the lifeline that he threw it was cut by people like me. Lutton ended his letter by writing 'no doubt the Medical Practitioners' Union (MPU) section of The Association of Scientific, Technical and Managerial Staffs (ASTMS) is waiting anxiously in the wings to take over when what Dr Marks predicts comes about'.[2] Fortunately he got that wrong too.

The Annual Dinner of the Barnet and Finchley Division of the BMA was due to be held in March and Shirley was now Chairman of the Division. The Member of Parliament for Finchley was Mrs Margaret Thatcher. She wrote to the Member for Chipping Barnet, Sydney Chapman, who was sponsoring the Annual Dinner at the House of Commons, asking him to convey to the guests

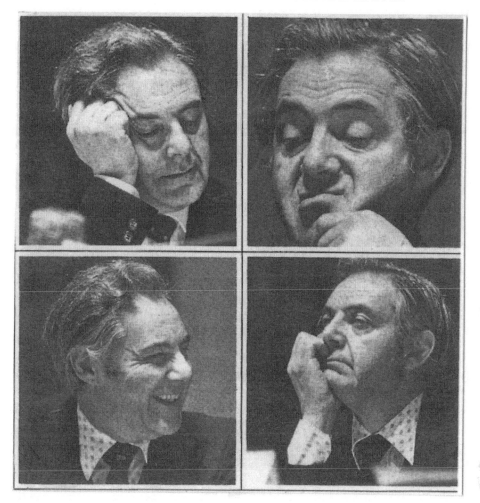

FIGURE 12.1 'The many moods of Marksism: Dr John Marks, Deputy Chairman of the Representative Body, puts on a good face to the changing aspects of the Conference'. © *General Practitioner* 6 July 1979.

'my warm regards and appreciation for the splendid work they do and especially for the way in which they uphold the highest professional standards. The lead they give in that respect is a wonderful example to everyone'.[3] The letter itself became a news item and was reported, under a photograph of Shirley, Sydney Chapman, and the BMA president, Dame Josephine Barnes.[4]

The dinner was a great success and a few days later Mr Chapman wrote to Shirley saying how much he had enjoyed it adding, 'above all I hope we keep in close contact in the future do not hesitate to get in touch if I can be of any help'.

He also thanked me for the copy of my booklet on local medical committees. I hope that he read it very carefully.[5]

MY FIRST OFFICIAL TRIP TO THE UNITED STATES

When Tony Grabham took office he found that nothing had been done about arranging an overseas meeting after the Hong Kong one. In the late autumn he sent for me and suggested that we should have a meeting in the United States and that I should go there to arrange it. I soon learned that there were six essential requirements for a successful meeting: a venue, speakers, travel arrangements, accommodation for delegates and others, costs, and also arrangements for accompanying wives. Social change and 'political correctness' caused the BMA problems as participants could be accompanied by people of either the same sex as themselves, or the opposite one. In other organisations those people became known as 'partners', but the BMA could not use that term because of its particular connotation in general medical practice. In the end we produced programmes for 'Accompanying Persons', which became the accepted term.

Andrew Blair, the travel agent for the Hong Kong meeting accompanied me to the States. We were joined by Barbara Middlemiss, the BMA official responsible for all meetings, who was a professional right to her fingertips. John Havard had a contact in San Francisco and so that was our first port of call.

I soon learned that those who arrange meetings are treated as VIPs. Flights, almost always business class, were provided free of charge by airlines that hoped to capture the business when the meeting took place. Similarly, hotels offered hospitality, and so I flew to San Francisco business class and started my stay in the Presidential Suite of the Fairmile Hotel, one of the most luxurious in the city. I inspected their facilities and through the good offices of John Havard and his friend Dr Jamplis, I had a meeting with the dean of the Medical School at Stanford University. I then moved to an equally luxurious suite at the Sir Francis Drake Hotel. Unfortunately, I soon realised that San Francisco was such a popular conference centre that there was a waiting list of a least four years for conference facilities, which did not suit us.

We then flew to Miami, where we were met by not one organising committee but by two, each of which arrived at the airport with a fleet of limousines and a host of tough-looking gentleman who were quite determined that we would use their group. Unfortunately, the waiting list for facilities in Miami was as long as that in San Francisco, and so we returned home to report our failure to the chairman. Fortunately Stephen Lock, the editor of the *British Medical Journal*, was visiting the West Coast of America and he had a contact in San Diego. He managed to fix a meeting, which would be held there in the autumn of 1981.

A COUPLE OF SOCIAL OUTINGS

When I left Dublin in 1947 I vowed that I would never return having seen enough poverty and squalor there to last me a lifetime. However, in April 1981 I was sent to Wexford to represent the BMA at the Annual Meeting of the Irish Medical Association, which still had strong links with the BMA. Shirley and I arrived in the evening and when we turned up for the first plenary session the next morning we found ourselves sitting in an empty hall. Ultimately a passer-by informed us that the meeting took place in Irish time, which ran considerably behind clock time. At the end of the day we were invited to an informal dinner and at the end of the second day we attended a formal black tie dinner given by the President and Council of the Association. It was a great meal, and the alcohol flowed. I was relieved to see that at last the table was clear of bottles, whereupon someone put their hand under the table and produced another crate. I have no recollection of what followed.

In July Shirley and I attended a Royal Garden Party at Buckingham Palace. We were lucky that the weather was good. The Queen looked positively radiant. It was an interesting experience.

A LITTLE LOCAL DIFFICULTY

Although I was getting increasingly involved in medical politics I was still a general practitioner providing services in Borehamwood. In line with my philosophy of concentrating services in high-quality premises we decided to reduce our surgery hours at Manor Way surgery and improve those at the main surgery in Theobald Street, which we had developed into a first-class group practice centre with money borrowed under the Government's Group Practice Loans Scheme from the GP Finance Corporation. We obtained the necessary permission from the Family Practitioner Committee in Hertford and made the changes. A petition opposing them received over 2000 signatures, while Dr John Marx [sic] was quoted as saying, 'it is the correct way to run medicine. Both Labour and Conservative governments have agreed doctors should have joint practices with branches [sic]'.[6] The Deputy Mayor criticised us[7] while the Town Council called on the local Member of Parliament, Mr Cecil Parkinson, to persuade the doctors to change their minds.

A copy of a letter written on 16 June 1981 by the Administrator of the Hertfordshire FPC, Mr Buck, to the Clerk of Elstree Town Council, weeks before the stories appeared in the local press, came into my possession. It pointed out that the FPC had no powers under the regulations made by Parliament to require a doctor to open or reopen a surgery or branch surgery. It continued, 'A number of persons who signed the petition were interviewed and it was apparent that not all those who had signed a petition were patients of [our practice]'. It also said that the doctors believed that the service they could give at the branch surgery could only be improved by damaging the overall service given by the practice.[8] It is obvious that members of the Town Council must have known of Mr Buck's letter long before the nasty stories appeared, but denigrating doctors is always more popular than trying to educate the public into proper use of health care facilities.

I BECOME CHAIRMAN OF THE REPRESENTATIVE BODY

The ARM in 1981 was held at the Brighton Centre, a huge hall very suitable for the Conservative Party or Trade Union Congress, but far too large for the BMA's 600 representatives. The only incident of note was an invasion of the hall by a group of militant anti-abortionists, who staged a sit-in in front of the platform, whose occupants took no notice of them. A group of burly junior hospital doctors lifted them up and deposited them on the pavement outside. One very important motion was passed, condemning the misuse of psychiatry in the Soviet Union and requesting that the BMA raise the matter with the World Medical Association.

The election of the Chairman of the Representative Body takes place every third year. Within living memory there has never been more than one candidate: the sitting Deputy Chairman. He takes office at the end of the meeting and reigns for three years. At Brighton I stood for election unopposed and when I became chairman the *Jewish Chronicle* was quick to lay claim to me as a founder member of the Borehamwood Synagogue and a current member of the Edgware Reform Synagogue, the Israeli Medical Association and the London Jewish Medical Society.[9]

THE WORLD MEDICAL ASSOCIATION GENERAL ASSEMBLY

Tony Grabham and I represented the BMA at the 34th General Assembly of the World Medical Association in Lisbon in the autumn of 1981. In spite of its grandiose title, in law the Association was merely a limited company set up in the State of New York and bound by its laws, in the same way as the British Medical Association is a limited company under British law. In 1979, a recommendation from the BMA Council to the RB that the Association should withdraw from World Medical Association (WMA) because of its deficiencies as a world organisation was rejected by the representatives.

Steve Biko had died in detention in South Africa, and Tony Grabham had spent a long time investigating the involvement of doctors in the case. He was convinced that the South African Medical and Dental Council (the equivalent of the British GMC) had mishandled the affair, and he was told by the chairman of the Council of the Medical Association of South Africa (MASA) that he was in no doubt there was a prima facie case of unethical conduct against the doctors involved.

In 1981 MASA was not a member of the WMA, but there was a strong move afoot to re-admit it at the General Meeting. Tony and I were instructed to oppose it. The voting strength of a country at the WMA assembly was proportionate to the subscription that it paid, not to the number of doctors that it represented. The USA had 35 votes; the BMA had two. We proposed a compromise resolution to put off the decision for two years and send a fact-finding mission to South Africa. It was defeated by the combined vote of Brazil, West Germany, Japan and the United States, which between them held sufficient votes to overcome any opposition. A dozen African doctors representing Nigeria and Ghana walked out in protest and Liberia, Egypt, Ethiopia and Togo announced their intention of leaving.[10] Prior to the discussion on South Africa I spoke in favour of the BMA's resolution condemning the misuse of psychiatry in the Soviet Union. I reminded the delegates that in 1978 at Manila the WMA itself had condemned the use of psychiatry as a means of controlling political dissidents, and it was sad and disgraceful that the matter should arise again with particular reference to the Soviet Union.[11] In my speech I reported that all the founder members of a Working Commission on the misuse of psychiatry in the Soviet Union had been imprisoned, exiled or forced to emigrate. Our motion was passed without dissent.[12]

A couple of weeks later Tony and I reported on the meeting to the BMA Council. I described the voting system at the WMA as 'diabolical' and that although there was a great need for a world forum in medicine I doubted whether the WMA was the right one. Council agreed to consider withdrawing from the WMA at its next meeting.[13]

THE MEETING IN SAN DIEGO

The Overseas Clinical Meeting was to be held at San Diego in October 1981. Shirley and I decided that as our fare to the States was being paid we would have a holiday linked to the meeting, a pattern that we subsequently followed whenever possible. We arranged to go first to Las Vegas, then to the Grand Canyon and then on to Phoenix, where my father's cousin and her family lived. What we had not bargained for was President Reagan's reaction to a strike of air controllers, which started in August – he sacked the lot. As a result, planes were diverted, cancelled, or despatched irregularly. We did our trip in a roundabout way, which involved going through Phoenix airport on three separate occasions. In Las Vegas we saw an intoxicated Sammy Davis Jr literally dragged off the stage. We slept in a huge bedroom with an enormous mirror in the ceiling, and I made sufficient money playing poker against a machine to pay for our dinner. At the Grand Canyon we made our first, and last, helicopter flight. It turned out to be a magnificent holiday.

In San Diego the keynote address was to be given by Alistair Cook KBE, the distinguished broadcaster. He accepted our invitation on one condition, that we paid him no fee but provided him with a first class ticket between New York and San Diego. The Chief Officers, the senior BMA officials and their wives had a very interesting dinner with Mr Cook the night before the meeting started.

The meeting was opened by our President Sir John Walton and we were welcomed by Dr Brad Cohen, President of the Californian Medical Association, and Dr Thomas Lyons, President of the San Diego County Medical Society. After Alistair Cook had delivered the keynote address on 'The doctor in society', I gave the vote of thanks and the socialising began.[14]

According to *American Medical News*,[15] one purpose of the BMA convention in San Diego was to explain the workings of the British medical system to American physicians. It added that 'the difference between GPs and specialists is so marked that the BMA had designated a speaker to explain each'. I described general practice in United Kingdom and how it worked in the NHS and Tony Grabham talked about the role of the consultant. That was in line with the sensible policy that the Association had for dealing with overseas meetings. All the senior members of the Association who had no choice but to be there on duty, and whose expenses were funded by the paying members of the conference, were expected to 'sing for their supper'.

There was a heated debate on the role of women in medicine. The former president of the BMA, Dame Josephine Barnes, stormed out of the meeting saying 'being a woman did not affect my career'. Dr Mary White, a member of the Council, accused female complainers of using sexual discrimination as an excuse. Being married to a woman doctor I had a special interest in this matter, and I was one of the very few men present. I said, 'The sad fact is that medical associations are dominated by male chauvinist pigs', but according to the report there was unrest when I added 'the saddest thing I heard recently was a young woman who said she had to choose between her career and her uterus'.[16]

At the end of the meeting we drove via Big Sur to San Francisco, from where we flew home. The meeting had been a success and the holiday had been a great success. All we had to do now was to prepare for the BMA's sesquicentennial celebrations in 1982.

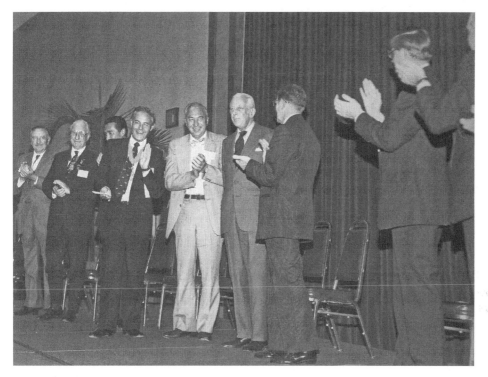

FIGURE 12.2 With Alistair Cooke, BMA Overseas Meeting, San Diego, California 1981. © British Medical Association.

FOOTNOTES AND REFERENCES

1 Illman J. A new threat to the BMA? *General Practitioner.* 1980 Feb 8.
2 Lutton CC. BMA decline: new threat from an old problem. *General Practitioner.* 1980 Mar 28.
3 Handwritten letter dated 13 March 1980 on 10 Downing Street notepaper from Mrs Thatcher to Mr Chapman.
4 *Barnet Press.* 1980 Mar 21: 2.
5 Handwritten letter dated 19 March 1980 and addressed to Dear Shirley and John from Sydney Chapman MP.
6 2000 back the demand for Manor Way evening surgery. *Borehamwood Post.* 1981 Jul 7.
7 The people who 'can't afford to be sick'. *Borehamwood Post.* 1981 Jul 30.
8 Letter dated 16 June 1981 from Mr Buck, Administrator of the Hertfordshire Executive Council, to Mr Orton, Clerk to Elstree Town Council.
9 All in the family. *Jewish Chronicle.* 1981 Jul 24.
10 Stride RS. Africa in by a whisker. *Doctor.* 1981 Oct 10.
11 Jolliffe J. Medical congress ends by condemning Russia. *Guardian.* 1981 Oct 3.
12 Marks J. Cause for concern: the Commission that was wiped out. *World Medicine.* 1981 Nov 14: 77–8.

13 MacCormack M. BMA ponders merit of staying in WMA. *General Practitioner*. 1981 Oct 16.

14 Programme of the BMA Congress San Diego, 19–22 October 1981.

15 American physicians are given an explanation of British system. *American Medical News*. 1981 Nov 6.

16 Bishop M, Britton D. Barnstorm performance. *Doctor*. 1981 Oct 29.

CHAPTER 13

AIDS and the
BMA

ACQUIRED IMMUNE DEFICIENCY SYNDROME (AIDS) WAS UNKNOWN
before 1981. In 1986 AIDS became headline news[1] and Norman Fowler, Secretary
of State for Social Services, outlined the measures the Government was taking to
combat the spread of the disease. A Cabinet Committee on AIDS set up under
the chairmanship of William Whitelaw, the Deputy Prime Minister, held its first
meeting on 11 November.[2] The Council of the BMA advised that patients with
HIV antibodies and those with full-blown AIDS were entitled to confidentiality
and that blood could be tested only with the patient's full consent.[3] Its advice
was based on the long-established view that it was vital not to drive sexually
transmitted diseases 'underground'. Historically, the management of sexually
transmitted diseases (STD), then known as the venereal diseases (VD), were
covered by the Venereal Diseases Regulations passed by Parliament during the
First World War.[4] They guaranteed absolute confidentiality for anyone seeking
treatment for one of those diseases. As a result, control of venereal diseases in
Great Britain was better than most other places in the world.

THE BMA TAKES A LEAD

In February 1987 I and other representatives of the Association gave evidence on
our attitude to AIDS to the House of Commons Social Services Committee. We
were attacked there by Nicholas Winterton MP as 'promoters of promiscuity',
not because of our attitude to AIDS but because of our policy on confidentiality
regarding the prescribing of the contraceptive pill to girls under the age of 16 by
doctors. We rebutted Mr Winterton's perpetuation of the myth that AIDS was

confined to homosexuals.[5] The press became interested, and among other daft ideas put forward was a demand that HIV positive people should carry cards announcing the fact.[6]

In March 1987 the BMA published a booklet, *AIDS and You*,[7] which set out in simple words and explicit cartoons how HIV was spread and what precautions young sexually active people should take to avoid it. It was the brainchild of Dr John Dawson, the highly gifted Assistant Secretary of the BMA responsible for science, education and ethics. Although the pamphlet provoked outrage among the more reactionary and bigoted members of the profession, 60 000 were distributed to various organisations.

Years later it won a Plain English Award which was presented to me at the English Speaking Union by Michael Cashman, an actor starring in *Eastenders* and a well-known homosexual activist.[8]

In May 1987 the BMA Council approved the establishment of The BMA Foundation for AIDS, also inspired by John Dawson.[9] Its functions were to educate the public and the professions about AIDS and to counteract the wild hysteria surrounding the subject. Sadly, John Dawson died a couple of years later from cancer of the prostate.

THE BRISTOL ARM – THE BMA'S BAD DECISION

The ARM that year was held in Bristol. The debates on AIDS were a procedural nightmare and according to the medical commentator 'Scrutator' they were more confused and unruly than any that he had witnessed in two decades of observing annual meetings. In spite of my warning against hysteria, and my urging the representatives to debate the issues like scientifically trained doctors who should listen, think and then vote in what they believed to be the best interests of their patients and the community, the meeting degenerated into chaos. In winding up the debate I said quite bluntly, 'The motion is bad: reject it', but the representatives decided by 183 votes to 140 'that the testing of HIV antibodies should be at the discretion of the patient's doctor and should not necessarily require the consent of the patient'. Whilst the votes were being counted the question was raised as to whether a two-thirds majority was needed, a requirement when any change of established Association policy was being considered. The chairman ruled that such majority was not necessary, and so by a small majority the BMA had a new policy on testing for AIDS.[10]

This new policy provoked a justifiable furore in the press from one end of the country to the other, with headlines like 'Secret AIDS test storm'[11] and 'Fury after the BMA agrees on secret AIDS tests'.[12] The National Council for Civil Liberties condemned the decision and suggested that the Association should

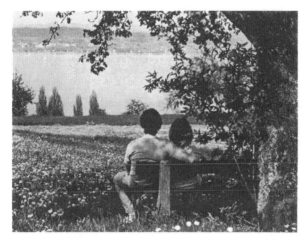

A·I·D·S

AND YOU

An illustrated guide

British **M**edical **A**ssociation

FIGURE 13.1 Front cover, *AIDS and You* 1987. © British Medical Association.

start a programme of educating its members. The legal situation was far from clear, some lawyers believing that taking a person's blood for a purpose for which he had not consented would constitute an assault.[13]

During the autumn there were hysterical articles in the press about doctors with AIDS. When I wrote a letter to *The Times*[14] pointing out that doctors too were entitled to confidentiality the tabloid newspaper *Today*, under the headline 'Medical madness', demanded that doctors who were HIV positive should not work[15] and that all doctors be tested for HIV.[16]

That meeting was James Kyle's last one as Chairman of the RB and the newly elected Chairman, Benny Alexander from Manchester, was as concerned about the problem as I was. We both knew we had to reverse the decision on consent at the next RB meeting to be held in Norwich, or give up our offices, as we felt unable to represent such a self-defeating and damaging policy.

As a first step we managed to persuade the Council, backed by advice from Michael Sherrard QC,[17] to 'decline to implement' the RB policy. A bye-law in the BMA company articles gave the Council that right if it considered that a resolution of the RB was 'undesirable in the interests of the Association and its members'. The Bristol resolution on AIDS certainly was such a resolution.[18] In my experience of over 40 years I cannot remember another time when that procedure was used. However, there was a proviso – Council's decision had to be brought to the next RB Meeting.

FURTHER OPPOSITION TO THE COUNCIL

The Consultants Committee of the BMA, and particularly its surgical members and their constituents, were very unhappy with the BMA's opposition to testing without consent, partly due to their misunderstanding of the risks to themselves. It sought a second legal opinion from Mr Leo Charles QC, who concluded that the patient's consent must precede any physical contact by the practitioner with the patient. He said, 'The resolution passed at the ARM in 1987 is inapplicable. It would expose the practitioner to legal liability in both the civil and criminal courts'. The Medical Defence Union had obtained yet another opinion, which took the same view. The GMSC had supported the BMA Council's decision not to implement the 1987 Resolution, and at the Conference of Local Medical Committees a motion to censure the committee for its actions was moved and heavily defeated. The wrecking amendment was moved by Dr Outwin of Doncaster, the man who put my name forward in the famous 'Chambers crisis'.[19]

Meanwhile, in the broader community even more hysteria was being generated. It was widely reported that an orthopaedic surgeon who had worked in Redditch had died of AIDS in an Exeter Hospital. I was quoted as saying 'Although there is a theoretical risk there has not been a single case in the whole world of a patient who has been found to be HIV-positive as a result of contact with a health worker'.[20] The Foundation for AIDS launched three videos advising family doctors about the management of HIV testing[21] which received a certain amount of press coverage.[22] In May an ex-Minister Sir Rhodes Boyson, speaking on the BBC, labelled homosexuality as unnatural and claimed that AIDS would die out if homosexual practices were wiped out. That was reported in the *Daily Express*, but to be fair to that newspaper it also reported that I accused Sir Rhodes of being hysterical.[23]

On the 20 May I was interviewed in depth on Channel 4 News by Peter Sissons. The station was responding to a report prepared for the Chief Medical Officer which recommended voluntary testing of pregnant women, prisoners, and eventually heterosexual men through GP surgeries in an attempt to establish how widespread the HIV virus was in the general community. The Government had had the document for more than two months but had taken no decisions on it. That same story was quoted elsewhere.[24] Mr Sissons wanted to know why surgeons were not being protected by having every patient tested for HIV before operation. I explained to him that, because of the latent period of up to three years during which people who were infected with the virus tested as 'HIV negative', they would escape detection but could still infect others. Therefore surgeons had to rely on normal methods of infection prevention in order to be safe. We then got on to prisoners and once more he was quite aggressive, finally demanding to know why prisoners who could not possibly be HIV-positive were being locked up with those who might well be infected and had not been tested. I said, 'If you and I were locked up for a year and I was HIV-positive I could not infect you unless we had homosexual sexual intercourse'. The interview ended immediately but my grin was shown on the screen, his horrified expression was not.

THE ARM 1988 AIDS DEBATE AT NORWICH
Sadly my close friend Dr Benny Alexander developed a malignant cerebral tumour shortly after his election. For most of the medico-political year he was out of action and his Deputy, Dr Alexander (Sandy) Macara, did most of his work. However, showing unbelievable bravery and courage, Benny insisted on dealing with the AIDS issue himself.

A motion was received by the Agenda Committee criticising the Council's decision not to implement the 1987 resolution. I took the view, and persuaded the Agenda Committee to agree, that this was a motion of no confidence in the

Council (and its Chairman). As such it would have to be taken immediately after the Chairman's annual address, when I would be on a high, and furthermore it would be clearly separated from the scientific and clinical debates on AIDS which were scheduled for two days later.

The censure motion was moved by Dr James Appleyard, a consultant paediatrician who, in 1972, had been one of the prime movers in the refusal by junior doctors to pay the GMC retention fee. He was supported by Dr Pickersgill, a general practitioner from Norwich and a popular member of the local Division and the Organising Committee of the meeting.

The Council's decision was backed by the mover of the 1987 resolution, Dr RA Keable-Elliott, because in his opinion that motion's wording was flawed. Literally interpreted, it meant that a doctor could take blood from a patient without his permission. (What a shame he had not thought of that the previous year, it would have saved a lot of bother!) He was supported by the Chairman of the Medical Academic Staffs Committee and the chairman of the GMSC. The motion was defeated, to quote the *British Medical Journal*, 'with no need for the vote to be counted'.[25] We then had to wait two days for 'the real debate'.

On the Wednesday morning a divisional representative, Dr Surendra Kumar from St Helens, proposed that 'HIV testing should be performed only on clinical grounds with the full informed consent of the patient'. Dr Keable-Elliot then suggested an amendment, a classical example of BMA verbosity – 'HIV testing should be performed only on clinical grounds with the specific consent of the patient. There may be individual circumstances when a doctor believes that in the best interests of the patient it is necessary to depart from this rule, but if the doctor does so he or she must be prepared to justify this action before the courts and the General Medical Council'. It was seconded by Mr Kyle, who had chaired the 1987 debate, and was by supported by the leaders of the main committees. It was reported that I begged the Representative Body to pass it.[26] As it was a statement of the obvious, was absolutely in line with my views, and saved the face of the Association and those involved in the Bristol fiasco, how could I do anything else? It was passed and the 'AIDS crisis', yet another potential disaster of the BMA's own making, was over.

In the following years AIDS became a major international health problem and parts of Africa have been almost decimated by it. However in the United Kingdom it has been reasonably well contained, partly due to the public education on 'safe sex' instigated by *AIDS and You* and other publications, by the quality of the services provided, and by the maintenance of the confidentiality of those seeking treatment. Furthermore, following the discovery of antiviral drugs, the condition is now treatable, which it was not when the BMA temporarily took leave of its senses.

FOOTNOTES AND REFERENCES

1 Bureau of Hygiene & Tropical Diseases. *AIDS Newsletter*. 1986 Mar 25; **Issue 4**.

2 Berridge V. *AIDS in the UK: the making of policy 1981–1994*. Oxford: Oxford University Press; 1996: 104.

3 Howard N. Patient priming is vital to blood test for HIV virus. *Doctor*. 1987 Jan.

4 Public Health (Venereal Diseases) Regulations, 1917.

5 Clash over AIDS. *New Scientist*. 1987 Feb 26.

6 Mclean A. 'Civil liberties at risk' as AIDS toll mounts. *Scotsman*. 1987 May 7.

7 British Medical Association. *AIDS and You*. London: British Medical Association; 1987.

8 Plain English award for 'AIDS and You'. *BMJ*. 1988 Jan 9.

9 Smith H. BMA launches new AIDS trust. *General Practioner*. 1987 May 15.

10 'Scrutator' was the nom de plume of Dr Gordon McPherson, Deputy Editor of the *British Medical Journal*.

11 Shock decision at BMA meeting: secret AIDS test storm. *Western Morning News*. 1987 Jul 3.

12 Fury after BMA and agree on secret AIDS tests. *Aberdeen Press and Journal*. 1987 Jul 3.

13 Wynn Davies P. AIDS testing: the doctor's legal dilemma. *Law Magazine* 1987 Jul 24: 29.

14 Marks J. BMA view on doctors with AIDS. *The Times*. 1987 Nov 13.

15 Medical madness [editorial]. *Today*. 1987 Nov 14.

16 Make every doctor take AIDS test [editorial]. *Today*. 1987 Nov 16.

17 Michael Sherrard is the brother of my younger brother's wife. The members of the BMA's staff who consulted him in the first instance were unaware of that fact. When I was informed I went out of my way to make sure that all concerned were made fully aware of the fact.

18 Woodfield G. Doctors shy from secret AIDS tests. *Liverpool Daily Post*. 1987 Oct 1.

19 Second opinion sought: *BMJ*. 1988 Jul 2: 7

20 Matthews L, Edwards R. Don't panic appealed to patients: alert over AIDS doctor. *Birmingham Daily News*. 1988 Apr 1.

21 BMA Foundation for AIDS. *Talking about AIDS*. Report. 1988.

22 Pallot P. Health services staff: AIDS video advice to doctors. *Daily Telegraph*. 1988 Apr 6.

23 MP calls for war on AIDS. *Daily Express*. 1988 May 2.

24 Extended AIDS test urged. *Guardian*. 1988 May 21.

25 'Scrutator.' The week in Norwich. *BMJ*. 1988; Jul 16: 208.

26 'Scrutator.' The week in Norwich. *BMJ*. 1988; Jul 16: 223–4

CHAPTER 14

A Royal
sesquicentennial year

THE BMA WAS FOUNDED IN WORCESTER BY CHARLES HASTINGS ON 19 July 1832, and 1982 was therefore its sesquicentenary. The Duke of Edinburgh had been the first non-medical President of the Association in 1959, and once it was known that the Prince of Wales had consented to be the President for 1982 his 'election' as President-elect at the 1981 meeting was a mere formality.

The presidency of the BMA is a titular role and theoretically at least it is completely apolitical. The post is usually held by a distinguished clinician who normally has a link with the town in which the Annual Meeting is being held. In 1980 the town was Newcastle upon Tyne, and the presidency was held by the eminent neurologist Sir John Walton. When his successor was taken ill before assuming office Sir John did a second year as President, and during the Prince of Wales's presidency Sir John carried out most of the presidential duties thus being, in effect, President for three successive years.

The Adjourned Annual General Meeting starts with the formal installation of the new President by the outgoing one.[1] The President then gives his address, and is thanked by the chairman of the RB.

The AAGM of 1982, held at the Royal Festival Hall, was most eventful. A reporter on *General Practitioner* described, correctly, under the heading 'Who wrote to the Prince?' how the Prince opened his speech. None of the 'nationals' made any mention of what was potentially an extremely embarrassing situation.

He began 'Last year I had a letter from a member of the medical profession who said that his fellow members were pleased that I was honouring them by

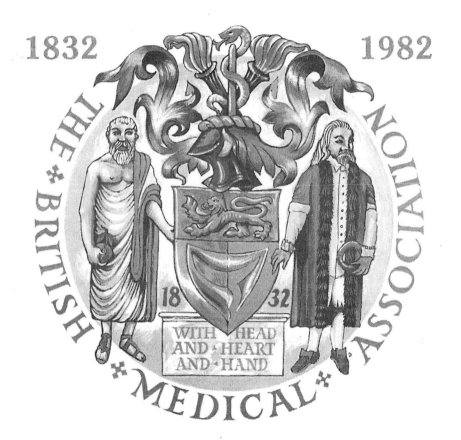

FIGURE 14.1 The programme of the Adjourned Annual General Meeting, 7 July 1982, showing the official BMA Crest ('The two old men holding hands'). © British Medical Association.

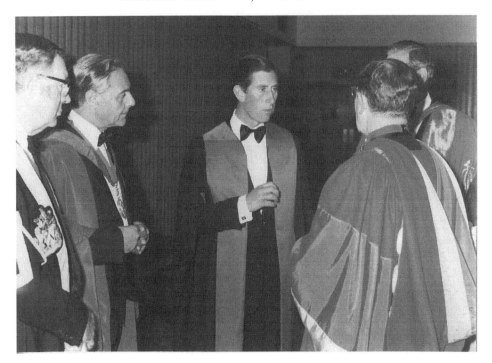

FIGURE 14.2 Meeting the Prince of Wales prior to his installation as President of the BMA, Royal Festival Hall, 7 July 1982. Left to right: Dr Tony Keable-Elliott, me, the Prince of Wales, Sir John Walton and Dr John Havard. © British Medical Association.

accepting the presidency of the BMA, despite the risk of my public image being tarnished when I was seen to be taking an active interest in the Association's affairs. The letter went on to say that he was concerned it would only serve to alienate me from the majority of doctors in my own age group and confirm the worst fears of my critics of all ages.' The Prince continued, 'the letter ended by reminding me that the initials BMA stand for "bigoted, moribund and apathetic"'.[2]

Sitting beside the Prince I could see the audience of about 2000 people, many of them doctors and their families, looking horrified and shocked at what they had heard. I knew I had a very difficult situation to deal with – I had to justify myself to the audience who would expect me to defend the reputation of their Association, without offending our new President.

The Prince continued by praising the devotion to duty of those doctors working in the NHS and in the Armed Forces serving in the South Atlantic, and expressed his fears about the erosion of professional standards. He went on to describe what he called the difficulties faced by the Sikh community in Britain, complaining that Sikh women could not go to see a male doctor and that there were no Sikh women doctors.[3] That statement did not match the experience of a large part of the audience. He then went to criticise the Association's negative approach to 'complimentary medicine'.

I started my response by thanking the Prince for his address, and then went on to say that any Association that elected a Cockney Jewish grammar school boy to its highest political office could not possibly be bigoted. I assured him that the letter B stood for British and that the BMA members were proud of that. The audience began to look less miserable. I then pointed out that 'M' stood for Medicine but also for membership, and a recent increase in our membership figures showed that we were by no means moribund. The audience looked even happier. Finally I told our President that if he sat in my chair he would very soon learn that the Association was far from apathetic. This was greeted with a great cheer and much applause. I had justified my position as a spokesman for the Association.

My troubles were far from over. The reception after the meeting was to be held in a large open area of the Festival Hall, and each member of the audience had been charged £15 for the privilege of eating there. There was a small area reserved for the Prince and those who were to be invited to meet him, which did not include many of the very eminent Past Presidents of the Association, presidents of Royal Colleges and other medical VIPs. John Havard gave me the job of leading a queue of these ladies and gentlemen away from the protected area. The leader of the queue was John Richardson, Past President of the Royal Society of Medicine and current President of the GMC, to whom the Prince had just presented the BMA's highest honour, its Gold Medal. He, like the rest of them, was not pleased.

The behaviour of the members was quite unbelievable. There was food, but the service was slow and those waiting literally grabbed the food off the waiter's trays as they came out of the kitchen. My three children, then in their teens, were there and they came up to me yelling, 'Daddy you must see this'. They took me to see members who had actually invaded the kitchens in their search for food. Many people left in disgust and at the end of the evening a lot of food was left uneaten.

The following morning John Havard and I were instructed to complain to the management of the Festival Hall and we arranged a meeting that turned into a tirade by the other side against our members, to which we had no defence. We left the meeting feeling very humble and extremely ashamed. Fortunately, the only newspaper article that made any reference to the meal merely complained about the size of the portions.

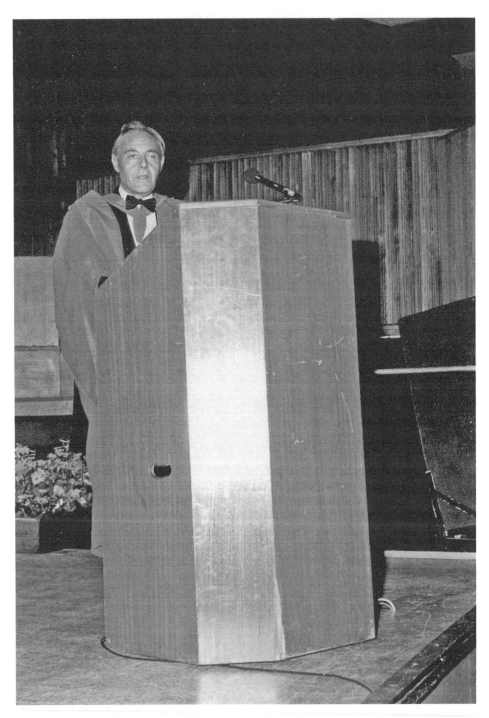

FIGURE 14.3 Replying to the 'Bigoted, Moribund, Apathetic' address. © British Medical Association.

On 19 July the official 150th birthday party was held in Worcester. The local Division organised a special commemorative meeting at the technical college, and an actor, Stephen Hancock from the television series Coronation Street, was dressed up to look like Hastings himself.[4]

A CONFERENCE ON WOMEN DOCTORS

The following weekend I chaired a large meeting in BMA House devoted solely to the problems facing women doctors. The speaker that made the most news was my wife, who warned the Conference that women would be just part of the medical proletariat 'if women don't represent themselves and declare their own rights'. She urged women doctors to stand for their LMC or become BMA representatives. She told the meeting that when she was working for a pittance in the mid-1950s one of her senior male partners said that he did not approve of women doctors and insisted that she saw no male patients.

When the meeting adjourned for lunch we made our way from the Council Chamber to the room in which lunch was being served. The women all stood aside so that I could open the door for them. In the afternoon I reminded them of the incident and said 'the profession is still dominated by middle-aged men who will open all doors except the ones you want opened'. I took unofficial votes – one of them showed strong support for part-time training during the two years hospital part of vocational training for general practice. There was considerable press interest in the conference and its discussions.[5,6,7,8]

The following month, with Tony Grabham, John Havard and our wives, I went to Hawaii for the Council Meeting of the WMA. We tried, again unsuccessfully, to get a discussion on voting rights going, and we were brought face to face with representatives of the Medical Association of South Africa.[9] The meeting was quite useless but we had a marvellous holiday afterwards, touring the various Hawaiian Islands. I think Maui is the most beautiful place I have ever seen, while Honolulu is one of the ugliest

REPRESENTING MINORITY GROUPS

The problems concerning representation of minority groups such as women doctors and overseas doctors within the Association which I had met at my first ARM in 1966 had not been resolved. They were grossly under-represented on the Council and committees of the Association. There were two organisations that did not have direct access to negotiating machinery – the long established Women's Medical Federation (WMF) and fairly new Overseas Doctors Association (ODA). The BMA set up a conference to discuss the problem,

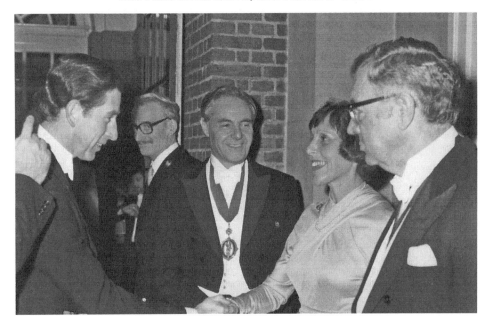

FIGURE 14.4 Greeting the Prince of Wales before the Council Dinner, BMA House, 1982. Left to right: the Prince of Wales, an unknown BMA employee, me, Shirley Marks and Dr Tony Keable-Elliott. © British Medical Association.

but before the meeting the Chairman of the ODA, Dr Karim Admani, told a journalist that the conference was mere 'window-dressing'. Dr Dorothy Ward, President of the WMF, took a more positive attitude. There was a considerable difference of opinion as to whether there should be seats on the negotiating committees and the Council restricted to overseas doctors and women. Dr Mary White, a member of the BMA Council, said that women should not be subject to positive discrimination because it implied inequality. Dr Hamid Hussein, himself an overseas doctor, also wanted no special privileges.[10]

I ran the meeting as two separate conferences but both of them came to the same conclusion – minority groups did not want special privileges. A confidential questionnaire filled in at the women's conference showed that this was the view of ninety one percent of the participants.[11]

On the 14 December the BMA Council gave a formal dinner attended by the Prince of Wales, who proposed the traditional toast, 'The Common Health', and *The Times* published a long extract from it. He made a great plea for unorthodox medicine and pleaded doctors to treat disorders of the whole person, involving not only the patient's body but his mind, his self-image, his dependence on physical and social environment, as well as his relation to the cosmos.[12] I am sure that, like me, most of the audience agreed with that part of the speech.

Tony Grabham responded and then proposed the health of 'The Guests', to which Secretary of State Norman Fowler responded. The guests included many distinguished past and present leaders of British medicine, but I was particularly happy to see among them three of my contemporaries from Edinburgh, Air Marshal Sir David Atkinson, Lieutenant General Sir Alan Reay, and Sir James Fraser, the current President of the Royal College of Surgeons of Edinburgh.[13] Not bad for one cohort!

Although the calendar year ends on 31 December the 'Presidential year' extended into 1983. On 15 March the Prince of Wales, who had already attended meetings of the Council and the two senior negotiating committees, was on the platform at a meeting of the Hospital Junior Staff Committee. Seated between the Chairman of the Committee, Dr Michael Rees, and me he took an active part in a discussion on medical manpower planning.[14] Later in the year he hosted a reception at the State Apartments in Kensington Palace, which turned out to be a very interesting and informal event. It is fair to say that, allowing for the obvious limitations imposed by his Royal status, and in spite of his controversial speeches, he served the BMA well during his year as President.

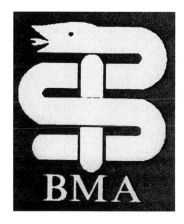

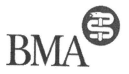

FIGURE 14.5 The first BMA logo, Hissing Sid, 1985. © British Medical Association

FIGURE 14.6 The current BMA logo. © British Medical Association.

FOOTNOTES AND REFERENCES

1 Court Circular. *The Times*. 1982 Jul 8.
2 Who wrote to the Prince? *General Practitioner*. 1982 Jul 16.
3 The Prince fears erosion of health standards. *The Times*. 1982 Jul 8.
4 Auld Lang Syne time for the BMA. *Doctor*. 1982 Jul 22.
5 Thomas J. Speak up or keep silent. *Doctor*. 1982 Aug 5.
6 Mihill C. GPs vote for option on part-time training. *Doctor*. 1982 Aug 5.
7 Walton P. Male chauvinism is alive and kicking. *Doctor*. 1982 Sep 16.
8 Newman L. Women doctors' problems. *The Times Health Supplement*. 1982 Aug 6.
9 Constitution of world body obscene. *Pulse*. 1982 Oct 16.
10 Cave S. BMA set for minority debate. *Pulse*. 1982 Oct 30.
11 Kenmard N. Minorities to leave BMA unscathed. *Pulse*. 1982 Dec 18.
12 Prince Charles: drugs – the patient has had enough. *The Times*. 1982 Dec 16.
13 See *The Times* 1982 Dec 15 for a complete list.
14 Medical manpower in the Year 2000: Prince Charles hears juniors' views. *BMJ*. 1983; **286**: 1073.

CHAPTER 15

International problems and political speculation

MY FIRST MAJOR COMMITMENT IN 1983 HAD NOTHING TO DO WITH the NHS or the BMA but was related to Soviet anti-Semitism. As a member of the Medical Committee for Soviet Jewry, which had been founded to assist Soviet doctors and allied professionals who were facing academic victimisation, I was a signatory to a letter in *The Times* drawing attention to their plight and urging the Soviet Government to refrain from persecuting them.[1] A week later it was announced that Mrs Thatcher had written a letter to Mrs Shcharansky supporting the efforts being made to free her husband, the eminent physicist Anatoly Shcharansky, who had been on hunger strike for 14 weeks and was being forcibly fed. In her view Shcharansky's release by the new Soviet leadership would be a step towards better East–West relations.[2] I went to a meeting in Golders Green attended by Mrs Shcharansky and the Euro MP for North West London, Lord Bethell, who arrived armed with a special message of support from the Prime Minister.[3] I condemned the use of force feeding, describing it as 'a revolting process'. In 1986 the Soviet authorities released Anatoly Shcharansky and I was privileged to meet him. I felt humbled by the experience and expressed the hope that the BMA's campaign might have been of some help to him.[4]

In April I attended the Annual Conference of the Royal College of Nursing in Bournemouth. The nurses were in dispute with the Government over their pay. Their president, Mrs Sheila Quinn, said that it was absolutely necessary that the Review Bodies, which the Government had promised to set up for nurses, be functioning by April 1984. She threatened to use political force to influence the next general election. One point of contention was the Government's determination to include nursing auxiliaries in the proposed Review Body machinery. I told the delegates that the BMA had backed the RCN view that nursing auxiliaries should be excluded.[5] Although the Chairman of the RCN Council welcomed my intervention some of the nurses thought my offer 'condescending'.[6]

At the Senior Hospital Doctors Conference Mr Dick Greenwood, a consultant surgeon, said that 'with the National Overseas Doctors Sponsorship Organisatision controlling foreign graduates' entry into Great Britain there should be another scheme to sponsor their return. He spelt it out: 'SOD OFF'. A storm of protest broke out, one doctor accusing him of using National Front language. I reminded the meeting that the BMA was opposed to racism, and several overseas doctors supported me. Dick Greenwood maintained that he worked with a lot of immigrants, was not racist, and that people did not appreciate his sense of humour.[7] Those people included me.

THE ARM IN DUNDEE

The ARM that year was due to be held in Dundee, a town linked with Nablus, a Palestinian town strongly associated with the Fatah movement, which was rabidly anti-Israeli. The PLO flag was flown over the front door of the Town Hall, and I told our secretariat that I would not walk under that flag and would enter the building only through the back door. That would have produced a very embarrassing situation, but the problem was solved by the Council sending all the flags that flew in front of the building to the dry cleaners.

There was a tiny Jewish community in Dundee and I arranged an inter-denominational service to be held on the evening preceding the meeting in the in the local parish church. The Lord Provost and other civic and academic dignitaries attended and Rabbi Malcolm Weizman, Minister to the smaller Jewish communities, participated. Afterwards, everyone was invited to a reception by the Dundee Hebrew Congregation where I again expressed my pride in my Jewish heritage.[8]

The big medico-political controversy of the year centred around a report *The Medical Effects of Nuclear War*, prepared by the Board of Science[9] and discussed by the Council at its meeting in March. The document considered all the evidence available and came to the conclusion that there was no effective civil defence against nuclear attack, which directly contradicted the Government's policy. At the Council meeting Tony Grabham asked whether the Council wished him to take a definite line on behalf of the Council at the RB. Tony Keable-Elliott thought the BMA should keep out of politics and stick to medicine and a number of other members agreed. On the other hand Stuart Horner, Chairman of the Community Physicians, said that his Executive Committee had not intended to be political when they proposed non-cooperation with civil defence, and he believed that people would be looking for a clear policy from the BMA. In an interview with the press after the Council meeting I expressed my determination to ensure that the nuclear war issue got a fair hearing and that sufficient time was allocated to it.[10] I then said, 'Moving on to the next business is a rare procedure now although a few years back it was more common, and it needed both the agreement of the Chairman and a two thirds majority to succeed'.

However, according to one medical newspaper that's exactly what happened. 'Having duly congratulated itself on its excellent report on the medical effects of nuclear war and expressing its horror at the effects of a nuclear attack, the conference proceeded to bury it as thoroughly as a barrel of radioactive waste. The delegates were determined to do nothing that would embarrass their leadership.'[11] In my view the Association had succeeded in bringing the realities of nuclear war home to the population without taking a 'political' stand, but we were made aware that the Government was not at all pleased with us.[12]

Passing to the next business produced another crisis when a group of what were then described as 'coloured doctors' walked out in protest over what they considered racial discrimination. In fact their motion about racialism was called for debate at 5.20 p.m. when the motion's proposer was not in the hall. We presumed that he had gone home. I tried to arrange to have the subject debated the following day but the representatives refused to change the standing orders of the meeting to allow it. Dr Deb Bose, an overseas doctor who had been awarded the Fellowship of the Association at the meeting, said that 'racialism' was an inappropriate term. In his view it was sometimes 'overseas doctors' who were already long-term residents in Britain who discriminated against more recent arrivals.[13]

THE MEETING IN TORONTO

In September we attended a joint meeting of the BMA and the Canadian Medical Association in Toronto. Shirley and I were particularly pleased to be going there because our daughter Laura was doing a Masters Degree in Education (MEd) at the University of Windsor, Ontario. Having obtained a degree in Psychology at the University of London and then qualified as a teacher at the prestigious Institute of Education she then found it almost impossible to get a job as a probationary teacher. She ultimately landed one in a very strict faith school, but when she tried to introduce progressive ideas she got into trouble. Life became very tedious for Laura and a friend suggested that she apply for a Commonwealth Scholarship. She got one, and she chose to go to Windsor.

Laura visited us in Toronto and we arranged to spend a weekend with her.

Windsor, although in Canada, is in reality a suburb of Detroit across the river in the United States. There were no flights from Toronto to Windsor on Saturday and so we flew to Detroit, going through United States immigration at Toronto airport. On Sunday we took a direct flight back to Toronto and then set off on a journey across Canada finishing up in Vancouver.

Many months later we were looking at our passports and found that we still had the exit documents in them that had been issued in Toronto – we appeared never to have left the United States. I wrote to the Embassy in London explaining the situation and returning their bits of paper. We received no acknowledgement whatsoever and were rather apprehensive about our reception by their immigration officials if and when we returned there.

A HYPNOTIC AFFAIR

In his Presidential Address the Prince of Wales had criticised the Association over its attitude to alternative medicine and so a Working Party was set up under the chairmanship of Professor Jimmy Payne, an eminent anaesthetist. In October I chaired a workshop on hypnosis, which Jimmy attended. Dr Bernard Shevlin of Stoke-on-Trent, a general practitioner participant, had treated more than 2000 patients with hypnosis, which he claimed was safer than tranquillisers.[14] I too had considerable experience in the use of hypnosis, having been trained in the technique and being a member of the British Medical and Dental Society for the Study of Hypnosis. I had used the method in Borehamwood for 'anaesthetising' dental patients and treating asthma, eczema and anxiety states.

I challenged Dr Shevlin to demonstrate the technique on three members of the audience. The paramedical newspaper *Current Practice* reported how Dr Shevlin failed to induce a trance in the three volunteers, adding that several members of the audience were hypnotised while watching the demonstration.[15]

MORE PROBLEMS WITH THE WMA

Towards the end of the year I went to a meeting of the WMA Council in Venice. The BMA had decided that, failing a resolution of the constitutional issue, we would withdraw from the WMA at the General Assembly in 1985. However, discussions about the constitution failed to make any progress whatsoever. The Italians were terribly concerned that too many new doctors were being trained in Europe and that there was a real risk of medical unemployment. They wanted the matter discussed but the lawyers reminded us that the organisation was registered in New York for charitable reasons and that any discussion on the subject of employment would have broken American anti-trust laws.[16] In spite of the lawyers I managed to get the item on the agenda but nothing significant happened.

STRAWS IN THE WIND

In September 1983 Tony Grabham had almost nine months to run before his Chairmanship of Council ended, but according to the magazine *Doctor* speculation about the succession was rife within the BMA.[17] The article claimed that Mr Grabham was worried about his succession and had had secret talks with Tony Keable-Elliott in a move to swap jobs. It also claimed that John Ball, a former Chairman of the GMSC, might seek election to the top post. The article then continued 'another possible contender is the popular but self-effacing North London general practitioner John Marks but any move towards making him chairman would have to come from his backers'. There was also speculation about the forthcoming election for the chairmanship of the Consultants Committee and the article suggested that Dr Brian Lewis might win. Fortunately for me, Maurice Burrows, with whom I had good personal relationships, emerged victorious.

A few weeks later in its diary feature *Pulse* claimed that the idea of the job swap between the two Tonys 'first revealed in this diary in June' had been abandoned in the face of some opposition. The writer of the diary claimed to have heard that 'the smart money is now being placed on John Marks to become the next chairman'.[18] In February Tony Keable-Elliott announced that he would not be standing for re-election as Treasurer and also that it was 'probable' that he would be standing for the chairmanship of Council.[19]

FOOTNOTES AND REFERENCES

1 Black D, *et al*. Jewish doctors in the USSR. *The Times*. 1983 Jan 6.
2 Knipe M. Thatcher support for dissident. *The Times*. 1983 Jan 15.
3 Dissident's wife speaks out. *Borehamwood Times*. 1983 Jan 20.
4 Marks meets released Soviet dissident. *General Practitioner*. 1986 Oct 17.
5 Bassett P. Royal College of Nursing could use 'political forces' over pay. *Financial Times*. 1983 Apr 12.
6 Cousins J. Nurses' RB earns full Marks. *Hospital Doctor*. 1983 Apr 21: 4.
7 *Hospital Doctor*. 1983 Jun 6.
8 Goldman E. Kirk to kiddush. *Jewish Chronicle*. 1983 Jul 1.
9 British Medical Association. *The Medical Effects of Nuclear War*. Oxford: John Wiley and Sons; 1983.
10 Kent A. Nuclear report divides the BMA Council, but ARM chairman promises fair hearing. *Current Practice*, 1983 May 13.
11 Going through the motions. *World Medicine*. 1983 Jul 23.

12 The report became a very important source document and was quoted in written evidence to the Select Committee on Defence as recently as February 2006.

13 Lymn P. Coloured doctors walk out in protest. *Birmingham Post*. 1983 Jul 1.

14 Hypnotism 'safer' than tranquillisers. *Doctor*. 1983 Oct 6.

15 Unconvincing performance. *Current Practice*. 1983 Sep 30.

16 BMA likely to quit world medical group. *Glasgow Herald* 1983 Dec 12.

17 McCormack M, Bishop M. Job-swap idea may fill Council chair. *Doctor*. 1983 Sep 15: 2

18 Marks times BMA Chairman? *Pulse*. 1983 Dec 10.

19 Charles J. BMA Treasurer to step down. *General Practitioner*. 1984 Feb 10.

CHAPTER 16

Two crises and one election

THE YEAR 1984 STARTED WITH A BANG. AFTER A TELEVISION PROGRAMME criticising general practitioners' deputising services Kenneth Clarke, Minister of Health, issued a document setting out the Government's intention to restrict the use of such services by general practitioners.[1] There was a real problem: some of the deputising services were inadequate and the standard of some of their doctors and management left patients at risk. On the other hand many doctors in inner-city areas who were single-handed and lived away from their premises found it difficult to get cover when they wanted leave or a night or weekend off duty. I believed that without deputising services general practice in the centre of large cities would not survive, a view I had clearly expressed twenty years before on the Isle of Man.

There was great anger among general practitioners over the way the document had been released without consultation and Kenneth Clarke's obvious intention of imposing the changes regardless of what the doctors thought about them. As far as the BMA was concerned there was another problem – the BMA ran a Central Advisory Service Committee (CAC), which had a direct link with one of the deputising companies, Air Call. On the other hand the hierarchy of the Royal College of General Practitioners was keen on the idea of controlling deputising services and had a policy that all deputies must be principals in general practice, or be eligible to be principals. Thus this dispute again brought to the fore the sharp division between the BMA and the Royal College of General Practitioners, and I knew where my prime loyalties lay.

Doctors are notorious for not attending meetings unless they feel deeply threatened but a meeting of around 200 angry family doctors in Woodford

Bridge, Essex voted, with only two dissenters, that in the event of unacceptable controls being imposed the BMA should declare an official dispute and advise its members to take appropriate action. My remark that 'I have been a member of the College since it was founded and I bitterly resent its meddling in politics. I have let the college know my views and I suggest you do the same' was cheered. Shirley, a member of the College Council, asked the 30 or so RCGP members present if they agreed with the College or the BMA. All voted for the BMA.[2] I also attended a meeting in Croydon, where 120 doctors supported the BMA stance, and the next day I went to Wembley where another 200 doctors took the same view.[3]

On 28 February I took part in an Extraordinary General Meeting of my Faculty of the College, North and West London, which meets at the College headquarters. More than 60 members turned up to hear the College Secretary, Dr Bill Styles, also a member of that faculty, defending his, and the College's, position. After Dr Styles had spoken I said 'this College must be told once and for all that terms, conditions and remuneration are none of its business'. This was greeted with 'thunderous applause', and the meeting gave overwhelming support for a proposal from the floor that the GMSC should handle the entire dispute.[4]

A meeting of the Royal College Council heard its chairman, Dr Irvine, say that the consultation document sent out by the College to its 11 000 members had shown a substantial measure of support. The College went further than that, calling on the Government to ensure 'as soon as possible' that all deputies should be principals or eligible to be a principal. Drs. Irvine and Styles both received standing ovations.[5,6]

I led a delegation to see Mr Clarke which included Dr Lionel Kopelowitz, Chairman of the BMA's Central Advisory Committee. We made it clear to the Minister yet again that only the GMSC could negotiate for general practitioners.[7] In the end a compromise was reached, but the requirement that deputies should be at least eligible to be principals, so dear to the College, was not incorporated into the regulations.

In spite of political differences there were always attempts to maintain reasonable personal and social relationships and on 16 May the Chairman of the Council gave a dinner at BMA House at which Kenneth Clarke was a guest. I took the opportunity to give him a copy of my booklet on LMCs as I thought it would improve his understanding of general practice. I had a nice letter of thanks from him promising to read my pamphlet as part of his recess reading.[8] I don't know whether he did or not.

Because of a problem with purchasing their house Richard, his wife Hilary, their sons Oliver and Joe, and the mother's help all moved into Brown Gables in the spring and stayed for six months. The arrangement worked unbelievably well. In April we announced the engagement of our elder daughter, Helen, to Mark Hainbach, a Dublin businessman. Mark's father Kurt was a trained textile engineer. He had escaped from Austria in 1938 and made his way via London to Dublin, where, in due course, he established a successful business manufacturing knitted linenware clothes. Kurt had married Ella, a Scottish Presbyterian woman, and ultimately they all converted to Roman Catholicism. Sadly, Kurt died when Mark was only 14 years old. Helen and Mark provided us with two more grandchildren, Katherine (always known as Katie) and Matthew. That finally put paid to my antipathy towards visiting Ireland!

THE ANNUAL REPRESENTATIVE MEETING, 1984

Manchester was the venue for the ARM of 1984. Apart from the election for the Chairmanship of Council, which I shall deal with separately, everything went fairly smoothly except for two debates, one on an investment trust, and the other on the arms race.

Early in his chairmanship Tony Grabham had negotiated with a firm of insurance brokers with a view to providing special financial services to BMA members. A joint venture, BMA Services Ltd, known as BMAS, was set up and I was one of its first customers – they arranged a mortgage for my new house in Elstree. A unit trust that BMAS had been recommending to members included shares in the tobacco industry. I had warned them that this was wrong and would be resented by some of the members but I was told it was impossible to establish a tobacco-free trust. The matter had since been raised at the Junior Members' Forum, but more importantly the community physicians were very angry. Dr Gabriel Scally told the representatives that the involvement in such a trust would embarrass the Association and compromise its authority when speaking out against smoking. Tony Keable-Elliott, Treasurer of the BMA and a director of BMA Services, upset the representatives by urging them to vote against the motion, which he said was based on 'fundamental misconceptions'. The voting appeared to be very close, but I had noted that several members of the Council of the BMA who were not representatives had voted, and such votes were invalid. I ordered a new vote and a count showed the motion carried by a large majority, 169 to 99.[9] Tony Grabham expressed his pleasure that members were prepared to put the interests of patients above their own financial interests and said that BMAS would have to look at the problem again. They found such a trust, which was highly successful for many years.

A proposal from the Bath Division calling for 'a massive and progressive reduction in world arms spending, both nuclear and conventional, with a diversion of the resources freed to health care and welfare at home and in the developing countries' was passed by more than a two thirds majority. According to one reporter I greeted the vote with a muttered 'good lord'.[10] That was another decision that did not improve our standing with the Government!

Our activities also displeased the right-wing *Daily Express*. In a sarcastic editorial it referred to our annual jamboree pontificating on all sorts of issues. – 'Down with boxing'; 'Down with smoking (naturally)'; 'Up wit [*sic*] state spending on health' (naturally); 'Down with nuclear arms'. We were advised to cease our frenetic lobbying for favourite causes and the editorial ended by suggesting that the BMA should carry a warning 'Conferences can damage your image'.[11] The following week the newspaper published my reply under the heading 'The remedy is yours'. I pointed out that 150 debates that related to the wellbeing of our patients had taken place, and the newspaper, not the BMA, decided which were given prominence in print. I suggested that perhaps the newspaper itself should carry a warning: '*Express* editorials can limit your understanding of BMA Conferences'.[12]

THE CHAIRMANSHIP OF COUNCIL

Tony Grabham's chairmanship would expire at the end of this meeting, at the same time as I was due to leave the chairmanship of the Representative Body. Tony Keable-Elliott's three-year term of office as Treasurer also came to an end. It had been obvious for years that there would be a contest between Tony Keable-Elliott and me for the 'top job' and we both felt quite confident about the outcome.

We had very different medico-political backgrounds. I had been 'a BMA man' for my entire medico-political career dating back to 1966, and had also been deeply involved in 'GP politics'. Tony on the other hand was essentially a 'LMC/GMSC man' and had only become involved in BMA affairs after he had been elected as Chairman of the GMSC in 1974. Both of us, as Chief Officers, were entitled to attend all the 'craft' committee meetings and their conferences. I was careful to attend most of them, especially those that represented the minority groups, because I believed that doctors in the Armed Forces, occupational medicine and other small 'crafts' desperately needed the support of the profession as a whole. Tony attended infrequently; he was busy keeping the Association solvent. However he had the support of most of general practitioner members of Council, well organised by the GMSC negotiators. I was to be nominated for election by the Chairman of the consultants, Maurice Burrows, and seconded by the Chairman of the medical academics, Jimmy Payne a Professor of Anaesthetics. With many junior doctors and others supporting me I had been pledged at least 38 votes, more than enough to win.

The election of the Treasurer of the Association is by members of the RB and takes place almost at the start of the meeting. Council elects its Chairman after the RB has finished. On the Sunday afternoon before the start of the ARM Tony Keable-Elliott and I went for a walk. I pointed out that if he did not stand as Treasurer, there would be an inexperienced one for the next three years. I told him that I had sufficient votes to guarantee my election and I really needed him to remain in office as Treasurer and colleague. Neither of us made any public comment, but when he was nominated for the treasurership on the Monday morning, and elected unapposed, the situation became clear to everyone.

At the end of the ARM the Council met under the chairmanship of the President. I was elected unopposed, although years later I discovered that an eminent general practitioner wished to stand against me. Mr James Kyle, a surgeon from Aberdeen, became the new Chairman of the RB and my good friend Benny Alexander was elected as his Deputy.

The press dealt with my election in a variety of ways.[13,14] The *British Medical Journal* gave it one paragraph.[15] *BMA News Review* published a special edition related to the Annual Representative Meeting, with photographs of Tony and me on its front cover under a caption 'Marks and Spender'and articles about us inside.[16] *The Jewish Chronicle* published the story complete with photograph[17] and I was invited to complete a form with a view to my inclusion in the Who's Who section of the *Jewish Yearbook*.[18]

There was one sour note. A week before the ARM I had given a long interview to Judith Charles. She wrote an article headed 'Leader not in the interests of GPs' in which she said that my election 'can ironically be seen as a symbol of the decline of GP power in that organisation'. She based her conclusion on an incident the previous year when I was booed at the LMC Conference because I argued against the views on medical manpower expressed by the leaders of the GMSC. The rest of the article was factually correct in its analysis of my career and Tony's, particularly the part played in my election by the smaller crafts within the Association, which she dismissed as 'the odds and sods'. She ended her article with a statement that '[John Marks] has fulfilled his desperate personal desire to lead the BMA'.[19]

The word 'desperate' was neither justifiable nor correct. Another journalist, Mike MacCormack writing in *Hospital Doctor*, said that ambition played a comparatively small part in my elevation to the chairmanship of the BMA Council, and described how I had fallen into the job because the Chairman of the Representative Body always emerged as a strong candidate for it. He, and Judith Charles, would not have known how I had been persuaded by others to oppose my close friend Benny Alexander for the deputy chairmanship of the RB six years earlier. He also quoted me as saying that when I give up the chairmanship I'd like to be remembered as having played a part in converting the BMA from a relatively inefficient talking shop into an efficient representative organisation of all branches of the profession, able to maintain the position of the profession and the standards of the health service.[20]

THE GMC ELECTIONS

I had been elected to the GMC in 1979 and elections were held again in the summer of 1984. I was so busy with other things that I did not bother to submit an election address. When the results were declared my name was absent from the list of new members. With hindsight it was fortunate for me that I was not elected because the next five years turned out be very busy ones and I would have had no time for the GMC. The election attracted considerable attention in the medical press because of the extremely low turnout – thirty-four percent.[21,22]

I START MY NEW JOB

The duties of the Chairman of Council extend far beyond the formal business of chairing the Council and other recognised medico-political activities. I was very fortunate to inherit a wonderful secretary, Mrs Joan Fairburn, and when she retired Dale Westerway was a worthy successor. The week after my election, in addition to chairing a meeting of the Council Executive, I attended a meeting of the Council for Postgraduate Medical Education (CPME), the Standing Medical Advisory Committee (SMAC)[23] and the board of BMAS.

Within a fortnight I was chairing my first working party, which was considering the Griffiths Report on management in the NHS. The Secretary of State had appointed Sir Roy Griffiths, Deputy Managing Director of Sainsbury's, as Chairman of a committee to prepare a report on management in the NHS. Its recommendations[24] included the establishment of a strong general management board at the centre, a strengthening of the regional structure, and the involvement of clinicians more closely in management decisions. Their recommendations were at first guardedly welcomed by the *British Medical Journal*[25] but the Association was concerned that managerial decisions should not override those of clinicians. In the end the Government imposed changes, and by and large the professions co-operated.

The next month I attended the Annual Meeting of the Irish Medical Organisation in County Mayo, and a couple of weeks later I was the guest of honour at a luncheon given by the Board of Deputies of British Jews at their headquarters across the road from BMA House. It was attended by the great and the good in the profession, and a bevy of politicos of all hues including a former Minister of Health, Dr Gerard Vaughan.[26] In my speech I remarked on similarities between the two organisations, each representing the interests of a small but well defined group of people and that living in a democracy we were classed as pressure groups.[27] I reminded the audience that I was the second Jew to have chaired the BMA Council, the first being Dr Solomon [Solly] Wand, a GP from Birmingham,[28] whose funeral I had attended in Birmingham just a few weeks previously.

As was the custom the BMA decided to hold a memorial service for Solly, who was a member of an Orthodox Jewish community in Birmingham. Such memorial services for senior BMA offices were usually held at St Pancras Parish Church, a few yards from BMA House on a Wednesday when the Council was in session. That guaranteed a good attendance, and the fare of many of the congregation was covered by the member's subsistence allowance. The nearest Orthodox synagogue to BMA house is the one in Great Portland Street, but as Solly's second wife was not Jewish the United Synagogue refused to allow us to have the service there or at any other of its synagogues. Fortunately, the Reform Jews were more understanding, and the late Rabbi Hugo Gryn welcomed us to the West London Reform Synagogue[29] and conducted a moving service, appropriate to the man's eminence, at which I paid tribute to his service to the profession.[30]

Also in November I attended my first meeting of the small informal gathering that called itself 'The Heads of Professions' at which I met the chairmen or presidents of organisations such as the Law Society, the Bar, the British Dental Association, the vets, the architects and so on. We discussed matters that affected all professions at a time when the Tory Government was making life difficult for most of them. There were no agendas and no minutes, but a great deal of useful work was done.

Three days later I left for Singapore as head of the BMA delegation to the Commonwealth Medical Association Council. The Chief Officers and their wives had an invitation from the Chinese Government to visit Chinese medical facilities after the meeting and to meet with the Chinese Medical Association.[31] On the morning that we were due to leave Singapore Shirley was taken ill, and there was only one direct flight from Kuala Lumpur to Beijing each week. The Chinese authorities were prepared to fly me there later via Hong Kong, but declined to pay for Shirley, so she and I stayed in Singapore until she recovered and we flew home.

THE LIMITED LIST

We arrived home to find ourselves in the middle of a major medico-political crisis. A year earlier the then Secretary of State, Patrick Jenkin, had endorsed the findings of the Greenfield Committee which had been set up by the Department of Health to investigate prescribing costs.[32] It had completely rejected the concept of a list limiting the drugs that general practitioners could prescribe. Kenneth Clarke, then Minister of Health, told Parliament then that 'we [the Department] are not convinced that such a list confining the judgement of doctors would be in the best interests of patients'.[33]

While I was in Singapore, in spite of the above statement and the long tradition of ministers consulting the profession in advance on proposals for changes in the NHS, Kenneth Clarke had given just two hours notice that Norman Fowler intended to introduce a limited list of drugs which would be available on NHS prescriptions. The objective was to save £100 million from the drug bill, which could have been saved in other, better ways. Michael Wilson, the newly elected Chairman of the GMSC, decided that the problem was within the devolved responsibility of his committee and started a public campaign against the changes before I returned to the United Kingdom. I took the view that the proposals were not in the patients' interests and would ultimately spread to other branches of the profession. In those circumstances, I had no option but to get involved in a campaign where I did not have overall control from the start.

Kenneth Clarke took the unusual step of making public a letter that he had written to me explaining the Government's proposals, and inviting my comments on them. It was released to the press before I had even seen it.[34] He described the enormous increase in both the number and cost of prescriptions, and that to save £100 million the Government was going to limit prescribing in two groups of drugs – treatments for dyspepsia and tranquillisers. He went on to say that many common remedies for conditions which did not require intervention by doctors were available over the counter and that, in reasonable quantities, they cost less than the statutory prescription charge, which was of course true. He insisted that 'an adequate range of cheap and effective generic drugs would be available when doctors felt that the clinical needs of individual patients generally require such medication'. The new Regulations would also limit the range of benzodiazepine tranquillisers to a small number of generic drugs. Attached to the letter was a provisional list of drugs 'it proposed to leave prescribable under the NHS'.

I issued a statement saying that the greatest danger was not what the Government was doing but what it could do, merely by altering the Regulations. 'If they got away with it there will be one health service for the rich and one

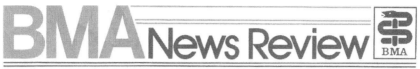

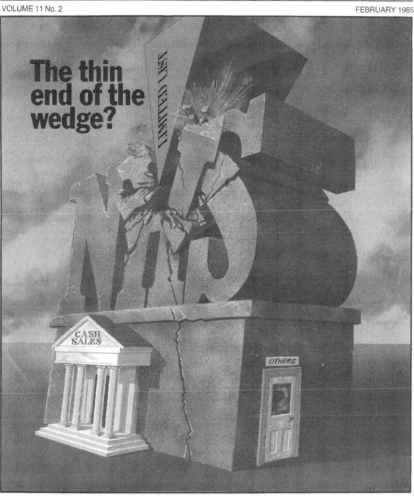

FIGURE 16.1 'The thin end of the wedge'. Cover of *BMA News* reporting on the Limited List. Possibly the beginning of the end of the NHS? © *BMA News*.

for the poor,' I commented. 'In my view that's the end of the NHS as I know it.' I also pointed out that the list was so limited as to be ludicrous, and I asked the unanswered question, 'Who drew it up?'[35] Opposition to the Government's proposals came from the medical profession and the pharmaceutical industry, which pointed out that the UK research and discovery programmes would decline.[36] *The Times*[37] ridiculed the BMA's concern for patients and claimed that our actions were motivated solely by self-interest. My reply dealt with each point in the leader, and reminded the readers that the BMA's actions prior to the introduction of the NHS in the 1940s, which occupied a considerable part of the article, were completely irrelevant. The current leadership of the profession had spent their entire lives working within the National Health Service and cared for it. The editorial had ended with the words 'They [the doctors] have to fail'. I replied, 'If we do it will not be the doctors who will suffer, it will be the poor, the elderly, the confused and the disadvantaged who will have to make do with a minister's nominated nostrums'.[38] Laurie Pavitt alleged, correctly, that this was the first time a minister had interfered with clinical freedom. He urged support for his Generic Substitution (National Health Service) Bill, which was due for a second reading on 8 February.[39]

A meeting of the Council Executive on 12 December suggested that doctors should not enter into discussions with the Health Departments on proposals to limit prescribing by regulation. Writing under the [not entirely correct] headline 'BMA bans doctors' aid in drawing up drug list', Nicolas Timmins reported my view that it was not possible to compile a national list which would not cause confusion and patient damage, but that we were happy to see local lists which could be overridden when the patient had particular needs.[40]

On 9 January 1985 two meetings took place and I managed to attend both. The first was a routine meeting of the BMA Council, which supported the Executive's view on the management of the crisis by a majority of 34 votes to 9.[41] *BMA News Review* produced an A4 coloured flyer that was included in the edition that was ready for dispatch to every member. Under the banner headline 'Stop press', it set out the Council's recommendations, which were that we should seek a meeting with the Secretary of State to present our objection to the scheme and offer to take part in fresh discussions on prescribing costs, and that individual doctors should not enter into any discussions with the health departments. We advised doctors to tell their patients how the proposals would affect them and encourage them to write to their MP.[42]

The second meeting, and in the circumstances the more important one, was a meeting of the Standing Medical Advisory Committee (SMAC), under the chairmanship of Dr Stuart Carne. As Stuart told *The Times* the advice the Committee gave to Mr Fowler was confidential. Nevertheless, the newspaper reported that the Committee told the Secretary of State that it was opposed to the plans to draw up a blacklist,[43] and similar stories appeared in other broadsheets.[44]

On the evening of the 16 January Shirley and I attended the Annual Dinner given by the Council of the Royal College of Nursing. The guest of honour was the Prime Minister, Mrs Margaret Thatcher. When she started her response to the toast of 'The Royal College of Nursing of the United Kingdom' she put on her reading spectacles. At that precise moment reporters entered the room – Mrs Thatcher angrily removed her glasses and said something like, 'I was not told the press was going to be here'. The minute she had finished her speech I also had to leave so that I could get to the BBC in time for a television interview condemning her Government's actions on prescribing. I enjoyed that.

I held a press conference with Michael Wilson and Maurice Burrows where we told the press of Clarke's deafness to any ideas but his own, and that clearly there would be both a white list of prescribable drugs and a blacklist of non-prescribable ones.[45] The GMSC contemplated taking legal action, and Sir Douglas Black, the Association's President, made an appeal to the European Commission to intervene.[46]

My local newspaper reported that I had appeared on the BBC2 programme *Newsnight*.[47] That broadcast generated considerable interest in the paramedical press because the newspaper *Doctor* described it as a debate and claimed that 'Kenneth Clarke wiped the studio floor' with me'.[48] Two weeks later, under the headline 'Debate over drugs plan was "parody"', I explained how Kenneth Clarke had refused to debate with me, and had insisted that I made a statement to which he could reply. I was not allowed to speak after that.[49,50] A series of letters in *Doctor* expressed their disapproval of the article.[51,52] While I wrote to every Member of Parliament[53] and met leaders of the opposition just prior to the debate in the House of Commons, Michael Wilson and Maurice Burrows tackled Tory backbenchers.[54] All to no avail: the Regulations came into force on the first of April.

During this time of great medico-political activity I had a few minor diversions. I was asked to be a judge at the Smith Kline and French Radio Award for 1984, which recognised excellence in broadcasts on health matters. I met several influential medical journalists socially at the presentation of the award in February 1985, always a useful thing to do. I was also asked to submit a biography for *Who's Who in World Jewry*, and I chaired a BMA dinner in honour of my predecessor Tony Grabham. The dinner was held at the Law Society as BMA House was being refurbished, the old Great Hall being converted into a new library.

I have heard members of the BMA and other organisations questioning the usefulness and cost effectiveness of all these dinners. Although the 'ordinary' members paid their own way at these events, and thoroughly enjoyed meeting their own kind, in my view the enormous exchange of information which took place between the leaders, now called 'networking', fully justified the cost of entertaining the guests.

Prior to my being elected as Chairman the Public Affairs Division of the BMA had instituted media training courses for the Secretary and other senior officials. The driving force was Pamela Taylor, the deputy head of the division. Soon after I became Chairman she approached me with the suggestion that senior elected officers like me and Michael Wilson should undergo similar training and I had my first dose of 'interview training' in December. Four months later an article appeared in *Doctor* under the heading 'On your Marks, get set for a new image', alleging that I was to be sent to 'Charm School'.[55] It claimed that my much more human face compared with my predecessor, 'super cool Tony Grabham', frightened some of the BMA hierarchy, and might be interpreted by many doctors and politicians as political naivety. It then asserted that I was chosen as Chairman because I was a genuinely honest man. The rest of the article was rehash of the alleged plot between the two Tonys and the revelation that Dr John Ball 'who was equally keen on the job, and strongly tipped, lost out because he left his bid too late'. That was indeed news to me.

FOOTNOTES AND REFERENCES

1 Rivett G. *From Cradle to Grave: 50 years of the NHS*. London: King's Fund; 1998.
2 Mihil C. East London doctors vote for industrial action. *General Practitioner*. 1984 Feb 23.
3 BMA tells doctors to take softly, softly approach on deputies: *Doctor*. 1984 Feb 23.
4 RCGP told to quit row on deputies. *Doctor*. 1984 Mar 8.
5 Charles J. Act swiftly on deputies' call. *General Pratitioner*. 1984 Mar 16.
6 Dr Shirley Nathan. Personal communication.
7 Deputising-BMA spells it out for Clarke. *Pulse*. 1984 Mar 16.
8 Letter from The Rt. Hon. Kenneth Clarke QC MP. 1984 May 24.
9 Vote snub to Keable-Elliott over tobacco investments. *Hospital Doctor*. 1984 Jul 24.
10 Bishop M. Good Lord! *Doctor*. 1984 Jul 12.
11 Quiet please, Doc! *Daily Express*. 1984 Jul 6.
12 Marks J. The remedy is yours. *Daily Express*. 1984 Jul 12.
13 New BMA leader's pledge. *Pulse*. 1984 Jul 14.
14 GP lands top BMA job. *Current Practice*. 1984 Jul 13.
15 BMA Council meeting. *BMJ*. 1984 Jul 21.
16 Albert T. Gamekeeper turned poacher. *BMA News Review*. 1984; 10(8): 14–15.

17 GP new BMA head. *Jewish Chronicle*. 1984 Jul 13.

18 Undated letter from *Jewish Yearbook*.

19 Charles J. Leader not in the interest of GPs. *General Practitioner*. 1984 Jul 13.

20 MacCormack M. Battling cockney who loves a fight. *Hospital Doctor*. 1984 Sep 6.

21 Thomas J. BMA orders probe into disastrous Council vote. *Doctor*. 1984 Aug 9.

22 Cameron J. General practice fails in election to the GMC. *General Practitioner*. 1984 Aug 21.

23 The Standing Medical Advisory Committee (SMAC) had a duty to advise the Secretary of State for Health on 'such matters relating to medical services as they thought fit', or were referred to them by the Secretary of State. It was abolished in 2005.

24 *NHS Management Inquiry Report* (Griffiths Report). London: DHSS, 1983.

25 Business management for the NHS? *BMJ*. 1983; **287**: 1321–2.

26 Luncheons: Board of Deputies of British Jews. *Daily Telegraph*. 1984 Nov 9.

27 Two of a kind. *Jewish Chronicle*. 1984 Nov 16.

28 John Marks honoured at lunch. *General Practitioner*. 1984 Nov 18.

29 Memorial Service, Dr S Wand. *The Times*. 1985 Jan 10.

30 Profession pays its tribute to the GPs champion. *General Pracitioner*. 1985 Jan 18.

31 Alternative talks. *General Practitioner*. 1984 Nov 9.

32 Informal Working Group on Effective Prescribing. *Report to the Secretary of State for Social Services*. London: Department of Health and Social Security; 1983.

33 *Hansard*. House of Commons. col. 144. 1983 Nov 22.

34 Health Minister's letter to the BMA. *Pulse*. 1984 Nov 17.

35 Marks J. The end of the NHS. *General Practioner*. 1984 Nov 16.

36 Campaign against medicines proposals. *Southern Evening Echo*. 1984 Dec 5.

37 Prescribing propaganda. *The Times*. 1984 Dec 13.

38 Marks J. Doctors' interest in best use of drugs. *The Times*. 1984 Dec 17.

39 Laurie Pavitt MP: a Labour cure for the ills of health service prescribing. *Guardian*. 1984 Dec 18.

40 Timmins N. BMA bans doctor's aid in drawing up drug list. *The Times*. 1984 13 Dec.

41 BMA votes to fight drugs limit. *Daily Telegraph*. 1985 Jan 10.

42 STOP PRESS – the threat to patient care. *BMA News Review*. 1985 Mar 9.

43 Timmins N. Government's medical advisors oppose plan for limited drug list. *The Times*. 1985 Jan 10.

44 Henke D. Advisors tell Fowler to drop NHS drugs ban. *Guardian*. 1985 Jan 10.

45 'Scrutator.' The week in Plymouth. *BMJ*. 1985; **291**: 67–74

46 Duncan N. Government may face court action on drug list. *Pulse*. 1985 Feb 2.

47 Franklin A. Doctor attacks prescription charge plan. *Borehamwood Post*. 1985 Jan 24.

48 Rapier sharp wit can't parry concern. *Doctor*. 1985 Jan 24.

49 Marks J. Debate over drugs plan a parody *Doctor*. 1985 Feb 7.

50 Ministers last stance means no reply on limited list. *Pulse*. 1985 Feb 7.

51 Buckman L. Clarke did the dirty on himself. *Doctor*. 1985 Feb.

52 Davies TC. The TV debate that never was. *Doctor*. 1985 Feb 21.

53 Dr Marks spells it out for MPs. *Pulse*. 1985 Jan 17.

54 GPs fight on to 11th hour. *General Practitioner*. 1985 Mar 15.

55 Bishop M, MacCormack M. On your Marks, get set for a new image. *Doctor*. 1985 Apr 25.

CHAPTER 17   Princess Diana opens the library and I have a rough ARM

THE ANNUAL REPRESENTATIVE MEETING OF 1985, MY FIRST AS CHAIRMAN, was held in the Guildhall at Plymouth. In 1985 the major political issue was the Limited List even though it had been in force for a couple of months. Representatives wholeheartedly supported the Council's stance and showed their disgust at 'government by dictat'.[1] My comment that 'the Secretary of State is a thoroughly bad employer' went down very well.[2] There were serious debates on the implementation of the Griffiths managerial report, the desirability of increasing the number of consultants in the health service, the sponsorship scheme for training overseas doctors, and other matters of more interest to doctors than the general public.

However, the most important debates of the meeting were on the Warnock Report on human fertilisation and embryology.[3] There was a small but fundamental difference of opinion between the Council and the BMA's Central Ethical Committee. The Council took the view that the prime objectives in fertilising a human ovum using in vitro techniques were two in number. The first was to produce a normal child within the context of an infertile family where infertility could not be relieved by other means. Secondly it could be used to produce a normal healthy child by the use of donated gametes or embryos in those at risk of transmitting hereditary disease. The Central Ethical Committee believed that 'the sole, solitary and lone justifiable purpose of fertilising a human ovum is to produce a child within the context of an infertile family.'[4]

I described the Committee's view as 'a very narrow one that risked bringing advances in vitro fertilisation to a halt'. I explained that improvements in technique meant that pregnancies had already been achieved by freezing fertilised ova at an early stage in their development with their later implantation into their own mother's womb. The Council had had the benefit of the advice of Professor Callum McNaughton, President of the Royal College of Obstetricians and Gynaecologists, who told it that the supply of spare ova had been exhausted and in many centres the only spare ones came from women who willingly donated them while they were undergoing sterilisation operations. The final outcome of the debate was that the Representative Body agreed that experimentation should be permitted on human embryos up to 14 days after fertilisation.

The next debate was on the equally emotive subject of surrogate motherhood. Dr Lotte Newman, a general practitioner from North London,[5] said that since surrogacy existed whatever the BMA decided it was better that it should be supervised, monitored and controlled by a proper licensing authority rather than be a haphazard arrangement for gain. In spite of strong opposition from the Chairman of the Ethical Committee, and the minimal opposition offered by me in line with the Council's existing policy, which opposed surrogacy, the motion 'that surrogacy should be permitted in selected cases with careful controls' was passed by 193 votes to 182. Both of these debates were widely and sympathetically reported in the national press[6,7] and in the opinion of at least one experienced writer these two debates demonstrated the honest conviction and real caring attitude of the Association and its members.[8]

For the first and last time four members of the Marks family attended an Annual Representative Meeting, my son Richard being there as one of the junior members' representatives and his wife Hilary as an 'accompanying person'. During the debate on alcohol the platform seemed to be completely uncertain as to the Association's policy on some particular detail. While confusion reigned on the platform, a junior member stormed onto it and insisted that the Chairman of the Representative Body send someone to find out what the policy was. The Chairman may have been embarrassed, but his embarrassment was not in the same league as mine when the intruder's actions were greeted by loud shouts from the junior section 'Marks for Chairman', meaning Richard, not John. Shirley, who was in the audience, said that my blushes were the best she'd seen for years.

The Meeting instructed the Council to press the Government for a significant increase in excise duty on all alcoholic beverages and a complete ban on promoting and advertising them. It then turned its attention to tobacco, welcomed the BMA's campaign against the drug, and supported a total ban on tobacco advertising. All this was too much for one representative, Mr JW Stevenson of Bromley, who failed in his attempt to persuade representatives that the BMA was spending too much time on banning things and too little attending to the real problems of the NHS.[9]

During the debate, which instructed the Board of Science to assess the medical and civil defence implications of nuclear winter in an appendix to its report, *The Medical Effects of Nuclear War*, the Chairman of the Meeting predicted a slackening of interest in nuclear war within the profession. This prompted Richard to write to the *British Medical Journal* criticising those remarks, which in turn spawned an article in *Pulse* under the heading 'Nuclear fallout in medical family'[10] claiming that the members of our family had agreed not to fall out nor comment on each other's views, implying that they were in conflict. They were! Richard and his rheumatologist wife Hilary suggested in the letter that doctors should send a donation to the Medical Campaign Against Nuclear Weapon's Hiroshima Day Appeal. Shirley and I observed a discreet silence.

I received a very nice letter from Professor McNaughton thanking me for my intervention defending the use of embryos for research purposes, and suggesting that without it the narrow view of the Ethical Committee might have prevailed. That would have given valuable ammunition to those parliamentarians who were opposed to any form of embryo research.

In 1990 a BMA working party had concluded that it was not desirable, nor possible, to prevent doctors being involved in surrogacy arrangements and had issued guidelines which included an assessment of the risks.[11] The passing of the Human Fertilisation and Embryology Act 1990 legalised the procedures. There must be literally thousands of women and children who may not know how grateful they should be to the College of Obstetricians and the BMA for the stance they took on embryo research, hereditary disease and surrogacy in those crucial years.

One of my first duties when I returned to London from Plymouth was to attend a meeting of the MSD Foundation. That was a charitable educational foundation for general practice supported by the drug manufacturer Merck Sharpe and Dohme (MSD) its director being Professor Marinker, who had been a general practitioner in Essex before becoming Professor of General Practice in the University of Leicester. My fellow trustees included Sir John Walton and Rabbi Julia Neuberger. I also entertained my 'bad employer' Norman Fowler, the Secretary of State, to lunch at BMA House. In those days politics were relatively civilised and lunches and dinners were a good way of keeping communications open between people who seriously opposed each other. I received a note from Mr Fowler thanking me for my hospitality, saying how much he enjoyed our discussion and hoping that we could repeat it. It was signed 'Yours Norman'.[12]

The Annual Meeting had engendered a great deal of interest in the BMA and its Chairman. *The Health and Social Services Journal* noted that along with the major [physical] refurbishment of the Association's headquarters the BMA had emerged unequivocally as a staunch defender of the NHS. The journal noted that one of the leading lights in this shift of attitude was the BMA's Chairman, 'whose ebullient style contrasted sharply with a somewhat stiffer approach of some of his predecessors'. It also reported that on at least one issue I had a very clear view: 'I think the ideas of the Royal College of General Practitioners on formal audit are nonsense, and we won't buy it'.[13] (There was nothing wrong with 'medical audit' – it was the ideas of the College that were nonsense. Years later my wife Shirley was being paid to audit general practitioners in Hertfordshire.)

I was asked by *The House Magazine* which describes itself as 'the unique weekly business publication for the Houses of Parliament and all those with an interest in policy and legislation' to write an article about the Association which appeared in January 1986. I started by quoting *The Times* article published on our 150th anniversary:

> To the British public the BMA virtually is British medicine. It suffers for a start from a constitution so democratic that given full rein it would paralyse decisions.[14]

I then described our role as a medico-political body but emphasised that scientific and ethical matters were of great importance to our members. I described the background to the Limited List and explained our opposition to it. I reminded the readers that:

> the first set of regulations banned 1800 drugs. The vast majority were unknown to practising doctors, and included drugs that were obsolete when I was a student in the 1940s. Furthermore, because of the haste with which the list was introduced it had many spelling errors and other mistakes. To correct these blunders and to make it legal a second set of amending Regulations had to be issued almost immediately. Yet another set of Regulations had been introduced rapidly to define an 'appropriate non-proprietary name' in order to frustrate those clever doctors who prescribe proprietary drugs by listing each and every item that they contained . . . I am glad that I do not have to explain that Newspeak to the patient.

The article ended with a quotation from a speech by Baroness Trumpingon who said in the House of Lords:

> With regard to the discussion between doctors, [*sic*] in hindsight it could have been better handled and it will be better handled in the future.[15]

I added 'Let us hope she is right!' Time has shown that she was not.

I was interviewed by a local journalist whose article appeared in *The Times* and *Post Newspapers*, which circulate over a large area of Northwest London and Southern Hertfordshire, including Mrs Thatcher's constituency of Finchley. I reminded the readers that within the Government's policy of reallocating resources, Barnet was one of the highest donor regions in the country and as a result of that policy Barnet General Hospital had done hardly any non-urgent surgery for almost four months.[16]

In a Government reshuffle Kenneth Clarke was replaced as Minister of Health by Barney Hayhoe, who spent his first week in office meeting representatives of the various professions. Along with the leaders of the craft committees I spent over an hour with him and gained the impression that he would consult the profession before taking any actions – an attitude exactly opposite to Ken Clarke's.[17] A few weeks later the BMA, the Royal College of Nursing (RCN) and the Institute of Health Services Management (IHSM) published a report on health service funding[18] which they had commissioned from the Centre for Health Economics at York University. Based on its findings we asked the Government to spend £100 million extra on the service, which did not include an allowance for pay awards nor for the £1.7 million that had been set aside to meet the repairs and maintenance. Norman Fowler invited Ken Jarrold, President of the IHSM, Trevor Clay, General Secretary of the RCN and I to meet Barney Hayhoe and the Chairman of the NHS Management Board to discuss the matter. The meeting took place[19] but no money was forthcoming.

A FLURRY OF OVERSEAS MEETINGS

The Joint Clinical Meeting with the Egyptian Medical Association, which had been arranged during Tony Grabham's chairmanship, took place in October 1985. A group of doctors and their travelling companions – 90 people in all – did a pre-conference trip on the River Nile on a boat called the *Horus*. Every one of them was stricken with gastroenteritis. We were still at home at the time and I well remember the grinning face of Richard Baker reading the story on the BBC News. The overseas meetings were carefully arranged so that the work was done in the morning, and I particularly remember a brilliant lecture by Professor Harold Ellis on ancient Egyptian medicine. The afternoons were kept free for sightseeing. The evenings were taken up with formal dinners when we entertained our Egyptian colleagues, Government officials, and others.

I managed to persuade a group of British doctors to join me on a visit to Ismalia. The town itself was barely recognisable, the French club had gone, and there was no trace of the Moascar garrisons or my Medical Reception Station.

The whole day was a great disappointment to everyone, but especially to me.

Shirley and I had booked a Nile cruise, one of our fellow passengers being Dr Lionel Kopelowitz, a member of the BMA Council but also President of the Board of Deputies of British Jews. He was an enormous security risk, and we were 'escorted' by Egyptian military frogmen, who made sure their presence was noted. In spite of that, our trip was a great success.

Jill Draper replaced Barbara Middlemiss as the BMA official responsible for arranging meetings. A decision had to be made about the next overseas meeting, and we had received invitations from the Indian and Malaysian Medical Associations. Many factors had been to be taken into consideration: the content and nature of the scientific meeting, accommodation and travel arrangements, the safety and well-being of our members and their accompanying persons, the political significance of the meeting, and the cost to those members of the Association who were participating. The Association itself was not involved in the finance because all overseas meetings had to be self-supporting.

It was decided that Jill, Andrew Blair, Shirley and I would visit Malaysia and India. We flew to Kuala Lumpur, where our first task was to select a hotel. We looked at many but the Shangri-La was head and shoulders above the others. We met officials of the Malaysian Medical Association, all of whom spoke excellent English and many of whom had trained in Britain. Shirley was dispatched with Andrew to visit potential resorts where delegates could spend time before or after the meeting, and she repeated that function several times in the future. It was quite obvious to all of us that a successful meeting could be held in Kuala Lumpur.

The four of us then travelled to Delhi and were taken to the Taj Palace Hotel. Shirley and I were allocated a top-ranked suite and a butler whom we nick-named Creepy. The minute we walked into the hotel he would appear as if from nowhere – we were sure that he was warned by the doorman. He said he was available to do anything that we wanted, but when Shirley suggested that he do the ironing he declined gracefully. In fact he did precious little, and if his presence was meant to boost our egos and incline us towards choosing India for our meeting, the mission failed. We decided to have a holiday before getting down to the formal business and so we did a tour of the Golden Triangle. We spent Christmas Day in Udipur at the Lake Palace Hotel, and gave a Christmas treat to a young British couple who were backpacking: we let them use our bath.

In Delhi we attended the Annual Meeting of the Indian Medical Association, which was a very interesting experience, marred to some extent by a complete lack of punctuality that I found difficult to manage. The Minister of Health was due to open a meeting of the Indian College of General Practitioners, which we also attended. A few minutes before the meeting was due to start there was a panic because the Minister could not be found. I was approached and asked if I would deputise for him and give an opening address of about 40 minutes but to my intense relief the Minister appeared and I could relax. After he had given his address he and the doctors on the platform had a public and ferocious disagreement. I thought at the time that perhaps we should do the same thing in United Kingdom – it might improve attendance at the RB.

We were invited to the wedding of the daughter of one of the Indian travel agents who would have been involved if the meeting took place in India. The opulence was almost unbelievable – there were flowers strewn all over the hotel floors and down the staircases, the young couple were on golden thrones, and there were vast quantities of top-class food. I found it very difficult to reconcile what I saw there with the lean-to shacks that I had seen at the back wall of the hotel.

We returned to London and reported to the Annual Meetings Committee which decided that the meeting would be held in Kuala Lumpur and that arrangements would be made so that those who wanted to go to India before or after the meeting could do so.

MORE AT HOME

The week beginning 13 January 1986 was a busy one for me. I did a full day's work in the practice on the Monday and Tuesday morning surgery. On Tuesday afternoon I met some of the professional advisers to discuss our evidence to the Review Body, and later in the afternoon I had a meeting with the Medical Defence Union (MDU). I flew to Edinburgh the following morning for a meeting of the Association's Scottish Council in Edinburgh, flying back to London for a formal meeting at the Royal College of Nursing. The following morning I attended a meeting of the GMSC, in the early afternoon I was at the Board of BMAS followed by a meeting with Jill and Andrew, and in the evening I had dinner at the British Dental Association. The next day I did a full day's work in the practice, and was on duty that night. I realised that I had no option but to give up even more clinical work.

A few weeks later I was invited to yet another luncheon at the Board of Deputies. There the guest of honour was Mr Neil Kinnock, the Leader of the Opposition. I had a serious conversation with him on the state of the health service on which he seemed very well informed.

OPENING THE NEW LIBRARY

The BMA had taken over its new library from the builders on 17 July 1985, but it had not been 'officially opened' and a decision had to be made as to who would do it. Following discreet inquiries it was agreed the Princess of Wales would honour us by opening it on 20 February 1986. She was greeted on her arrival by the Mayor and Mayoress of the London Borough of Camden, and I accompanied her throughout the entire visit. Mrs JG Links, the daughter of Sir Edwin Lutyen, who had designed BMA House, was also presented to Her Royal Highness.[20]

After the Princess had unveiled a plaque commemorating her visit I gave her a tour of the library, which was videoed. The record shows quite clearly that she and I walked down the central aisle and then disappeared. It also recorded the increasing anxiety of the officials as we failed to reappear. What happened was quite simple; the Princess had spotted a book on ophthalmology on one of the shelves, asked me what it was about, and then headed off down the side aisle

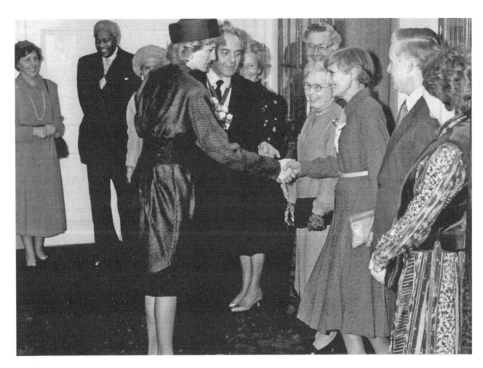

FIGURE 17.1 Greeting the Princess of Wales at the opening of the BMA library, 28 February 1986. From right to left: Mrs Shirley Marks, Lord Pitt (President of the BMA), Lady Pitt, the Princess of Wales, me, Mrs Dorothy Kyle, Dr Tony Keable-Elliott, Mrs Gillian Keable-Elliott, Mrs Anne Havard, Dr Stephen Lock and Mrs Shirley Lock. © British Medical Association.

to look at it and other books. While we were there we discussed a few other medical matters, and then we returned to the main corridor.

I next took the Princess down to the members' main recreational room, the Hastings Room, named after our founder, and introduced her to the members of Council and their spouses. I then lead her out into the quadrangle where about 500 children of staff members gathered. Although she had been friendly and animated with the adults in the Hastings Room, the transformation when she came in contact with the children was remarkable – the best description I can give is that she 'blossomed'. It is a matter of public record that she spent 45 minutes at BMA House, 20 minutes more than the scheduled time.[21] That same day her Lady-in-Waiting, Mrs George West, wrote me a letter saying that the Princess of Wales had asked her to thank me for making her visit a particularly interesting occasion, and expressing her appreciation at the helpful information that I had provided for her on both the history of the building and the development and use of the library. That was a perfect ending to one of the memorable days of my life.[22]

THE ANNUAL REPRESENTATIVE MEETING 1986

This took place in Scarborough. Although I had never been there I remembered the town from my childhood because it had featured in a series of famous posters on the theme 'Scarborough is so bracing', issued by the London and North Eastern Railway (LNER). Apart from the by now routine attack on the Government for underfunding the NHS[23] and a debate over the clash between the BMA and the GMC over the latter's response to Gillick, the major item discussed was alcohol and particularly the relationship between alcohol and driving.

The previous year the RB had impetuously demanded a total ban on the promotion and advertising of alcoholic beverages. The Council had considered that decision in the cold climate of reality, and recognised the impossibility of achieving it. As I told the representatives, the word 'promotion' in our previous policy meant that nothing could be done to encourage others to drink, and that even offering someone else a drink would be an offence.[24] Furthermore, there was the internal dilemma of what to do about the BMA's Charles Hastings wine club, and whether to continue serving alcohol in the members' dining room. I personally objected strongly to the Association's being linked with a wine club, particularly as Charles Hastings himself was believed to be a total abstainer, but I was always in the minority on that subject.

As a result of a procedural error by the Chairman the Meeting became chaotic and I had to intervene in the debate and make a statement as to what the policy was and John Havard had to explained it 'with clarity' to the press[25] – we would call on the Government to launch an effective and sustained campaign aimed at reducing alcohol-related problems. We urged the introduction of random breath tests, which led to a vicious attack from trade protectionists acting for the alcohol industry. Under a headline 'B-test demand by BMA' the *Morning Advertiser*, our daily newspaper when I was a child, reported that the chief executive of the National Union of Licensed Victuallers had described our call for random breath tests outside pubs as 'a waste of taxpayer's money'.[26] Sadly no government has ever had the guts to implement such a policy – it would have saved thousands of lives over the years.

THE COMMONWEALTH MEDICAL ASSOCIATION

In October we visited Cyprus for the 12th Commonwealth Medical Conference on 'Community Medicine' (at which one of the speakers was Professor Sir Donald Acheson, Chief Medical Officer of the Department of Health and Social Security), and the 4th Pan Cyprian Medical Congress. However, the main reason for our journey was a meeting of the Council of the Commonwealth Medical Association (CMA). The CMA was established in 1962 at a time when an increasing number of Commonwealth countries were gaining their independence and overseas branches of the British Medical Association were being replaced by national medical associations (NMAs).

Two years after our previous visit to Cyprus in 1972 it was invaded by the Turks and Northern Cyprus was set up as a separate state. On this visit the Greek part of the island appeared to us to be much more prosperous than it had been – the Turkish part was out of bounds. The meeting of the CMA Council had only one item of importance to consider – should it go on or should it be wound up. The amateur Secretary Mr Tony Grabham was replaced by the professional Secretary John Havard and it was decided to keep the organisation running for another three years, when a meeting would be held in London to coincide with a meeting of Commonwealth governments.

1987 JAMAICA AND DURHAM

In January 1987 Shirley and I, along with Jill Draper, the BMA Conference Secretary, and our travel agent, visited Jamaica and Washington DC to choose a venue for a clinical meeting to be held in October 1989. Little did we know what else would be happening in the United Kingdom in October 1989!

We spent five days in Jamaica and two in Washington DC, and then had to decide between two very different venues. Jamaica is a developing country and had already been visited by the BMA in 1974. The climate, although hot, is pleasant and the main language is English, though many people speak a patois among themselves. Furthermore, the Medical Association of Jamaica was originally a branch of the BMA and maintained close contact with it. Two parties were held in our honour and at one of them almost every member of the Council of the Medical Association turned up. Conference facilities and decent hotels existed in Kingston and Ochos Rios, there were many 'tourist attractions', and both the Department of Tourism and its Director were extremely helpful throughout our trip. We were sure that if we selected Jamaica as the venue the co-operation would be excellent.

On the other hand, Washington DC is a capital city with many famous places to visit and the climate in October is pleasant. There are many excellent conference facilities and the Convention Bureau was very helpful. We met the District of Columbia Medical Association, and visited the National Institutes of Health (NIH) and everyone was very enthusiastic about a proposed visit by British doctors. Unfortunately we soon realised that the costs would be far too high, and the trip would be far too expensive for many of our members. We decided that the meeting would be held in Ochos Rios, Jamaica.

While we were in the States Shirley and I took the opportunity to visit Durham, North Carolina, where our son Richard was an Assistant Professor in Anaesthetics at Duke University Medical School. His wife Hilary was pregnant with our first grandchild. In March 1956 when we had announced the birth of Richard, we would not have noticed a similar announcement of the birth of Hilary, the first daughter of Bernard and Valerie Sinclair of Buckhurst Hill. Bernard was a pharmacist and like us the Sinclairs were struggling to establish themselves. The two children met many years later and married in 1981.

After spending a couple of pleasant days in Durham we set off for the airport on the evening of Monday the 19th in brilliant sunshine. When we arrived there Hilary announced that our plane had been cancelled. We refused to believe her, but she was right.

The problem was that there had been a massive snowfall in the centre and north of the United States, and planes were not moving. British Airways were most helpful; they said that if I could get to any gateway city they would get me home. That proved to be impossible. By now I was panicking. I was due to lead the delegation to the Review Body on the Wednesday, with a pre-meeting on the Tuesday evening and I did not think my colleagues at the BMA would appreciate their leader being absent because he had left his return to the UK till the last minute. The Review Body was about pay, and many doctors considered that the prime function of the BMA was to maintain their standard of living.

We managed to get a flight to Newark, which was partially snowbound, and after running around the airport with our luggage we got onto a Virgin Atlantic plane for London. It never got there – it was diverted to Prestwick. We managed to get a flight from there to London and I made the pre-meeting by the skin of my teeth. I did not tell any of my colleagues about my adventure; I don't think they would have appreciated it.

AN INTERESTING TELEVISION BROADCAST

In March 1987 I took part in the BBC television programme *Watchdog* where I was questioned by viewers from all parts of the country on the health service and related matters. One questioner had been removed from her doctor's list, was very unhappy about it, and was even unhappier that she could not find out why. I explained to her that she could leave the doctor's list without any questions being asked and that although removals by doctors were very rare, and always followed a complete breakdown in personal relationships, they too were entitled to confidentiality. Other questions concerned home visits, immunisation and so on. I received a letter from the producer saying how extremely lively and informative the programme had been, that 'it got our highest ratings of the week' and asking if I would consider appearing in a future programme.[27] A few weeks later I took part in a radio discussion on health called 'The Politics of Choice'. I was beginning to be recognised by the media as an authority on health service matters, which stood me in very good stead years later. Not a bad advertisement for Pamela Taylor's charm school either!

FOOTNOTES AND REFERENCES

1 Jessop M. Angry doctors showed disgust at 'government by dictat'. *General Practitioner*. 1985 Jun 28.
2 Fowler's bad for health says top Doc. *Sun*. 1985 Jun 25.
3 Committee of Enquiry into Human Fertilisation and Embryology. *Report* (The Warnock Report) (Cm. 9314). London: HMSO; 1984.
4 'Scrutator.' The week in Plymouth. *BMJ*. 1985; **292**: 72–3.
5 Dr Newman was later President of the Women's Medical Federation and then President of the Royal College of General Practitioners.
6 Timmins N. Doctors to support surrogate motherhood and human embryo research. *The Times*. 1985 Jun 26.
7 Doctors overturn surrogate policy. *Scotsman*. 1985 Jun 26.
8 'Scrutator.' The week in Plymouth. *BMJ*. 1985; **292**: 72.
9 'Scrutator.' The week in Plymouth. *BMJ*. 1985; **292**: 90.
10 Nuclear 'fall-out' in medical family. *Pulse*. 1985 Aug 17.
11 Woodman R. Test tube baby clinics welcome surrogate charter: childless couples get fresh hope. *Liverpool Daily Post*. 1990 Mar 15.
12 Letter from the Secretary of State for Social Services. 1985 Aug 7.

13 Halpern S. BMA into healthcare battle zone. *Health Soc Serv J*. 1985 Sep 19: 1164.

14 Marks J. The British Medical Association. *House Magazine*. 1986 Jan 31: 23

15 *Hansard*. House of Lords. 1986 Jan 28.

16 Winner D. Waiting lists are stretching to eternity. *Times and Post Newspapers*. 1986 Feb 6.

17 BMA makes friends with new Minister. *General Practitioner*. 1985 Sept 20.

18 Bosanquet N. *Public expenditure and the NHS: recent trends and the outlook*. London: IHSM/BMA/RCN; 1985.

19 Medical staff and managers demand doubling of money for NHS growth. *Guardian*. 1985 Oct 31.

20 *BMJ*. 1986 Mar 1.

21 Princess of Wales visits the BMA. *General Practitioner*. 1986 Feb 28.

22 Letter from Buckingham Palace. 1986 Feb 20.

23 Timmins N. Angry doctors declare NHS needs a massive infusion of funds. *The Times*. 1986 Jun 24.

24 McDermid A. Row over drinks has doctors reeling. *Glasgow Herald*. 1986 Jun 25.

25 'Scrutator.' The week in Scarborough. *BMJ*. 1986; **293**: 34.

26 Forse V. B-Test demand by BMA. *Morning Advertiser*. 1986 Jun 27.

27 Letter from John Stapleton, BBC Lime Grove Studios. 1987 Mar 19.

CHAPTER 18 .... The approaching
storm

IN JUNE 1987 AT A TIME WHEN THERE WAS A GREAT DEAL OF POLITICAL
concern about the NHS John Moore replaced Norman Fowler as Secretary
of State. By September, health authorities started closing beds to save money,
proposals for a new pay structure brought the nurses out on strike, doctors were
petitioning Downing Street and blood transfusion staffs were taking industrial
action.[1]

A DISPUTE OVER NHS FUNDING

I have already referred to the report commissioned by the BMA, The Institute
of Health Service Management and the Royal College of Nursing, on NHS
funding, published in 1985.[2] It had suggested that real spending had failed to
match the increased demands of the NHS, and that at least £300 million was
needed to be added to the NHS budgets.

At the Annual Representative Meeting of 1987 I warned the Government
of the problems of introducing a business ethic into medicine. I said, 'If we had
modern premises like Marks & Spencer, if our customers could get the goods
they want without delay like Marks & Spencer and Sainsbury's and, above all,
if the Government and the NHS treated its staff half as well Marks and Spencer
and Sainsbury's do, this country really would have an NHS which was the envy
of the world.'[3]

A few weeks later the Institute of Health Service Management, the Royal
College of Nursing and the BMA launched their second public campaign to
persuade the Government to increase the funding of the NHS. Once again

this was backed by a serious study under the aegis of the Centre for Health Economics at York. It was dismissed out of hand by the Minister of Health, Tony Newton.[4]

On Sunday 3 January 1988 I appeared at short notice on the BBC's *World This Weekend* programme. The interview took place against the background of two sad cases. The first case was the hole-in-the heart boy Matthew Collier, whose parents had been told five times that there were no beds available at Birmingham Children's Hospital. The second was the sad death of David Barber, whose heart operation was postponed five times and who died a few days after surgery. It was reported that I challenged the Prime Minister's oft-reported series of health service statistics with one of my own which showed that Britain was at the bottom of the league in Western Europe in terms of health service spending.[5] According to another journalist, Ian Aitken,[6] I told Tony Newton, the Health Minister, that his incessant talk about more and more, 'value for money' was pure nonsense. I continued, 'we're through the fat, we're into the meat, and now we are dangerously close to the bone'. Aitken quoted extensively from the current edition of the *British Medical Journal* in which there were eight articles dealing with various aspects of Government policy as it affected the health service. Five of the articles were 'intentionally, even assertively critical of Government policy' and he hinted that the BMA was not popular with Mrs Thatcher. The right-wing press ridiculed us – the *Sun* describing me as 'Dr Chump'.[7] On the other hand, we were supported by the Tory-dominated House of Commons Select Committee on Health.

John Moore had been off work for weeks with a viral pneumonia, but when he returned to work he launched his 'almanac' and 'a portfolio of health indicators'. Collectively these would be called the 'Health Index'. A few days later the Presidents of three Royal Colleges met John Moore to discuss the statement they had released a few weeks earlier claiming that the acute hospital services had almost reached breaking point and that additional alternative funding must be found.[8] When they emerged from that meeting and said that their fears had been allayed, the BMA leadership, which was unaware of the meeting, reacted angrily for two reasons. Firstly, we feared that the Government would use the Presidents' statement to support the idea floating around in the Prime Minister's Office and the Treasury for an insurance based health service, and secondly we had to ensure that the BMA and its main committees continued to be recognised as the only bodies which could represent the entire profession in negotiations with Government. Twenty-four hours later we requested and were immediately granted a meeting with the Secretary of State where we established our point.[9]

On the 25 January in an interview with David Dimbleby on *Panorama* the

Prime Minister came under some heavy fire about the state of the NHS. She used a classical political device to divert attention from the NHS scandal. She announced, quite unexpectedly and to the surprise of her Cabinet[10] that the Government was going to undertake a fundamental review of the NHS. Having made the announcement, political expediency required that not only the review, but also any implementation of its recommendations, should be completed in a very short timescale – before the next election, then three years away.

There was good historical precedence for her actions. Caius Petronius who died in 66 AD wrote:

> We trained very hard, but it seemed that every time we were beginning to form up into teams, we would be reorganised. I was to learn later in life that we tend to meet any new situation by reorganising and a wonderful method it can be for creating the illusion of progress, while producing confusion, inefficiency and demoralisation.

Unlike previous reviews, the terms of reference were never published and the names of those who served were never officially revealed. However it became known much later that it included Mrs Thatcher herself, John Moore, Nigel Lawson, and John Major. It drew on Professor Alain Endhoven's work published in 1985 describing an internal market for the NHS.[11] Right-wing thinkers like John Redwood and David Willetts at the Centre for Policy Studies were also deeply involved, as were some politically motivated doctors like Dr Clive Froggat, of whom more later.

On 3 February less than 2% of the nation's 470,000 nurses went on strike in response to a union call for action over a pay claim,[12] but hundreds more who tried to march into Parliament Square were held back by police. On that same day I held a press conference where I explained that the BMA believed that an injection of up to £1.5 billion into the NHS was needed. Our view was that this should come from taxation, which was the most effective way of running 'probably the most cost-effective service in the world'.[13]

In the middle of all these very important events I found time to attend the presentation of the 1987 Domestos Health Education Awards, whose overall winner, Ruby Etherington, had devised a healthy eating programme for children at a primary school.[14] I also presented a cheque for £200 to the East Anglian Regional Health Authority for its campaign to stop the sale of chewing tobacco.[15] Although some of my colleagues believed that what I was doing was a waste of my time, I considered it vital to keep the image of the BMA as a caring professional body in the public eye at every opportunity, and that my involvement in what was really a commercial promotional event was fully justified by the publicity it attracted. For the same reason I travelled to speak at the Dumfries BMA Division, where I took the opportunity to describe the Government's denial of the health service crisis as 'patently untrue'. It went down well.[16]

THE COUNCIL DINNER

The BMA Council had held a formal white tie dinner to honour its Chairman since time immemorial. Invitations were sent out early in the year for my dinner, which was to be held at the Dorchester Hotel on 2 March. We were amazed when we were informed late in the day that the Secretary of State declined to wear a white tie, and we had to reissue the invitations with a different dress code.

The toast of this affair has always been the same – 'the Common Health' proposed usually by the Chairman. I spoke at some length about the chronic underfunding of the health service and then the Secretary of State replied. He launched (or really relaunched) what one reporter described as 'a revolutionary new scheme to test the nation's health'.[17]

He confirmed that the Government was conducting a review of the health service, and said that he would welcome a submission from the BMA and that 'it will be given the most careful consideration'.[18] He referred to the House of Commons Social Services Committee's report which had supported our view on health service funding, and said that the Committee's request that another billion pounds should be spent on the NHS had failed to convince him. He wished to see 'a portfolio of health indicators – a health index' – and acknowledged the lack of Government information on health outcomes. I showed a cautious reaction to the scheme, commenting that the information systems were not yet in place to take on board such a proposal.[19]

AN ALCOHOLIC DIVERSION

I was invited to appear on the *Today* programme on 12 March to discuss drinking drivers and to support the BMA's policy of random breath tests, especially near to pubs and clubs. The evening before the broadcast I had a speaking engagement at a 'black tie' dinner at the Birmingham Division of the BMA, and I drove there, anticipating that my wife Shirley would, as usual, drive back. However, on the way up she felt slightly unwell and we decided that I would drive both ways. Therefore I had just one drink.

Near our home in Elstree there is a particularly hazardous series of bends, and at about two o'clock in the morning I drove round them very gingerly.

Suddenly there was a ringing of bells and a flashing of lights, and I was forced to stop by a police car. A very young female police officer asked me to pull over, and produced a breathalyser. She enquired as to whether I knew what it was, and I told her I had been breathalysed before. (My car was hit by a drunk driver when visiting a patient in Borehamwood late at night and because both drivers must be tested, I was tested then.) I blew into the machine, and watched the tester's jaw drop. I knew that this was an 'illegal' random test so I asked her why she had stopped me. A deep voice in the background said, 'You crossed a white line Sir'.

I suspect the reality was that a senior office had spotted a car being driven very slowly at two o'clock in the morning by a man in a dinner jacket with an unconscious woman beside him, and had said words like 'Got one for you' to the trainee. When I attended the interview for the *Today* programme at around eight o'clock the interviewer and I had great fun at the police expense, but I got home my point that 'illegal random breath tests' like mine happened quite often, and that it was desirable that they should be legalised to prevent more road deaths.[20]

I was also involved in the vexed question of whether doctors should report drivers with a serious alcohol problem to the Driver Vehicle Licensing Centre (DVLC). I said that I would only consider doing it if the patient refused to contact the DVLC and after talking to the family and seeking specialist advice.[21] A misquotation in another medical newspaper gave me a second bite of the cherry.[22]

BACK TO MORE SERIOUS MATTERS

In February John Moore had told a joint meeting of the National Association of Health Authorities and the Society of Family Practitioner Committees that he would like to see the information on Family Practitioner Committee (FPC) lists about doctors services increased, and he wanted GPs to provide consumers with practice leaflets. He then went on to say he 'saw no reason why family doctors should not advertise provided they restrict themselves to factual information'. At that time we were already involved in discussions on that subject with the GMC and the Office of Fair Trading (OFT). I said that the BMA firmly supported practice leaflets but was utterly opposed to any form of advertising.[23] Prophetically, the article referred to the power of the OFT to refer matters to the Monopolies and Mergers Commission, which it did.

On 20 April we again gave evidence to the Select Committee on Social Services. We told them that we did not oppose general managers but were concerned about health authorities, which contracted services out to the public sector. We admitted that throughput of patients in hospitals was going up, but added that some patients had to return because they had been through too the system too quickly.[24] This was euphemistically referred to as the 'revolving door'.

Following the announcement of the review, the BMA expected to be asked to submit evidence, particularly in view of John Moore's statement, but when no invitation was forthcoming we submitted evidence anyway. Our evidence was published on 4 May and included as Annexes the two memoranda of evidence we had submitted to the Social Services Committee Inquiry into the National Health Service's resources. It showed that the Association had examined schemes based on Social Insurance, earmarked taxation, and an 'internal market' and had rejected them.

The 'conclusions' of our evidence included two vital paragraphs which made it clear that we believed that funding the Service by taxation was the most efficient way of doing it as it gave best value for money, and that a relatively small percentage increase in funding would undoubtedly resolve many of the present difficulties of health authorities. In our view it would be a serious mistake to embark on any major restructuring of the funding and delivery of health care in order to resolve the present difficulties.[25]

THE ANNUAL REPRESENTATIVE MEETING IN NORWICH
Apart from the debate on AIDS, which I have dealt with elsewhere, the major debates were on the funding crisis in the NHS and medical advertising. In my opening address I said, 'while it would be an exaggeration to say that the NHS is in imminent danger of collapsing, there is a major crisis in health service'. I described the Service as one of the greatest social experiments in history and one that, by and large, had been a success. Referring to the Government's current review of the Service I said that we had investigated alternative methods of funding and organisation and had concluded that most of them were peripheral to the real problem, and I reiterated our view that it should continue to be funded by taxation. The motion confirming our commitment to the NHS was passed with one dissident vote.[26]

The Representatives agreed that advertising by doctors was not in the best interests of the patient[27] but that decision received very little publicity. One journalist managed to link two completely unrelated debates under the headline 'Doctors warn of AIDS cure adverts'. However, he did quote me accurately as saying, 'Advertising is self-aggrandisement and touting. Those who write the best advertisements are not necessarily the best doctors'.[28]

The 40th anniversary of the NHS (and of my qualification) occurred while the RB was in session. To mark the occasion I cut a huge birthday cake with 40 candles.[29] As part of a series of broadcasts on Radio 4 entitled 'Pillars of Society' the eminent broadcaster Polly Toynbee presented a programme on the BMA. When I told the meeting of the impending broadcast the announcement was greeted with 'good-natured guffawing'.[30]

I have already referred to the magazine *You* which accompanied *The Mail on Sunday* and contained a feature spread over two successive weeks called 'Doctors at the birth'.[31] It reported that 80 of the 1948 Edinburgh cohort were due to meet in Edinburgh for our 4th reunion. Under eye-catching headlines such as 'The Millionaire' (Bill Graham) and 'The Cheeky Chappie' (me) it gave potted biographies of some of us.[32]

A NEW SECRETARY OF STATE

On 25 July 1988 Kenneth Clarke took over John Moore's Health responsibilities, and after a further year, during which he handled Social Security, Moore fell into political obscurity. From the outset, Clarke determined that he would be measured by his toughness, or at least by the public face of it. He resolved to tackle the job in a very different way from John Moore, who he accused of 'masterly inactivity'. He claimed that when wild allegations were made about disasters in the NHS he went out and replied to them, not allowing the public to listen to 'babies are dying' stories without finding out what it was about and rebutting them.[33]

A SMEAR CAMPAIGN

During the winter of 1988–89 the Government's review of the health service was continuing in secret. Over the weekend of 15 and 16 October 1988 a series of articles appeared in some of the Sunday newspapers, which supported the Government. Their headlines included, 'Curbs urged for lazy doctors'[34] and 'Sacking threat to lazy doctors'.[35] These reports, by political correspondents, not health correspondents, spoke of a crackdown on GPs who were too quick to prescribe drugs and refer patients to hospital and a 'tough medical audit' by Health Department officials who would, it was forecast, bring to heel those consultants who were not fulfilling their contracts.

I held a press conference three days later, accompanied by the leaders of the GPs and the consultants, Michael Wilson and Paddy Ross. I told the journalists, many of whom were specialists in health matters, that I had already written to Kenneth Clarke seeking his help to put the record straight. I said, 'There appears to be a deliberate attempt by someone to denigrate the work of doctors and undermine their standing in the public's eyes'. I thought the attacks might be part of a 'softening up' of the public, as 'It is much easier to see the doctor who can't get you into hospital as the problem [rather] than the hospital not having the money'. (During the following year my prophecy would be shown to be absolutely correct.) We had considerable press coverage which was, in the main, sympathetic.[36,37] Needless to say, the Department of Health had 'no immediate comment'.[38] As *The Lancet* commented later, all this took place against a background of Government figures which showed that record numbers of patients were being treated by those same lazy doctors.[39]

A MINOR DISAGREEMENT

On 8 January 1989 I lead a delegation to the Secretary of State to discuss the junior doctors' request that there should be an immediate ban on rotas which required them to work for more than 84 hours a week. A haematologist from Poole, Dr Jeremy Lee-Potter, represented the consultants. The Secretary of State rejected the request, but said he would urge health authorities to employ more consultants in an attempt to reduce the excessive hours worked by some doctors. Minister of Health David Mellor demonstrated the classical governmental hypocrisy of this issue, saying that it was up to the profession rather than ministers to stipulate the maximum length of continuous duty for doctors. Kenneth Clarke ruled out any legal ban on doctors' working hours on the grounds that 'they would be impossible to enforce'.[40] (In the early Twenty-first Century the EEC introduced a 48 hour week for all workers.)

OUR CHECKLIST AND THE REVIEW OF GENERAL PRACTICE

There had been various 'leaks' of the proposed White Paper, and those of us who saw them could not believe they were genuine, as we sincerely believed that the internal market would be a prescription for the ultimate privatisation of the service. We became aware that there were radical proposals including hospitals 'opting out' of the health service and general practitioners being given budgets to pay for their patients' hospital care. In the first week of 1989 we issued a statement emphasising that any changes in the principles of the NHS would need new legislation and that the BMA would exercise its right in a democracy to tell the public the implications of the changes.[41] We also published a checklist against which the public could judge the review and we sent that list to the Prime Minister and Kenneth Clarke.[42] Over the next couple of weeks the profession's leaders went out of their way to emphasise that they had no wish to have a confrontation with the Government. Michael Wilson, the Chairman of the GMSC, said, 'at the moment it is consultation by leak to see how we jump in one way or the other to certain proposals' and I said that 'doctors wanted to avoid any confrontation with the Government'.[43]

Running parallel with the review of the NHS was a review of general practice. This had started as long ago as 1986 with the publication of *Primary Health Care: an agenda for discussion*.[44] The objectives that it set – more consumer responsive services, higher standards of care, the promotion of health and the prevention of disease, greater choice for patients, better value for money, and clearer priorities for the service were completely non-controversial. However, to achieve those aims the Government proposed controversial changes in the general practitioners' contract and their remuneration. All of this was completely within the delegated responsibility of the General Medical Services Committee and its Chairman, and I played no part in any of the discussions or negotiations at any time.

Unfortunately, very little progress was being made and there was increasing antagonism between the Department of Health, ministers, and the general practitioners and their leaders. For my own experience and from my study of history I knew that, in the final analysis, the only sanction that general practitioners had was to give notice of resignation from the Service. We had no way of knowing how the negotiations would be influenced by the current review of the health service as a whole, nor if they would be subsumed by them. I was extremely worried that the two matters would become linked and that Kenneth Clarke would then be able to convince the public that any opposition to his proposed reforms linked to money and not to a difference in perception about patient care. (He tried that in an inappropriate setting and got an extremely unpleasant reaction – see below.) However, the general practitioners' negotiations continued long after the question of the 'reforms' of the NHS had been passed into law.

THE WHITE PAPER LEAKS

I have already referred to leaks about the White Paper. By chance the new Secretary Designate of the BMA, Dr Ian Field, had arranged for the entire leadership of the BMA to spend a weekend at Stratford-upon-Avon to discuss the whole future of the Association. Robin Cook, the Shadow Secretary of State got hold of a late draft of the White Paper, which he proceeded to distribute widely. When we first looked at our copies we thought they were a hoax. The idea of an internal market, similar to the American health maintenance organisations (HMOs), and hospitals being able to opt out of the NHS, smelt strongly of privatisation. However, we took the matter very seriously, and I decided as a matter of principle that we would be very wary in our response to the White Paper because we realised there was going to be a long struggle against a Government that was used to getting its own way. Public relations were going to be crucial, and we could not afford any mistakes.

FOOTNOTES AND REFERENCES

1 Rivett G. *From Cradle to Grave: fifty years of the NHS*. London: King's Fund; 1998: 358

2 Bosanquet N. *Public expenditure and the NHS: recent trends and the outlook*. London: IHSM/BMA/RCN; 1985.

3 Robinson F. Tories told to put NHS in business. *Doctor*. 1987 Jul 2.

4 Moore W. Health Minister attacked over NHS funding. *Health Serv J*. 1987 Oct 22.

5 McGregor-Health S. Row flares again as a top doctor urges more NHS cash. *Glasgow Herald*. 1988 Jan 4.

6 Aitken J. Why the doctors are grinding their scalpels. *Guardian*. 1988 Jan 4.

7 Dr Chump (Editorial). *The Sun*. 1988 Jan 6.

8 Statement by the Presidents of the RCP, RCS and RCOG. Crisis in the National Health Service. *BMJ*. 1987; **295**: 1505.

9 Duncan N. BMA fears Government secret review of NHS. *Pulse*. 1988 Jan 23.

10 Balen M. *Kenneth Clarke*. London: Fourth Estate; 1994: 160.

11 Enthoven AC. *Reflections on the Management of the NHS: an American looks at the incentives to efficiency in health service management in the UK*. London: Nuffield Provincial Hospitals Trust; 1985.

12 Fletcher D. Hospital strike backed by only 2% of nurses: *Daily Telegraph*. 1988 Feb 4.

13 Timmins N. Doctors call for injection of extra £1.5 billion into NHS. *Independent*. 1988 Feb 4.

14 Domestos winner. *Modus*. 1988 Apr.

15 £200 award to chew on. *Cambridge Evening News*. 1988 Feb 2.

16 McAuley E. Chronically underfunded, says BMA Chairman. *Dumfries Courier*. 1988 Feb 26.

17 Bell C. Moore's almanac for health and care. *Western Daily Press*. 1988 Mar 3.

18 Fundamental principle of NHS not in doubt says minister. *BMJ*. 1988; **296**: 803.

19 BMA responds to Moore's 'health index' proposals. *Medical Monitor*. 1988 Mar 14: 1.

20 Albert T. So there! *BMA News Review*. 1988 May.

21 Shop drink-drivers only as a last resort. *Doctor*. 1988 Mar 10.

22 Only 'shop' persistent drink-drivers. *General Practitioner*. 1988 Apr 22.

23 A doctor's dilemma. *Health Serv J*. 1988 Mar 10.

24 Davies P. The BMA: taking account of conventions. *Health Serv J*. 1988 Apr 28.

25 British Medical Association. *Memorandum of Evidence to the Government Internal Review of the Health Service*. London: British Medical Association; 1988.
    The relevant paragraphs of the Memorandum of Evidence were:

Para 12.2: 'Whilst many of the alternative systems have shown superficially attractive features, we have always been led to the inescapable conclusion that the principles on which the NHS is based represent the most efficient way of providing a truly comprehensive health service, whilst at the same time ensuring the best value for money in terms of the quality of health care. They also enable the cost of health care to be controlled to a much greater extent than has been achieved with other systems, as has been shown by experience of other countries.'

Para 12.4: 'A relatively small percentage increase in funding would undoubtedly resolve many of the present difficulties of health authorities, and it would be a serious mistake to embark on any major restructuring of the funding and delivery of health care in order to resolve the present difficulties. The BMA would be vehemently opposed to any measures which would undermine or in any way adversely affect the basic principles on which the British National Health Service is founded. It believes strongly that it is in the best interests of the health of the nation that the Government should examine this conclusion extremely carefully before it takes any decisions about introducing other and relatively untried systems of health care which have not stood the test of time to the extent that the NHS has done over the past 40 years.'

These two paragraphs alone justified any future reaction by the profession to proposals which could destroy that basis for the NHS.

26 Christie B. Doctors defend principle of free health system. *Scotsman*. 1988 Jul 5.
27 'Scrutator.' The week in Norwich. *BMJ*. 1988; **297**: 230.
28 Mihill C. Doctors warn of AIDS cure adverts. *Today*. 1988 Jul 5.
29 *Medical Monitor*. 1988 Jul 18.
30 Davalle P. Radio choice: state of the union. *The Times*. 1988 Jul 7.
31 Tyler R. Doctors at the birth. *You Magazine – Mail on Sunday*. 1988 Jun 12 & 19.
32 The full list was 'The Millionaire' (Bill Graham); 'The Fighter' (Rosemary Davie); The Army Man (Sir Alan Raey); 'The Nurses Champion' (Bob Duthie); 'The Man in Hell' (Ian Grant Fraser); 'The Eye Expert' (Steve Drance); 'The Dropout' (John Bullman); 'The Belonger' (Douglas Bell); 'The Executive' (Bruce Scott); 'The Missionary' (Peter Green); 'The Local Worthy' (James Bruce Smith); 'The Man in Heaven' (Hamish Maclean); 'The High-Tech Man' (George Goodman); 'The Bowls Player' (Edward Lunn); 'The Beauty' (Bridget Fraser nee Evans); 'The Gas Man' (Alistair Gillis); 'The Air Force Man' (Air Vice-Marshall Sir David Atkinson) 'The Glamour Boy' (Dennis Lamont); 'The Friendly GB (Euan Kennedy); and 'The Radiologist' (Jake Davidson').
33 Balen M. *Kenneth Clarke*. London: Fourth Estate; 1994: 161.
34 Curbs urged for lazy doctors. *Sunday Telegraph*. 1988 Oct 16.
35 Sacking threat to lazy doctors. *Mail on Sunday*. 1988 Oct 16.
36 Prentice T. Government campaign against doctors alleged. *The Times*. 1988 Oct 20.
37 BMA slams stories about lazy doctors. *Belfast Telegraph*. 1988 Oct 20.
38 Doctors hit back at slur 'campaign'. *Birmingham Post*. 1988 Oct 20.
39 BMA's indignation at jibes in the press. *Lancet*. 1988 Oct 29.
40 Sherman J. Clarke rejects doctor's rota call. *The Times*. 1989 Jan 10.
41 BMA stands firm on principles of NHS. *Independent*. 1989 Jan 6.

42 Sherman J. Worries over profit motive in health reforms: BMA fears end of routine care. *The Times*. 1989 Jan 6.

43 Leaders reject conflict. *Doctor*. 1989 Jan 12.

44 Department of Health and Social Security. *Primary Health Care: an agenda for discussion*. (Cm. 9771). London: HMSO; 1986.

CHAPTER 19

A storm breaks:
The White Paper

ON THE EVENING OF 30 JANUARY 1989 I ATTENDED A RECEPTION GIVEN by the National Association of Health Authorities. Everyone observed the social niceties although I suspect that most of them knew then, as I did, that the White Paper was to be published next day and was likely to be very controversial. I was invited to the Department on Tuesday afternoon to see a private copy of the White Paper[1] and to give my views on it. I told Kenneth Clarke that although I personally thought it would be a disaster, I would not comment officially until the members of the BMA had had a chance to read it and make their views known through their democratically elected representatives.

That evening the review was published in a blaze of media glory. A million pounds was spent on a staff video, and Kenneth Clarke went down the Thames to a laser-lit closed circuit telecast from Limehouse to 2500 doctors and managers in six cities. The White Paper had the emotive title of *Working for Patients*, but the front cover referred to 'The Health Service', not 'The National Health Service.' Even more importantly, the White Paper was merely an outline of the Government's proposals – the details were to be set out in a series of eight working papers which, Kenneth Clarke told Parliament, were to be were to be published in 'in the course of the next week or two'. (They were not published until 20 February.) That evening I told innumerable interviewers what I had told Clarke – that the BMA would study the White Paper and consult its membership before coming to any conclusion.

Kenneth Clarke held a road show in Birmingham and the most hostile questions he received were from doctors. He declared that the BMA in his 'unbiased opinion' had never been in favour of change of any kind 'on any subject whatsoever' for as long as he could remember.[2] He or his advisers must have known that that was an untrue statement – I was involved in Keith Joseph's first reorganisation of the NHS and I have already pointed out that I had risked my medico-political future in getting it accepted by the profession. He also knew that senior members of the BMA, including Paddy Ross the Chairman of the Consultants Committee, were currently helping the Government in the Resource Management Initiative (RMI), an attempt to measure how resources were allocated and utilised. What mattered at that stage was that those ministerial allegations fitted the press stereotype of the profession, and received widespread publicity. At that stage the Council of Association and I maintained a dignified silence in line with our established policy.

It is worth glancing back to see how the proposals set out in the White Paper came about. In 1982 a Tory think tank proposed that the NHS should be replaced with an insurance-based scheme. It was leaked to *The Economist*[3] and the outcry which followed ensured its rapid demise.[4] In 1985 Professor Alain Enthoven from the Stanford Business School, who was involved in reshaping health care organisations in United States, published an article suggesting an 'internal market' for the NHS.[5] He emphasised the necessity for a small pilot study to ascertain the viability of such a radical change in the NHS. In fact, years later in 1999 when he gave the prestigious Rock Carling address 'In Pursuit of an Improving National Health Service' he said that the 'Big Bang' approach to health services reform, be it internal market or PCTs, was a mistake. He also said that significant change in the NHS that has noticeable effects at the bedside couldn't be implemented in 'political time', that is, before the run-up to the next election. He further argued that the failure to instigate pilot studies contributed to the problems of the 1990s![6]

The basis of the Government's case set out in *Working for Patients* was that efficiency in the health service could only come about through competition, in the so-called internal market, an unknown, untried and untested concept in a National Health Service. It also introduced two new concepts – 'self-governing hospitals' and 'fund-holding general practitioners'. Even at this stage journalists were interested in the effects the changes would have on their own community.[7]

In an interview with medical journalist Clare Ogilvie I remarked that 'the BMA is the greatest defender of the NHS, much more so than any Government to date'. She wrote 'some may see this as Dr Marks' last great battle. But this he rejects saying, "the NHS is no battleground". Rather, he is looking for a sensible answer from the Government'.[8]

OTHER MATTERS

In spite of the crisis in the health service I still had to attend to other matters affecting the BMA and my personal life. On 9 February John Havard and I went to Utrecht, along with our wives, for a meeting of European doctors. I got home on Saturday and the following day I drove to a meeting of the BMA's Welsh Council, which met in Llandridnod Wells, in the centre of the country. Transport between the north and south of Wales is very difficult at the weekend, but no town in South Wales was acceptable to the northerners as a meeting place and vice versa, and so for many years the meeting had been held in Shrewsbury which has reasonably good access to both parts of the principality. After a while someone realised that Shrewsbury was in England, and demanded that the meeting be moved, and Llandridnod Wells, the pole of inaccessibility, was the best compromise that could be reached. The following day I briefed the other 'Heads of Professions' about our problems and a few days later I attended a dinner at the Royal College of Nursing, where further networking took place. Subsequently, I had a private and very unofficial meeting with Robin Cook, and I also managed to put in an appearance at a dinner organised by The British Life Assurance Trusts (BLAT).

One of the most important meetings I attended was at Guy's Hospital the night before the BMA Council meeting. That hospital was to become crucial in the Government's plans for self-governing hospitals, and was often referred to as the 'flagship' of the reforms. The professor of surgery there was Ian McColl, soon-to-be Lord McColl. He was a prominent member of the Conservative Medical Society and was in close touch with the Government. Ironically he is also credited with having advised Barbara Castle during the private bed crisis 14 years earlier. The discussions that evenings were brisk, but I got the impression that opinion was completely divided and future events would show that I was right.

THE BMA'S RESPONSE

The Council of the Association had most unusually set aside two days, 1–2 March 1989, to debate the proposed reforms. A special edition of the *BMA News* appeared the next day. On its front page under the heading 'These plans will destabilise the NHS', I explained the Council's views in outline, a fuller report being carried on other pages. Also on the front page was a report of a speech by a major contributor to the debate, a member who had been directly elected by English doctors – Sir Henry Yellowlees, the immediate past Chief Medical Officer of the Department of Health. He vehemently attacked the White Paper, admitting 'I never trust a politician', and he castigated Mrs Thatcher's claims in her foreword to the White Paper that 'all the proposals in this White Paper put the needs of patients first' and that, 'the patient's needs will always be paramount'. 'These [claims] could not possibly be true', he said. 'We must have some positive attitude of our own: possibly we need a standing group to look at these.'

I revealed that following local initiatives by divisional secretaries and chairman huge meetings of doctors 'the like of which we have not seen since the GP charter days of 1964', had been held all over the country. They had overwhelmingly concluded that the proposed changes would not benefit patients and would diminish – not improve – their choice of secondary care. I urged all doctors to study the document, form their own opinions, and attend the local divisional meetings at which the Council's official report would be studied. I also urged them to write to their own MP, which many did.

Council took two major decisions. Firstly it arranged for a Special Representative Meeting to be held on 17 May, the first such meeting for 12 years. Secondly, and as far as I was concerned equally importantly, it authorised the expenditure necessary for the fight against the 'so-called reforms', the label I attached to the Government's proposals at every opportunity.[9] Tony Keable-Elliott was no longer Treasurer, and the post was held by Alistair Riddell, a general practitioner from Eastergate in the poorer part of Glasgow, who was as committed to the NHS and as opposed to the Government's proposals as I was.

That same day Kenneth Clarke condemned the BMA's 'woolly objection to change'. He said that 'like most trade unions they are backward looking and have rejected the need for reform to make the health service still more effective in delivering care'.[10] However, I now had a clear mandate from the Executive of the BMA to challenge the Government and Mr Clarke and I suspected that we would be supported by the Representative Body, often referred to colloquially as the 'Doctors' Parliament'[11] when it met in May. The Chairman of the Representative Body has a similar role to the Speaker of the House of Commons. He is the senior elected member of the Association, with the exception of the President who has no political role whatsoever.

Pamela Taylor, the head of public affairs at the BMA, was interviewed by her own professional journal *P. R. Week*.[12] She refused to reveal details of our campaign (I'm sure they were not yet decided) but she did say that it would involve media advertising, parliamentary lobbying, leaflets and posters aimed at patients in GP surgeries. She emphasised the strength of our resources and our considerable income.

TWO PUBLIC RELATIONS GAFFES

On the 7 March 1989 Health Minister Mr David Mellor criticised the BMA's opposition to the National Health Service, accusing it of behaving like 'Dr No'. (According to one newspaper report years later it was me personally who was known by Government ministers as Dr No, not the Association.[13]) In a counter attack on the White Paper, Dr Dawson, a BMA Undersecretary, said 'the idea that we are Dr No is laughable'. An excellent response. Unfortunately, he then made remarks to the effect that Mr Mellor was like Dr Goebbels. It was reported that 'the BMA chairman of Council, Dr John Marks, who is Jewish, was clearly upset at the remark and urged everyone to forget it'. Later Dr Dawson issued a grovelling apology.[14] Sitting on the platform of the Council Chamber and facing the speakers during debates I sometimes heard things that others didn't. I had certainly heard Sir Henry Yellowlees make a similar remark on March 1, but fortunately very few others heard it and after Henry and I had a private joke it was quietly buried. From then onwards we took great care to see that John Dawson stuck to his own expertise, which was science and education, and the problems surrounding AIDS.

Unknown to me, in August 1988 the Public Affairs Department staff, in intelligent anticipation of a difference of opinion between the Government and the BMA, had engaged the services of an advertising agency, Abbott Mead Vickers. They were unaware that my daughter Laura was a member of the staff of the agency, and there was consternation when I was told. I made sure that no attempt was made to hide the relationship, and everyone agreed that she must take no part in the campaign. For their part the principals of the agency only agreed to being involved with our campaign after we had convinced them that our motives were to help the public and not merely to indulge in 'Government bashing'. Once we started working together we did become quite an efficient team.

As the leader of an organisation covered by trade union legislation I had to be careful not to appear 'party political', but equally, it was a fact of life that the policy of the BMA Council coincided exactly with that of the Labour Party, and I had already given notice that we would use any legal democratic device to prevent the reforms becoming law. On 8 March, armed with the Council decisions to oppose the White Paper, I had my first official briefing meeting with Robin Cook, Shadow Secretary of State, and thereafter I regularly briefed him and Harriet Harman, the Shadow Minister. Over the next few weeks I attended divisional meetings in a variety of cities, and went to Belfast to address the Junior Members Forum. At these, and every other opportunity, and I attacked Kenneth Clarke's 'so-called reforms'.

Two days after John Dawson's outburst the Presidential Dinner of the Royal College of General Practitioners took place at their headquarters in Princes

Gate, and the guest of honour was the Secretary of State. I arrived at the dinner with Professor Sir Dillwyn Williams who was President of the Royal College of Pathologists, and he and I were door-stopped by reporters and television crews. We said our usual party pieces concerning the reforms and went into the building for dinner. The two of us were seated together on the top table near to the President, my close friend Dr Stuart Carne, and Kenneth Clarke. Everything went well until in the middle of his speech Kenneth Clarke said, 'I do wish the more suspicious of our GPs would stop feeling nervously for their wallets every time I mention the word reform'. I could not believe my ears. Dillwyn Williams went deathly pale, and you could have heard a pin drop. I thought to myself what a stupid thing to do – all the academics present at the dinner, and general practitioners all over the country, would be seriously offended. Only when I read Malcolm Balen's book did I discover, unbelievably, that his choice of phrase was deliberate.[15] Such a gross political misjudgement was of great assistance to me in my efforts to convince the profession that we were dealing with a serious threat to both the profession and the NHS.

DINNER AT THE CARLTON CLUB

In normal times there were good lines of communication between the Department of Health and the BMA, and indirectly with the Secretary of State and ministers. By the middle of the spring these had completely broken down. Sir Arnold Elton, President of the Conservative Medical Association was, like many others, becoming extremely worried about the effects that the BMA's campaign was having on the Tory Party's image. He arranged a very private dinner at the Carlton Club, where the only people present were Sir Arnold, Kenneth Clarke, John Havard and me. As I walked up the stairs and saw countless Tory prime ministers looking down I expected the walls to fall in on me. In a small private room we had an excellent meal with cultured conversation about everything and anything but the NHS. When we got down to business I begged Kenneth Clarke to have a properly evaluated pilot study in one region. His response was 'You buggers would sabotage it!' What a way to deal with a respectable profession.

He must have known that I was involved in Keith Joseph's reorganisation and had gone out on a limb to get the profession to accept it. He, or at least his officials, must also have known that we had asked Keith Joseph to have a pilot study to see if it would work. He refused it because the changes had to come in on 1 April 1974 to coincide with the reorganisation of local government, and that one of the essentials of those reforms was that health authorities and local authorities were to be 'co-terminous'. In the event that reorganisation failed miserably because no one had tried it out and spotted the flaws.

Only years later did I discover how obsessed Clarke was with the BMA. He told Nick Timmins 'the one thing we had to do was knock the BMA off its pedestal . . . we had to pull them into the mud with us and make it clear that this was just another trade union, actually one of the nastiest I had ever dealt with, and battle it out'.[16] He told a surprised Cabinet that there was nothing in the White Paper that the BMA could remotely accept, and that there was going to be a monumental row with the doctors. It would be like picking up every tablet of stone in the British Medical Association's book and smashing it on the pavement in front of Tavistock House. He thought that some members of the Cabinet blamed him for making the row.[17] He also forgot that our 'tablets of stone' included our support for the National Health Service and whatever else he did he failed to smash that.

'THE WAR PARTY'

The Council of the BMA set up a special working party of the Executive, labelled by the media 'The BMA War Party', which met at least fortnightly. We did not conform to the fuddy-duddy image of the BMA that I had joined, nor the one that Clarke and others cherished. He regarded the doctors' representatives as he regarded many union leaders: with a large dose of scepticism. They were, he considered, representative only of their own self-interest and not of their members' views. However, the BMA had successfully taken steps to improve its image with a series of high-profile campaigns on smoking, drinking and seat belts in cars, and was no longer seen by the public as the 'British Money Association'.[18] Another Conservative politician, Nicholas Ridley, bemoaned the fact that doctors had largely taken the place of the vicar in the community.[19] My insistence over many years that the BMA must be seen as a professional scientific body interested in the wellbeing of patients and the community was paying off. Furthermore, several of us had acquired the skills to promote our cause in the press, on the radio and television, and elsewhere.

On 16 March I attended a dinner meeting to celebrate the centenary of the prestigious Hampstead Medical Society. It was held in the Great Hall of Gray's Inn and the other speakers were Sir Ian Todd, President of the Royal College of Surgeons, William Slack, Dean of the Faculty of Clinical Sciences at University College and Middlesex Hospital's Medical School, and Stuart Carne, President of the Royal College of General Practitioners.[20] Sir Ian said that the Government was doing its best to divide the medical profession with its White Paper and that such a division should be avoided. I emphasised that doctors were being pursued like teachers and opticians, the panacea of competition being offered rather than the specifics of professional standards, and reminded the audience that during the debate in Parliament on the compulsory use of seat belts Mr Fowler had voted against it and the Prime Minister had abstained.[21]

A few days later I hosted the annual dinner given by the BMA for the presidents of all the Royal Colleges.[22] This had been arranged long before we had any inkling of what was to be the White Paper, and was of course completely apolitical. However the conversation always seemed to come back to Kenneth Clarke and his so-called reforms and the evening served as a sounding board for ideas.

THE PAMPHLETS

At a press conference on 30 March Michael Wilson and I announced that 11 million pamphlets and 40 000 posters, 'A Message from Your Doctor', would be distributed to general practitioners over the next few days. They carried our slogan 'An SOS for the NHS' and explained the proposed reforms and why the profession opposed them. Needless to say Kenneth Clarke called them 'disgraceful'.[23] General practitioners would be asked to display the leaflets in their waiting rooms, and also to explain the problem to patients if and when they were asked. I defended the leaflet against charges that it was unfairly slanted against the White Paper, and in what was described by veteran health correspondent Peter Pallot as 'an open challenge to the Government' I said, 'it will be interesting to see whether people believe doctors or politicians'. Kenneth Clarke of course was saddened, as always, to see the BMA was prepared to put out what he described as 'such alarmist nonsense'.[24]

The picture accompanying the article was quite amusing. It showed a very serious and rather anxious Michael Wilson and alongside him was me with a grin on my face and with two fingers raised. Those two fingers were close together and those who knew me recognised that I would be speaking and that was how I emphasised points when I spoke in public. Unfortunately, the impression given by the photograph was that I was giving a rude signal to Kenneth Clarke. I definitely was not, but in any case the picture did no harm to me or to the campaign.

That night I flew to Northern Ireland for a meeting of the Association's Junior Members Forum to enlist their support, and a few days later I went to Bristol where more than a hundred young doctors attended a meeting to launch their campaign against the White Paper. Describing the meeting as 'part of a growing chorus of criticism from nurses, doctors and politicians' a regional newspaper reported how one young doctor had said that everyone he had spoken to who had read the White Paper was against it.[25]

MORE FAVOURABLE PUBLICITY

We then had a public affairs coup. The Public Affairs Division arranged a conference of NHS consumers and patients' support groups that took place in BMA House on the 12 April. It was chaired by Mr Brian Redhead of Radio 4's *Today* programme, and was attended by the representatives of 50 charities and other organisations concerned with patient care. I told the conference that the aims of the White Paper – to put patients first, extend patient choice and devolve responsibility – were laudable, but unfortunately I did not believe the changes proposed by the Government could conceivably achieve those aims. 'They will lead to a fragmented service and destroy the comprehensive nature of the existing service – an appalling situation to contemplate. The Government's proposed self-governing hospitals would cream off the best doctors or, alternatively, make a profit by using poorly trained staff on assembly line surgery and medicine. Health authorities would in future consist of the appointees of the Secretary of State and appointees of those appointees, so that the Government will have a direct line of control from top to bottom.'[26]

That came to be the consistent theme of our attack on the Government's proposals until the Act received the Royal Assent on 29 June 1990, the day after I demitted office. Katherine Whitehorn of the Patients Association, a well-known journalist and broadcaster, told the Conference that the reforms were a smokescreen intended to blur the awful truth of Western health care – that costs are spiralling out of control. No one wanted to be in charge of rationing. So the Government was fudging the issue.[27]

There was also considerable activity at a local level. My partner Laurence Buckman and other doctors in Borehamwood attended a meeting of the Borehamwood Pensioners Association, which sent a petition signed by over 500 people to their MP, Cecil Parkinson, who was a member of the Cabinet and had the ear of the Prime Minister. He had been invited to the meeting but did not attended. However he issued a statement saying that the action of some doctors in scaring the elderly about future health provision was in his view despicable and the way they are playing politics with the fears of all people was to be deplored. In turn I described Mr Parkinson's accusations as unbelievable, whilst Mr Spector, the Secretary of the Pensioners Association, found the letter 'rather disconcerting'. As so often turned out to be the case, the public believed us rather than the politicians. To be fair to Mr Parkinson he did come and meet all the doctors, health visitors, nurses and ancillary staff at our surgery on a Saturday morning in May, because almost all of them were his constituents. Unfortunately he upset the health visitors, and lost their votes, by suggesting that they were a relatively new profession, thus inadvertently demonstrating his ignorance of health matters. However, according to Malcolm Balen, at a Cabinet meeting later in the year Cecil Parkinson reportedly broke ranks and warned that the doctors were becoming more, rather than less, entrenched. Balen quoted Cecil Parkinson as saying that 'what made a number of Kenneth Clarke's colleagues uneasy was that you had the feeling he actually liked attacking people.'[28]

I used every possible opportunity to get our message over to the public. As a meeting of the Pharmaceutical Society I likened the review to 'a poorly constructed and leaky old tub', adding that 'any other master mariner excepting Master Clarke would put into port to make his ship seaworthy'.[29] An article in *The Times* by David Willetts criticising our leaflets[30] gave me an opportunity to write 'how much better it would have been if, instead of turning to economists like David Willetts when drawing up their plans, the Prime Minister had turned to those who know and use the service'.[31] Following an attack in the *Daily Mail* I wrote 'I suppose we should expect a Government which is attempting to introduce untried, untested and unworkable proposals to attack those who have actually read those proposals, who understand them and can see where they are leading'.[32]

In an interview with Victoria McDonald for the *Sunday Telegraph* I pointed out that 883 motions had been submitted for Special Representative Meeting and that the 600 or so representatives would be telling the Government that it did not have 'the medical fraternity's support'. That contradicted Mr Clarke's statement in the House that the Government had achieved a substantial change of opinion inside the health service.[33]

FOOTNOTES AND REFERENCES

1 Department of Health. *Working for Patients*. (Cm. 555). London: HMSO; 1989.
2 Balin M. *Kenneth Clarke*. London: Fourth Estate; 1994: 169.
3 *Economist* 1982; 25.
4 Russell W. Think tank puts cat among the pigeons. *BMJ (Clin Res Ed)*. 1982; 285(6346): 985.
5 Enthoven AC. *Reflections on the Management of the National Health Service*. London: Nuffield Provincial Hospitals Trust; 1985.
6 Enthoven AC. *In Pursuit of an Improving National Health Service*. London: Nuffield Provincial Hospitals Trust; 1999.
7 Wick A. NHS plans may have unpleasant side effects. *Borehamwood Times*. 1989 Feb 9.
8 Ogilvie C. Preparing for the BMA White Paper challenge. *Pulse*. 1989 Feb 18.
9 *BMA News* 1989 Mar 3 (special edition): 1.
10 Doctors prepare for battle over NHS plan. *Press and Journal (Aberdeen)*. 1989 Mar 3.
11 Vaughan P. *Doctor's Commons: a short history of the British Medical Association*. London: Heinemann; 1959.
12 Chomet W. BMA to fight NHS reforms. *PR Week*. 1989 Mar 9.

13 Marks J. Where are they now? (Bulletin). *Health Serv J.* 1995 Aug 31: 30.
14 Goebbels remarks an error says doctors' leader. *Shropshire Star* (Wellington). 1989 Mar 9.
15 *Kenneth Clarke*, op. cit.: 174.
16 Timmins N. *The Five Giants: a biography of the welfare state.* London: Harper Collins; 1995: 466.
17 *Kenneth Clarke*, op. cit.: 168–9.
18 *Kenneth Clarke*, op. cit.: 171.
19 Ridley N. *My Style of Government.* London: Hutchinson; 1991.
20 *The Times.* 1989 Mar 17.
21 Top surgeon: avoid a split on NHS plan. *Hampstead and Highgate Express.* 1989 March 24.
22 British Medical Association [dinner]. *The Times.* 1989 Mar 23.
23 O'Hanlon P. Doctors get protest leaflets. *The Times.* 1989 Apr 1.
24 Pallot P. Health services staff: Clarke attacks doctors plea to patients. *Daily Telegraph.* 1989 Apr 1.
25 Young medics vow to beat NHS change. *Bristol Evening Post.* 1989 Apr 7.
26 Pike A. NHS plans 'would bring in worst of US system'. *Financial Times.* 1989 Apr 13.
27 Radio host gets reform critics talking. *Doctor.* 1989 Apr 20.
28 *Kenneth Clarke*, op. cit.: 176.
29 Clarke is all at sea, says BMA chief. *Evening Standard.* 1989 Apr 7.
30 Willetts D. No faith in the doctors. *The Times.* 1989 Apr 7.
31 Marks J. BMA leaflets. *The Times.* 1989 Apr 17.
32 Marks J. Ill-advised change. *Daily Mail.* 1989 Apr 27.
33 McDonald V. NHS reforms: a cure for all ills? *Sunday Telegraph.* 1989 May 14: 23.

CHAPTER 20

The profession rejects the Reforms

THE SPECIAL REPRESENTATIVE MEETING (SRM)

A document that would form the basis for the debates at BMA divisions and the Special Representative Meeting (SRM), *Special Report on the Government's White Paper – Working for Patients*, was released by Council on 13 April 1989 at a well-attended press conference.[1] The front cover carried a message from me stating that it was possibly the most important document that the Council had issued in the last 40 years. I urged members to read it and, if possible, attend the divisional meetings at which it would be considered. I continued 'there you can influence the policy decisions which are to be made at the SRM, which in turn could well influence the future of the NHS'.

The report received extensive coverage in the press and on television and radio, but although the quality newspapers gave great prominence to our campaign, tabloids such as the *Sun*, the *Daily Express* and the *Daily Mirror* paid very little attention. The tabloids refuted our allegations that they were deliberately ignoring us, the News Editor of the *Sun* claiming that what his readers wanted to know was how much a pair of glasses would cost and whether eye checks were to be free. Senior editorial staff at the *Daily Mirror* and *Today* were too busy to comment, but Claire Dover, a medical reporter at the *Daily Express*, said that being a right-wing newspaper it took an open view on the Government proposals, adding that any right-wing paper must have a problem with this kind of story.[2]

The main recommendations put forward by the Council for consideration at the SRM were:

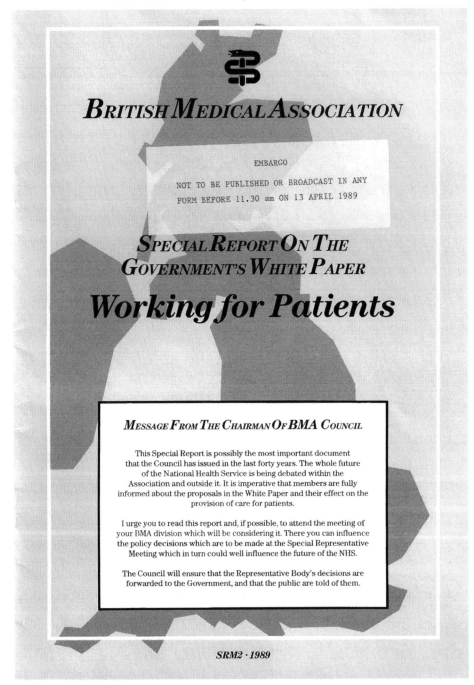

FIGURE 20.1 Special Report by the BMA Council on the Government's White Paper *Working for Patients*, 13 April 1989 (SRM2). © British Medical Association.

That the Secretary of State for Health be informed that:

I. Needs of patients must be paramount.

    a. The NHS should continue to be available to all, regardless of income and be financed mainly out of general taxation.

      Patient choice should be extended.

      Those who provide the services should be responsible for day-to-day decisions about operational matters.

      Health authorities should ensure that the health needs of the population for which they are responsible are met, that there are effective services for the prevention and control of diseases and the promotion of health, and that their population has access to a comprehensive range of high quality, value for money services.

    b. The Association is ready and willing to co-operate in introducing any proposals which have been fully discussed with representatives of practitioners working in the Health Service, and which can be shown clearly to be capable of achieving the aims set out in the Foreword and para 2.11 of the White Paper.

    c. The Association does not believe that the changes proposed in the White Paper would achieve those aims. On the contrary it is convinced that many of the proposals would damage the Service.

II. That having regard to the determination of the Secretary of State to introduce the proposals contained in the White Paper without adequate time for consultation and without any pilot studies or evaluation, the Association will continue to devote resources to inform the public and Members of Parliament of the damage which will be done to the National Health Service and of the consequences for patients.

BMA members reacted. Huge numbers of doctors turned up at local meetings to consider the Council's report, to draft motions for the SRM and to express their views on the whole subject. Not one single division of the Association supported the White Paper! Shortly afterwards I appeared on Sky Television's current affairs programme *Target*. At two angles of a triangle sat the two interrogators – the Labour MP for Grimsby, Austin Mitchell, and the right-wing Tory MP for Chingford Norman [now Lord] Tebbit. At the apex sat the victim – on this occasion, me. Norman Tebbit was extremely well informed and antagonistic, but I had been over the ground hundreds of times and I think I held my own against him and got our case over to the viewers.

    The SRM was held on 17 May at the Queen Elizabeth II Conference Centre, at a reputed cost of £75,000.[3]

In the keynote address I urged Mr Clarke to 'calm down, sit down, and slow down', because his timetable was reckless. I continued, 'having calmed down he should re-read our evidence to the review [where] we made a positive statement that experiments in methods of providing NHS services in a more efficient fashion, in a way which does not damage the NHS, are worth pursuing. The NHS is too important to be treated in a reckless way. If Kenneth Clarke does calm down, and sit down and slow down, he might be remembered as the man who devised the health service really capable of caring in the 1990s. Should the go-ahead, in defiance of all reason and his ideas fail, he will go down in history as the man who took the National Health Service and tore it apart.'[4] Although exact estimates of the number of doctors present vary, the *Independent* believed that there were 800 representatives in the hall, and noted that only three of them voted against the Council's proposition to 'advise all doctors not to co-operate with the implementation of the NHS White Paper pending negotiations over the plans with the Department of Health'.[5] The Treasurer, Dr Alistair Riddell, and I were particularly relieved at the instruction by the RB to 'devote resources to inform the public . . .'

The next day we unveiled the first of our adverts, which appeared in ten national newspapers. Along with Pamela Taylor I had spent many hours at Abbot Mead Vickers discussing our campaign and choosing advertisements and posters. One of the first drafts they produced showed a series of railway lines and railway points heading towards a distant hospital. At first sight it looked amazingly effective, but to me it recalled the photographs of the entrance to Auschwitz concentration camp that I had seen immediately after the war – it was instantly rejected. The adverts that did appear, including one showing patients being treated like cans of 'Clarke's processed peas' whilst another showed an old lady in a hospital 50 miles away from her home with the message, 'If the Government gets its way the local full-service hospital may soon be a thing of the past. Being ill will be a lonely business'. A third showed a complete list of the medical bodies supporting the Government – it was a blank page. All of the adverts carried the slogan I had devised: 'The NHS – underfunded, undermined, and under threat'. Needless to say Mr Clarke denounced them as 'misleading and unscrupulous'. He also said that we were deliberately trying to frighten patients.[6] That was partially true – if making people aware of a serious risk to something they held dear is 'frightening' that is what we were doing. The alternative was to do nothing, allow Mr Clarke and the Government to fragment the Service and impose the internal market, etcetera, with no political risk to them. That is not what I had been told to do by those that I represented.

Sue Marks, the BMA's Parliamentary Officer, had excellent contacts and together we arranged a series of meetings with Conservative Members of

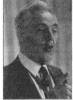

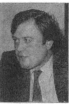

BMA News

May 19, 1989

BMA

BMA News Review

A special edition of
BMA News Review
sent to all doctors

The BMA gives its democratic verdict on the government's proposals to change the NHS.

'Calm down, sit down, slow down'

John Marks cautions...

...speedy Kenneth Clarke

OPINION
Future is in jeopardy

JOHN MARKS, chairman of BMA Council, sounded a warning in his keynote speech, and it was addressed to Health Secretary Mr Kenneth Clarke: 'Calm down, sit down and slow down,' he said.

These words of reproof at the haste in which the white paper was being rushed through were, said Dr Marks, what he would like to say to Mr Clarke.

'Having calmed down he should re-read our evidence to the review,' Dr Marks continued. 'We make a positive statement that experiments with

By Claudia Cooke

Every motion put before representatives was carried, often unanimously, most with overwhelming support, and the mood was calm but determined.

Speaker after speaker echoed the sentiments of Dr Marks when he said: 'What large retailing chain, or lage manufacturing industry would set up a management experiment and impose it on every branch before it was

shown to work? The managing director would not last long.'

Nor, implied the doctors, would Mr Clarke unless he slowed down and began to negotiate with the profession, as well as carrying out proper pilot

studies with proper evaluations before putting into effect his plans.

But underneath the fighting spirit of the meeting, it was clear that there were real fears about the effect on patients of implementing some of the white paper's proposals.

John Chawner, chairman of the private practice committee, speaking in favour of a motion

decrying market forces as a means of ensuring that health services meet population needs, recalled a visit to America: 'My own memory is of a patient lying on the steps outside the John Hopkins hospital with no doctor and no nurse coming out to see to him because he could not afford the health insurance...'

Representatives gave short shrift to the government's attempt to use medical audit as a management tool. They agreed that the BMA should advise all doctors not to co-operate with the implementation of the white

THE REASON for this week's special meeting – the first of its kind for 12 years – is that, not to put too fine a point on it, many of us believe that the whole future of the National Health Service is in jeopardy.

Two years ago we had a crisis in the health service – a result of the prolonged and chronic underfunding of the NHS by governments of all colours. Mrs Thatcher used a classic political device to divert attention from this basic problem – she announced a review.

It is that review which led to Wednesday's meeting. I believe that many of the review's proposals will lead to serious damage to patient care within the NHS.

FIGURE 20.2 Front page of *BMA News*, 19 May 1989, reporting the Special Representative Meeting of the previous day. I advise Mr Clarke to 'Calm down, sit down, and slow down'. © *BMA News*.

Parliament. The first contact involved having lunch with [Dr] Charles Goodson-Wickes, the MP for Wimbledon. At the end of our meeting I realised that I had an uphill struggle to convince any Tory of the merits of our case. Jerry Hayes, the young MP for Harlow, was due to come to BMA House the following morning when a bus and tube strike was taking place. He arrived on time, on his bicycle. I had several meetings with Jerry and I'm sure that he informed Kenneth Clarke or one of his minions about them, and what we discussed. That same afternoon I had interviews with Timothy Rasen and James Lester and found them equally unconvinced by our arguments. However, I developed a very good relationship with Sir David Price, the MP for Eastleigh, who looked, sounded, and acted like the Tory country gentleman that he was. Like Jerry Hayes, he was a member of the Select Committee on Health and was passionately devoted to the National Health Service because his wife had had a serious accident and had received a very high standard of care from the Service for many years. We met regularly for lunch at the Goring Hotel near Victoria Station and I know that he took our arguments on board.

I also had many quiet dinners with Dr Clive Froggatt, a prominent member of the Conservative Medical Society who had certainly been involved in the preparation of the White Paper and who I understood had the ear of the Secretary of State and almost certainly that of Mrs Thatcher. He made it quite clear that he was prepared to carry messages between Kenneth Clarke and me. We ate at very expensive restaurants and he was always driven back to Cheltenham, where his practice was, in a chauffeur driven Jaguar. He started an organisation called the NHS Reform Group to support the Government's proposals, but it appeared to be very ineffective. In May, the Social Services Committee published its first report on *Working for Patients*, which criticised the speed at which Kenneth Clarke was proceeding, drawing attention to major flaws in the document.[7]

AN UNWANTED INTERLUDE: I APPEAR AT AN INDUSTRIAL TRIBUNAL

In the midst of this major medico-political crisis I had to spend two days at an industrial tribunal in South London. In November 1988 John Havard had received a phone call from Uxbridge Magistrate's Court telling him that one of the Association's employees, John Hopkins, had been sentenced to three months imprisonment for taking indecent photographs of a nine-year-old girl. At the time he was the Assistant Secretary responsible for the Association's child abuse policy. He had been involved in the 'Cleveland Inquiry' conducted by Lord Justice Butler-Sloss the previous year, and had represented our views to outside bodies such as The National Society for the Protection of Children.[8] I consulted John Havard and together we met our lawyers. I took the view that retaining this man on our staff would make us look ridiculous in the eyes of both the public and our members, and would also be irresponsible. I dismissed him. Unbelievably, he sued the Association, of which I was in effect the managing director, for wrongful dismissal. Even more unbelievably, he got legal aid to do it. I spent a couple of very unpleasant hours in the witness box, but in the end the tribunal ruled in our favour. By chance there happened to be a 'stringer' sitting in the court who recognized a good story when he saw one, and it received wide publicity. The *Daily Telegraph*'s 'Child sex offender sacked as BMA's adviser on abuse'[9] compares favorably with the *Daily Mirror*'s 'Kid porn shame of BMA man',[10] but the prize headline appeared in the *Sun*, 'BMA's child-sex expert was kiddie porn beast'.[11]

STITCHING UP THE NHS

By now I was completely committed to the BMA and found it difficult to do any work with patients. On the afternoon of 5 June I had a meeting with a television production company, Vanson-Wardle Productions, which was preparing a programme on the proposed health service reviews for Channel 4. The programme, which was called *Stitching up the NHS*, did not appear until 28 August. It examined the perceived threats to the Service that would follow the implementation of a two-tier system. Partly filmed in the USA, where a market in health already existed, *Stitching up the NHS* examined the Government's proposals by talking to those who would have to implement them, including a series of 'ordinary' general practitioners, consultants, nurses and health visitors, all of whom condemned them. There were contributions from the professional advocates of change such as Dr Clive Froggatt and Lord McColl of Dulwich, who was managing the proposed opting out at Guy's Hospital. The opponents from within the NHS represented every group working in the service included Professor Jim Watson, a consultant's psychiatrist at Guy's Hospital; Christine Hancock, General Secretary of the Royal College of Nursing; Dr Maureen Dixon, Director of the Institute of Health Service Management; Rodney Bickerstaff, General Secretary of the National Union of Public Employees (NUPE); Shirley Goodwin, General Secretary of the Health Visitors Association; and me. Philip Hunt, the Director of the National Association of Health Authorities, was particularly concerned at the pace of change and the lack of resources to meet these. Much more telling were three contributors from America. Two doctors, Professor Victor Sidel, representing the American Public Health Association, and Professor Schneider, an obstetrician from the Medical College of Pennsylvania, pointed out how bad the American system was, how many people were excluded from it on the grounds of poverty and how competition drove standards down, not up. Attorney Gordon Borney emphasised how a lack of money led directly to a lack of treatment, and quoted a case resulting in a patient's death. Representatives of the Government promoting the reforms were conspicuous by their absence.[12]

On the 12 June the Association held a press conference to launch two further propaganda initiatives. The first was a video film featuring 'soap opera' celebrities such as Ishia Bennison, who played Guizian Osman in the popular television soap opera *Eastenders*. She recalled stories told by her family about the old days when you got treatment if you lived in the right place, had money or paid insurance. The video was to be shown at 30 public meetings through-out Great Britain, the first taking place at Bath on 22 June, to be followed by screening at Aldershot, Peterborough, and Aberystwyth.[13] The second initiative was a series of public meetings throughout the country, with a million leaflets being issued to advertise them.

Two days later I had a formal meeting with Kenneth Clarke which went on for a full two hours. I came out of the meeting saying that although there were still 'fundamental differences' over self-governing hospitals, drug budgets and plans for GPs to buy hospital care for their patients, we were prepared to look at the concept of 'money following patients'. However later that evening Clarke told another newspaper that he refused to offer any concessions over the reforms.[14] I immediately responded by saying we would continue our opposition 'every step of the way'.[15]

THE ANNUAL REPRESENTATIVE MEETING IN SWANSEA JULY 1989

I was looking forward to giving up the chair of the BMA Council having served my normal five years as Chairman. Long before the meeting a problem arose as to who would be my successor. I believed it ought to be Mr Paddy Ross, a consultant surgeon from Winchester who was Chairman of the Consultants Committee, but he was standing for the chairmanship of the Joint Consultants Committee, which in those days usually carried a knighthood. His two deputy chairmen, John Chawner and Jeremy Lee-Potter, were both competent and capable of leading their own craft, but I did not think either of them would be able to conduct the sort of campaign that the members of the Association wanted. I then heard rumours that Sir Anthony Grabham was contemplating standing for re-election. Both he and I were eligible for election under an obscure bye-law which said that, in exceptional circumstances and with two thirds of the Council voting in favour, a Chairman could be elected for a sixth year. Historically that had never happened.

I decided then and there that I would stand for a sixth year. I took the view that if I were replaced by Tony Grabham both the profession and the public would conclude that the BMA was 'caving in'. The medical magazine *General Practitioner* assumed a contest would take place, quoting a senior hospital consultant as saying 'we have to get the Secretary of State off the hook, and Dr Marks' macho approach was not the way to do it'. On the other hand it quoted a senior GP Council member as saying 'a majority of members feel at this stage that if he [Dr Marks] is replaced our campaign on the NHS will be misinterpreted.[16]

Throughout the first day of the meeting I was sitting impotently on the platform acutely aware of all the lobbying and pressurising there was taking place among the Council members. It was quite obvious that neither Tony nor I could possibly get a two-thirds majority. Unfortunately, Tony received a message that his father was very ill and he left the meeting. On the Thursday, the last day of the meeting, and the day of the Council election, the Secretary, Ian Field, read out the following message soon after the start of business:

'Following speculation in this morning's press, and to remove any uncertainty, Sir Anthony Grabham has asked me to let it be known that he is not a candidate for the chairmanship of Council of the BMA and he offers his full support to the current Chairman Dr John Marks in the profession's campaign against the Government's dangerous and damaging proposals from the National Health Service.'

The Swansea meeting demonstrated the profession's continued opposition to the so-called reforms and there was extensive press coverage. A Gallup poll on the fourth of July showed that three out of four people believed the reforms would result in cuts in services, 73% of those asked believed that the proposals were the first stage in NHS privatisation. Furthermore, and highly significantly, a majority of Tory voters believed the changes would result in cuts in services. Commenting on the poll, Kenneth Clarke declared that three out of four people were mistaken and plainly had not understood the reforms.[17]

According to the *Guardian* Kenneth Clarke admitted that the British Medical Association was winning the propaganda war against his proposals,[18] while John Warden, a well-known parliamentary correspondent, wrote in the *British Medical Journal* that Mr Clarke was more bruised and battered than ever and openly admitted that he was being forced onto the defensive by the weight of medical opposition to his reforms.[19]

A debate took place at the RB on a motion from Barnet and Finchley Division supporting the first pamphlet issued by the BMA, *An SOS for the NHS*, which had been denigrated by Kenneth Clarke and others. Shirley was the mover of the motion and analysed each point in the leaflet and showed that each of them was true. The meeting agreed overwhelmingly that the leaflet was absolutely accurate, and endorsed it.[20]

I had a good Annual Representative Meeting. It was reported that I received a rousing one-minute standing ovation for a trenchant speech and that I had defended the BMA against accusations from Mr Clarke of lying and obstructiveness. I said that what Mr Clarke wanted was first-class hospitals, preferably self-governing, with adequate funds, and second-class hospitals, presumably district general hospitals, without them.[21] Under the heading 'Clarke and doctors' leader fight it out over NHS facts' *The Times* used interviews that we had given to two senior journalists, Paul Wilkinson and Jill Sherman, to construct a 'debate' between the Secretary of State and me. Nothing new emerged.[22]

For procedural reasons part of the second day of the Swansea meeting was conducted as a 'Special Representative Meeting' devoted solely to the reforms. This academic difference was lost on the press and the medical reporters made

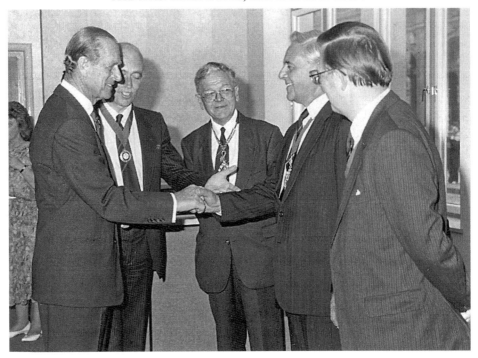

FIGURE 20.3 Opening of new BMA Scottish Office, 1 June 1989. Left to right: the Duke of Edinburgh, Dr Angus Ford (Chairman of Scottish Council), Mr David Bolt (President of the BMA), me, Dr Alistair Riddell (Treasurer). © *BMA News*.

no distinction between two parts. However, it gave me an opportunity to make a second set speech in which I urged the public to wake up to what was happening and to speak out against it.[23] I pointed out that although the BMA was a trade union it was also a scientific body which cared for patients and also for the general public health. I contrasted that with the Government's attitude by telling the representative, and through press reporters the public, that opposing the tobacco lobby was not as politically rewarding to the Government as doctor bashing. I said that the attitude of the Government to preventive medicine had been clearly demonstrated by its attitude to alcohol and tobacco. As far as alcohol was concerned there did not appear to be any strong movement towards introducing discretionary breath testing, and the failure to increase taxation on alcohol and tobacco was nothing short of disgraceful.[24] The constant reminder that we cared for patients and cared for their health was reflected in numerous polls showing that doctors were among the most respected members of the community, while politicians competed with car salesman and estate agents for the lowest position.

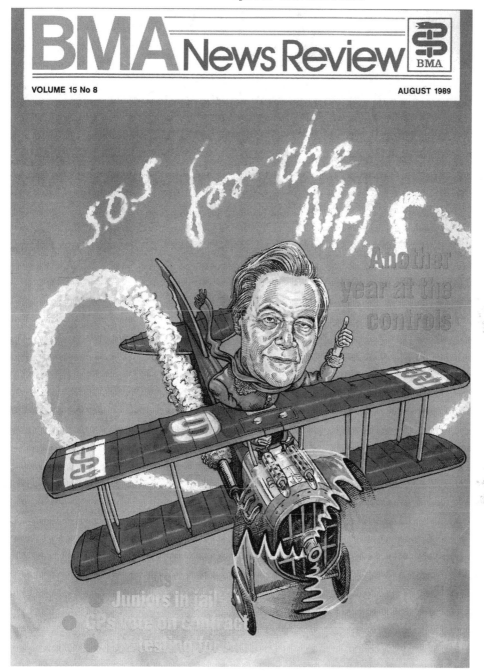

FIGURE 20.4 Cover of *BMA News Review* reporting my re-election for a sixth year as Chairman of Council, August 1989. 'SOS for the NHS.' © *BMA News*.

After the RB meeting the Council of the Association met in the afternoon and I was asked to leave the room. It was obvious that there was a long discussion about the chairmanship – I was finally invited back in and was re-elected by acclamation. Even my closest friends refused, and refuse, to discuss what happened behind those closed doors. However, the report of my election in *BMA News Review* revealed that Sir Henry Yellowlees, the former Chief Medical Officer had proposed my re-election.[25] The front cover of the next edition of *BMA News Review* showed me as the pilot of a First World War biplane behind which the words 'SOS for the NHS' were written in smoke. The original draft cover had shown two boxers – me and Kenneth Clarke – fighting over the NHS. I vetoed it as it conveyed exactly the wrong image.

There were some other interesting reactions to my re-election. *General Practitioner*, which had commented adversely on my election in 1984, said that it was good news for family doctors and good news for the NHS. It believed 'the BMA needs strong, no-nonsense leadership and that's just what it has got'.[26] On the other hand, the tabloid newspaper *Today* under a heading 'These heads should roll' included me in a list of people 'whose chopping would do the health and vitality of our nation no end of good'.[27] Ironically, the newspaper itself 'got the chop' six years later on 17 November 1995!

While I was in Swansea I was invited to address its small Jewish community. I talked about the role of the British Medical Association and my own involvement in the foundation and organisation of the small Jewish community in Borehamwood when it consisted of just 30 families.[28] I also addressed a sparse audience at a debate at Yakar, a Jewish educational centre in North West London. I gave the BMA view, Dr Richard Stone criticised the Government from a left-wing point of view, and Dr John Fry, an eminent member of the Royal College of General Practitioners, expressed his well-known view, which I suspect was the corporate view of the College establishment, that the BMA's attitude was too confrontational.[29]

Immediately after the Swansea meeting Clive Froggatt challenged the legality of the BMA's protests on the grounds that the law required a trade union to set up separate political funds voted for, and paid into, by their members. He alleged that the BMA was being overtly political and the leaflets we were issuing contained 'gross distortions of the truth'. He must have known he was talking nonsense but as *General Practitioner* commented, 'this move will please Health Secretary Kenneth Clarke who has made it clear he would like BMA members to mount a legal challenge to check on the anti-NHS reform campaign which the BMA has set up'. However, as Dr Field confirmed, we had contacted lawyers at every stage and had never crossed the line into party politics.[30] At the local level Sydney Chapman, the MP for Chipping Barnet, the same man who had hosted the Barnet Division dinner at the House of Commons and had expressed his admiration for the Association, accused us of misleading the public. It was reported, accurately, that he had met me and members of the Barnet Family Practitioner Committee and other health workers, but there was no evidence that he had convinced any of us that he was right.[31]

The results of the election to the GMC were announced soon after the ARM. I was elected, as were 23 others from the list of 32 that the BMA recommended. However, once again, the turnout was abysmally low – 33.7% in England and not much better in the other four constituencies.[32] The *Jewish Chronicle* was rather late in recording my latest achievement but two months later it appeared in its columns.[33]

FOOTNOTES AND REFERENCES

1 British Medical Association. *Working for Patients*. (SRM2). London: British Medical Association; 1989.
2 Chomet W. Tabloids ignoring us claim doctors. *P. R. Weekly*. 1989 Apr 20.
3 Bedford R. Rattling the rank and file. *BMA News*. 1989 May 19: 3
4 Cook C. *BMA News*. 1989 May 19: 1
5 Timmins N. Doctors advised not to co-operate in NHS plans. *Independent*. 1989 May 18.
6 Sherman J. Clarke attacks BMA 'scare' adverts on reforms. *The Times*. 1989 May 19.
7 Social Services Committee. *Resourcing the National Health Service: the Government's White Paper*, Working for Patients. London: HMSO; 1989.
8 'Secret' of BMA child officer. *Standard*. 1989 May 30.
9 Fenton B. Child sex offender sacked as BMA's adviser on abuse. *Daily Telegraph*. 1989 May 31.
10 Kid porn shame of BMA man. *Daily Mirror*. 1989 May 31.
11 BMA's child-sex expert was kiddie porn beast. *Sun*. 1989 May 31.
12 Stitching up the NHS. 1989 Aug 28.
13 Boseley S. Soap stars join doctor's fight. *Guardian*. 1989 Jun 13.
14 Timmins N. BMA tension with Clarke eases. *Independent*. 1989 Jun 15.
15 Sherman J. Clarke adamant in talks with the BMA. *The Times*. 1989 Jun 15.
16 Smith H. Top job may split BMA. *General Practitioner*. 1989 Jul 7.
17 Woodman R. Clarke rejects NHS poll shocker. *Western Daily Press*. 1989 Jul 5.
18 Brindle D. Clarke admits propaganda failing on NHS. *Guardian*. 1989 Jul 5.
19 Warden J. Letter from Westminster: Mr Clarke changes tactics. *BMJ*. 1989 Jul 22: 223
20 *BMJ*. 1989 Jul 22: 264.
21 MacDermid A. Poll shows three out of four back BMA on reforms. *Glasgow Herald*. 1989 Jul 5.
22 Wilkinson P, Sherman J. Clarke and doctors leaders fight it out over NHS facts. *The Times*. 1989 Jul 6.

23 *BMJ.* 1989 Jul 8: 130.
24 *BMJ.* 1989 Jul 8: 129.
25 BMA Council re-elect Marks for sixth year. *BMA News Review.* 1989 Aug.
26 Top Marks for BMA voters. *General Practitioner.* 1989 Jul 14.
27 These heads should roll. *Today.* 1989 Jul 14.
28 Marks L. Medical men talk small. *Jewish Chronicle.* 1989 Jul 29.
29 Few show they care. *Jewish Chronicle.* 1989 Jul 21.
30 BMA is 'breaking law', GP claims. *General Practitioner.* 1989 Jul 14.
31 MP says public misled on NHS. *Potters Bar Times.* 1989 Jul 6.
32 *BMJ* 1989; **229**: 224.
33 Doctors elected. *Jewish Chronicle.* 1989 Sep 15.

CHAPTER 21 .... # The campaign
                                          continues

ONE OF THE PROBLEMS THAT I FACE IN WRITING ABOUT THE NHS reforms is that at the same time general practitioners were in dispute with Kenneth Clarke over their proposed new contract. This did not directly concern me because under the BMA's Constitution that was a matter devolved to the General Medical Services Committee, its negotiators, and its Chairman, Dr Michael Wilson. Unfortunately the two issues were linked to some extent in the public mind. More importantly I was deeply concerned that if negotiations broke down the general practitioners might consider some form of retaliation. It would have been very damaging for our campaign against the 'reforms' if industrial action – strike action – was linked in the public's mind with general practitioners, and indirectly with the BMA as a whole. However, in early May Dr Wilson and his negotiating team won some concessions but a few weeks later a Special Conference of LMCs threw the deal out by 160 votes to 155. A ballot rejected a new contract by three to one but in the end Mr Clarke imposed the contract on them, a power that the Secretary of State holds.

THE ADVERTISING CAMPAIGN

On the 26 July 1989 we launched a fresh advertising campaign, at an estimated cost of £750 000.[1] Large posters were displayed on hoardings and it is estimated that in any one week more than 1000 posters were visible. One of the two posters featured a steamroller and read: 'Mrs Thatcher's plans for the NHS – don't let her steamroller the White Paper through. Write to your MP today'. The other showed an elderly woman hospital patient, seen in earlier newspaper advertisements, with a message: 'It's not a local anaesthetic if the hospital's 50 miles away. Don't let the White Paper destroy your local services. Write to your MP today'.

AN INDEPENDENT ANALYSIS

On 19 August *The Economist* published a long article headed 'Dangerous Doctors' suggesting that the doctors were proving more than a match for Whitehall.

> Scarcely a day goes by without another setback for the Health Minister Mr Kenneth Clarke [*sic*], and his deputy, David Mellor. On 10 August the House of Commons Social Service Committee published a withering report on the government's proposals for the National Health Service. It dismissed the government's timetable as unrealistic and warned that its main reforms might disrupt the whole service.
>
> Five days later the National Audit Office complained that far from possessing the expertise needed to implement the proposals, many district health authorities are ignorant of their costs and unable even to balance their books. Shackled with inadequate financial controls, they lack the information on which to base the most elementary planning decisions.

It went on:

> Ten years ago the BMA could not have taken on any government, let alone one as ideologically self-confident and politically experienced as Margaret Thatcher's. The Association was in the doldrums, firmly linked with such un-elevated activities as striking for higher wages and softer contracts. A hostile public dubbed it the British Money Association and its Secretary at the time was nicknamed 'Docker' Stevenson. Indignant doctors fled to the Royal Colleges, and membership fell to barely half the profession.
>
> Stung by adverse publicity and worried about diminishing cash, the BMA made a deliberate decision to revamp its image. Out went industrial disruption: in came well-publicised campaigns on smoking, drinking and seat belts. As it built up a patient-friendly image, disillusioned doctors returned to the fold. Membership is now back to more than three-quarters of the profession.
>
> Mr Clarke appears not to have noticed this revival when he set out on his campaign. His strategy – which was intended to pick out the leaders of the medical profession in small groups, isolate the BMA as the voice of the wallet-conscious backwoodsmen and winning the support of the Royal Colleges – was pitched at the BMA of 1979 [the year I was elected Deputy Chairman of the Representative Body

and Tony Grabham became Chairman] rather than 1989. The disastrous result was that all branches of the profession promptly united behind the Association.

The article also revealed that there was turmoil in Kenneth Clarke's Department. The role of the senior civil servants had been diminished and planning had been handed over it to a management executive dominated by outside businessmen. Furthermore, the Department:

> had little part in drafting the White Paper. *Working for Patients* was foisted on its civil servants by a high-level Cabinet committee dominated by the Prime Minister, heavily influenced by the Treasury, and advised by hand-picked experts like David Willetts. [I knew that to be true. At a one-to-one meeting with a very senior civil servant on another matter he had said to me, 'John there is a juggernaut running and none of us know how to stop it'.]

The article continued:

> [Kenneth Clarke] once tipped as a possible successor to Mrs Thatcher – he's now eyed nervously by many backbenchers.
>
> The BMA campaign has taken its toll on Conservative confidence. Some leading party figures fear that the reforms will be a medical and political disaster. 'What we have is a menu without prices' argued Sir Barney Hayhoe, a former Health Minister. Mr Nicholas Winterton, a Conservative member of the Social Services Select Committee, warned last week that the reforms could well cost the government the next election.
>
> But the likes of Sir Barney and Mr Winterton – not to mention a gaggle of timid backbenchers – should take lessons in politics from the BMA. The BMA's leaders are quite aware that the government cannot back down on the main thrust of its reforms: the introduction of an internal market . . . Quite what the BMA has in mind remains unclear.[2]

In the same edition, in a virulently anti-BMA editorial, the periodical suggested that Kenneth Clarke should run pilot studies. That answered the question posed in the article and was exactly what the BMA was crying out for, and what Kenneth Clarke refused to consider.[3]

A LITTLE INTERNECINE STRIFE
James Kyle, who had been Chairman of the Representative Body and who had since been appointed as Chairman of the Grampian Health Authority, gave

an interview to the Aberdeen *Press and Journal* in which he claimed that the doctors in the north and northeast of Scotland could benefit from the White Paper proposals. He accused doctors of showing the same innate opposition as they had to the introduction of the NHS, Keith Joseph's reorganisation, and the introduction of general management. For my part I claimed that talk about doctors resisting change was absolute rubbish. I also strenuously denied Mr Kyle's allegation that we were proposing pilot studies as a delaying tactic. Needless to say Mr Kyle stood by his comments.[4]

A POSTER TOO FAR

In late August the BMA issued two more posters. The first showed a driverless road roller with the caption 'Mrs Thatcher's plans for the NHS', and in smaller type underneath 'Don't let her steamroller the White Paper through'. The second was largely yellow with the following written in block capitals: 'What do you call a man who ignores medical advice? Mr Clarke'. Underneath in smaller letters, on a white background, were the words 'Doctors believe the NHS White Paper will damage patient care. Tell you MP you care'.[5]

Although Nick Timmins described our posters as 'of memorable brilliance'[6] there is little doubt in my mind that this poster was counter productive. It was perceived by many as being nasty and a personal attack on Mr Clarke, which of course it was. *The Independent* published a leading article under the heading 'The arrogance of doctors', which I described in a letter to the newspaper as 'intemperate'.[7] I claimed that 'to suggest that the BMA can make up people's minds for them insults their intelligence'. The advertisement had upset some

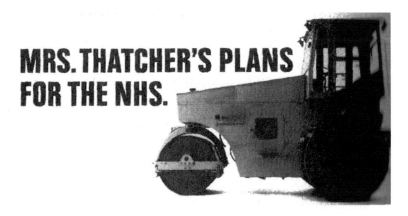

FIGURE 21.1 'Mrs Thatcher's plans for the NHS', August 1989. © British Medical Association/Abbot Mead Vickers BBDO.

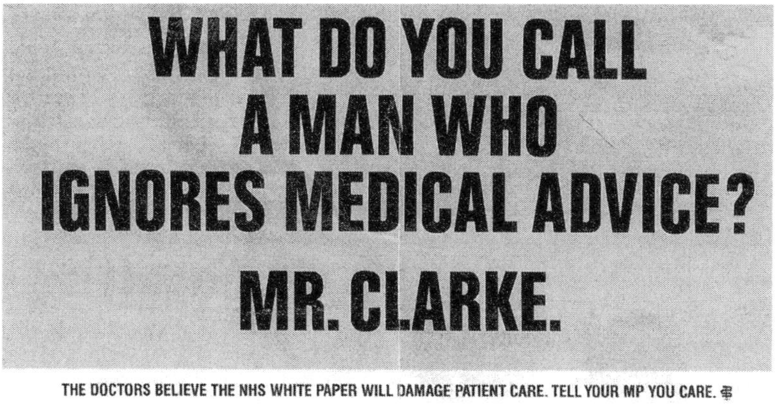

WHAT DO YOU CALL A MAN WHO IGNORES MEDICAL ADVICE? MR. CLARKE.

THE DOCTORS BELIEVE THE NHS WHITE PAPER WILL DAMAGE PATIENT CARE. TELL YOUR MP YOU CARE.

FIGURE 21.2 'What do you call a man who ignores medical advice', August 1989. A poster too far? © British Medical Association/Abbot Mead Vickers BBDO.

BMA members who did not realise the problems we had getting our message across, nor how inflexible Kenneth Clarke was. About 20 members resigned, but over the same period 2000 doctors joined or rejoined the Association. Ian Field said that Kenneth Clarke was the best recruiting sergeant that the BMA had ever had.

THE MEETING OF 27 SEPTEMBER

A meeting with Kenneth Clarke was scheduled for 27 September. Even Claire Dover, the health correspondent of the anti-BMA *Daily Express* told her readers the day before that things were not going well for the Government, and that even among Tory voters 44 percent disapproved of the White Paper proposals.

The main purpose of the meeting was to clarify the matter of general practitioner prescribing and general practitioner budgets. The following morning under the headings 'Prescription costs – GPs secure concessions from Clarke' Thomas Prentice wrote in *The Times*:

> 'The British Medical Association appeared to have won an important concession from the Government last night over the right of general practitioners to prescribe drugs regardless of cost.'[8]

Michael Wilson and I expressed our satisfaction with the outcome of the meeting.[9]

The following day Mr Clarke insisted that nothing had changed from the

NHS White Paper because he had not talked of cash limits, only of firm budgets. I pointed out that the crucial phase lay in a working paper accompanying the White Paper which said there would be legislation 'to require' authorities to keep to their drug budgets. I continued, 'Mr Clark, however, had since said that nothing had changed. If there is to be legislation for health authorities to keep to drug budgets, then cash limits must apply'. Ian Field, who had been present at the meeting, said the Association was prepared to accept that there had been a misunderstanding, but Mr Clarke's statements since the meeting gave the impression that was reneging on his promise to us. 'He gives us an assurance one day and the very next day seems to retract or contradict it.' Ian continued, 'If the legislation contains a requirement for authorities to keep drug budgets, we shall be shouting "foul" loud and clear'. Mr Clarke then issued a statement saying that he saw no point in reopening discussions on a matter that had already been resolved.[10]

I clearly recall that at one meeting, and I think it could have been that one, we discussed the part that computers would play in the reorganised NHS. I explained to him that a powerful sophisticated computer system would be required. I told him that our practice in Borehamwood was already partly computerised, and I was aware of the difficulties even at that level. Kenneth Clarke replied to me in words like, 'If you think I'm going to install some all singing all dancing all colour system you can forget it. Anything cheap and nasty will do'. In the event it did not do!

In September another poll showed that doctors were seen as the most trustworthy professionals. It also showed an increase in public disapproval of the White Paper since a similar poll in June.

At every opportunity I used the words untried, untested and unworkable as my mantra to describe the 'so-called reforms'. Those three words explained the situation simply and accurately to every member of the general public. I found television and radio appearances quite easy because I talked to the interviewer just as I would have spoken to a patient and as far as the viewers and listeners were concerned I appeared to be speaking directly to each of them.

I RETIRE FROM GENERAL PRACTICE

I had always taken the view that medical politicians should be involved in day-to-day clinical practice. The great advantage of using practising doctors as negotiators is that they can always tell the other side that their proposals would not work. 'I know that won't work because I have tried it', 'that cannot work because it conflicts with what is normal practice' and, particularly, 'that would be unethical' are arguments that the other side found difficult to refute.

Kenneth Clarke was probably unique in his total disregard for the BMA leaders' knowledge of clinical situations.

For my first four and a half years as Chairman I worked part-time in the practice. Although the BMA does not pay its senior elected officers, it does make up their loss of earnings. To make sure that the standard of care to our patients did not fall, we took in an extra partner, Dr Lawrence Buckman.

By midsummer 1989 it became quite obvious that I could not do both jobs properly, even on a part-time basis. To make life tolerable I took early retirement in September 1989, at least a year earlier than I would normally have done.[11] The practice gave a party in my honour and I had many letters of appreciation.

A BUSY FEW WEEKS

Just because I was involved in a struggle for the future of the NHS other responsibilities did not vanish. We were committed to having a Joint Clinical Meeting with the Jamaica Medical Association in November, and I flew to Jamaica for a weekend to discuss final arrangements for the meeting. While I was there my two-year-old granddaughter Katie was admitted to hospital in Dublin with meningitis. Her mother Helen was working and her father Mark was in America so Shirley left the practice and flew to Ireland.

On returning to the United Kingdom I went to Blackpool for the Conservative Party Conference, not the friendliest experience that I have ever had. I met Lord Hunter of Newington, who was to prove very helpful when the Bill was considered by the House of Lords. When I got back to London, I had one of my dinners with Clive Froggatt at Au Jardin De Gourmet, one of his favourite expensive restaurants.

Jill Knight MP (now Baroness Knight of Collingtree) and I held diametrically opposed views on the subject of abortion – she had supported the Corrie Bill and others – but both of us believed passionately in the National Health Service and she had led a backbench revolt against the imposition of charges for eye tests in 1987. I did not convince her that the BMA's campaign was worthy of support, but equally, she was very suspicious of Kenneth Clarke's proposals

JAMAICA AND SOUTH AMERICA

On 27 October 1989 we left for Jamaica. The meeting was held in the Americana Hotel at Ochos Rios and there were intensive clinical programmes each morning. During the afternoons, members had a choice of many sightseeing tours, including a visit to Noel Coward's and Ian Fleming's homes. We then had a break in Peru, visited the capital city Lima and Cusco in the mountains, before going on to Machu Picchu by train. That was of the most impressive sights I've ever seen. We sailed Lake Titicata, before boarding a bus for La Paz in Bolivia and then returning to the United Kingdom and its political crises.

FOOTNOTES AND REFERENCES

1 Brindle D. Doctors renew adverts attack to rile Tories. *Guardian*. 1989 Jul 27.
2 Britain: dangerous doctors. *Economist*. 1989 Aug 19: 19.
3 Still in search of a cure. *Economist*. 1989 Aug 19: 16.
4 Bremner S. BMA condemn reforms support: scathing attack on health chief. *Press and Journal*. 1989 Aug 18.
5 Hall C. BMA tells Clarke to heed NHS advice. *Independent*. 1989 Aug 29.
6 Timmins N. *The Five Giants: a biography of the welfare state*. London: HarperCollins; 1995: 471.
7 Marks J. Purpose of BMA advertising campaign. *Independent*. 1989 Sep 1.
8 Prentice T. Prescription costs: GPs secure concessions from Clarke. *The Times*. 1989 Sep 28.
9 Balyntine A. Retreat on doctor's budget. *Guardian*. 1989 Sept 28.
10 Timmins N. BMA accuses Clarke of reneging on drug pledge. *Independent*. 1989 Oct 5.
11 Marks to retire early. *Pulse*. 1989 Sep 30.

CHAPTER 22

The Bill
and reactions to it

THE NATIONAL HEALTH SERVICE AND COMMUNITY CARE BILL WERE published on the 22 November 1989 while we were still in South America. Although the Government denied that the market principles would mean an avalanche of bureaucrats and thousands more accountants, even it estimated that implementation would add at least £217 million to the cost of the service.[1]

The leaders of the health professions requested a meeting with the Prime Minister, but she refused to meet them. That led to an unprecedented move by leaders of the nurses', midwives' and doctors' professional organisations who organised a joint press conference which was widely covered by the national press and by regional newspapers, television, and the radio.

I told the conference it was a unique occasion with all the professional bodies coming together to express their frustration and anger that the NHS Bill showed no changes from the White Paper except pointless euphemisms and semantics.[2] Professor Dillwyn Williams, Chairman of the Conference of Royal Colleges reported 'we are convinced that the outcome of changes proposed in the White Paper will be at best uncertain and the worst extremely damaging'.[3] Miss Margaret Brain, President of the Royal College of Midwives, said that it was clear that real concerns – our worries about patient care – had not been heard.[4] The President of the Royal College of Nursing insisted that the Bill was continuing to address 'the wrong agenda'.[5]

There was no response from the Department of Health but a Gallup poll of general practitioners commissioned by *Doctor* claimed that only 16 percent of general practitioners said they would vote Conservative in the general election compared with 61 percent who had voted for the Tory Government at the last election. I commented 'the BMA is not a political organisation but if a group of highly intelligent people are treated with disdain and contempt those who do it must expect a reaction'.[6]

On 4 December 1989 *The House Magazine* published a series of articles which were written both by people who supported the legislation and by some who opposed it.[7] The first article 'A charter and a challenge' was by Kenneth Clarke, who claimed that the Bill would give the lie to all the talk of privatisation and that there was a great deal of enthusiasm among many people in the NHS for the changes. He then provided a list of the main provisions of the Bill. While the details of the changes were of interest to those deeply involved in the problems, they were of little concern to the man in the street. Similarly, they were not of great import to the vast majority of the Members of Parliament who would vote with the party Whip. Kenneth Clarke and I knew that the battle would be won or lost on what people thought, not what they read in parliamentary bills.

My contribution was entitled 'The BMA's view'. 'I qualified as a doctor on the day the NHS came into existence in July 1948 and it is not surprising, therefore, that I have a special affection for the service. After all these years I remain convinced that the NHS is one of the greatest social experiments in our history and I'm proud to have spent my life in it.' I pointed out that 'evidence from abroad suggests that real competition in the provision of health care forces standards down and cost up'. The editor of the journal chose to highlight part of my statement 'the Bill is a smokescreen designed to divert attention from the underlying problem of the NHS – years of underfunding'.

The last contribution was from Dr Rodney Grahame, a Consultant Rheumatologist at Guy's Hospital. He said, 'from the very time that the White Paper proposals were first leaked we at Guy's were subjected to a barrage of verbiage from management extolling the merits of self-government and fostering the notion that early involvement would be handsomely rewarded financially (although clearly this could only be at the expense of other hospitals). On the ground there was an all pervading feeling of inevitability and impotence. We were being managed without consent.'

Also on the staff at Guy's Hospital was Professor Harry Keen, a diabetologist with an international reputation who was passionately opposed to the Government's proposals. He organised a meeting of London consultants and academics to oppose it and ultimately went on to form the NHS Support Federation. He was a friend of my brother and I easily established personal rapport with him, so although we could never co-operate formally we made sure that each of us knew what the other was doing. I will refer later to Harry's activities.

In the end Guy's became one of the first self-governing hospitals and also became, for many of the doctors working there, a very unhappy place. Ironically, after yet another 'reform', Guys became the junior hospital in a partnership with its archrival St Thomas's Hospital.

THE YEAR DRAWS TO AN END

I received a letter from Virginia Bottomley, the Minister of State at the Department of Health, inviting me to talks about reducing junior hospital doctor's hours of work. The letter contained a series of statistics and also said that 'It remains our long-term aim to reduce average hours of duty to 72 a week, but this cannot be done overnight'.[8] Juniors claimed that her letter was an attempt to pre-empt their campaign which would involve 24 hour 'sleep-outs' in Bristol, Birmingham, and Edinburgh. The BMA pointed out that doctors who are tired run the risk of making mistakes, and made certain specific proposals to ease the junior's workload.[9]

As well as the problem of NHS reform Kenneth Clarke was fighting a second front. Since August ambulance crews had been banning overtime and rest day working in support of a pay claim. Their campaign was fronted by their Deputy Secretary Roger Poole who certainly did not fit the image of a militant trade union leader that Clarke was trying to paint. Like me he knew that an all-out strike would be damaging to his cause and that it was vital to get public opinion on his side. Clarke really wanted to separate ambulance drivers into two groups – those with paramedical training and those without it. In the long term this was a good idea, and in the long term I might have gone along with it, but there is an old Arabic proverb 'my enemy's enemy is my friend' and the ambulance dispute had enormous public support. I realised that supporting their dispute would do us no harm.

As the dispute dragged on, the public became more aware of how badly ambulance crews were paid and their sit-ins led to the police and the army being used to transport patients. This did not improve Kenneth Clarke's 'caring image' and by the end of the year public opinion was firmly on the side of the workers.

On the penultimate day of the year *Pulse* published a list of 'quotes you will always remember'. In my opinion the best was one by the Shadow Health Secretary Robin Cook: 'Kenneth Clarke's ability to think again appears to be as yet undiscovered – perhaps it's a gland that's calcified'.[10]

FOOTNOTES AND REFERENCES

1 Brindle D. Health changes to cost £217 million. *Guardian*. 1989 Nov 23.
2 United front show over NHS reform. *Birmingham Post*. 1989 Nov 30.
3 Fletcher D. Health reforms 'a prescription for cheap cure'. *Daily Telegraph*. 1989 Nov 30.
4 United front shown over NHS reform. *Birmingham Post*. 1989 Nov 28.
5 Health groups unite to fight Bill. *Nursing Standard*. 1989 Dec 7.
6 GPs turn backs on the Tories. *Doctor*. 1989 Dec 7.
7 The National Health Service. *House Magazine*. 1989 Dec 4.
8 Pallot P. Shorter week for junior doctors. *Daily Telegraph*. 1989 Dec 22.
9 Sherman J. Doctors to renew call for shorter working week. *The Times*. 1989 Dec 26.
10 The year-long verbal battle for the NHS. *Pulse*. 1989 Dec 30.

CHAPTER 23 .... The campaign continues: mysterious faxes and the Oxford debate

THE COUNCIL OF THE ASSOCIATION MET ON 3 JANUARY 1990 AND condemned Kenneth Clarke's refusal to consider any alternative proposals to his 'reforms' and deprecated the decision to bring in a Bill as an enabling measure. Such a Bill gave Clarke autocratic powers to fill in the details by Regulation which he could amend how and when he wished.[1] We also had a debate on the ambulance drivers' dispute. Clarke had made another public relations gaffe, saying that ambulance crews without training as paramedicals 'are professional drivers, a worthwhile job – but not an exceptional one'.[1] I told Council that 'the idea that moving an elderly lady from upstairs to go to hospital is something a taxi driver could do is an affront to ambulance personnel, and all caring professions'.[2]

The Council passed the appropriate resolution expressing grave concern at the prolonging of the dispute which was having a deleterious effect on patients.[3]

I also reported to the Council that we had lost 500 members in the autumn but we were so popular in the profession that overall our membership had risen by 3000.

At the press conference after the meeting I denied Mr Clarke's suggestions that the BMA had 'closed its tents and was going away'. 'Our opposition is not crumbling we are as opposed as we ever were', I said. I also denied rumours that more doctors were supporting the Government's plans, saying that there might be support by a minority of doctors but the majority were angry. I announced that we were planning a lobby of Parliament and expressed concern at the amount of money that was being spent on self-governing hospitals etc. without the necessary Parliamentary legislation.[4]

The Government received a further blow. A King's Fund Institute report said that in the United States the quality of care in the face of 'cost commitment containment pressures'[sic] depended on whether standards were regulated, and that reduced profit margins in private hospitals had resulted in patients who could not pay their bills being sent home.[5]

In Borehamwood at the weekend Dr Shirley Nathan presented the local ambulance crews with a cheque for £400, which had been collected by local supporters. Her picture with one of the ambulance men against the background of a large notice saying 'Borehamwood Ambulance Station – Emergencies Only Please' appeared above her remark 'I regret that the Secretary of State has not been able to make an acceptable offer to the ambulance crews'.[6]

Although the NHS reforms took precedence over everything else, I still had to continue with my other duties as Chairman of Council, and they were pretty extensive. I met Virginia Bottomley, the new Minister of Health, who had been a professional social worker, to discuss AIDS[7] and at the weekend I had to travel to Manchester to attend the consecration of Benny Alexander's tombstone. He had been a great friend, and had worked ceaselessly on behalf of the Association and the health service and, by the tenor of the addresses, had been a loved and respected member of the local community. On 24 January I gave a dinner for the medical press. I had always had a good relationship with the medical correspondents of the national press and also with the specialist medical press and they were relationships I fostered. In all the years that I was involved in medical politics never once did a journalist betray a trust – that is not to say that they did not write nasty things about me, but that was what some of them were paid to do. The next day I had a meeting of the AIDS trustees, and then left for Edinburgh, where I gave the prestigious Richard Scott Lecture sponsored by the University of Edinburgh Department of General Practice.

On 30 January I met with Nigel Duncan and Pamela Taylor, the Head and Deputy Head of the BMA's Press Department. They, along with Sue Marks, the BMA's Parliamentary Officer, made up the professional team that advised others and me on how to manage our campaign. They were superb.

I went up to Wolverhampton to speak at the annual dinner of the BMA Division that was attended by 70 doctors, the MP for Wolverhampton South, and the Chairman of the Local Health Authority. I made two points – the changes would create 'a cascade of patronage from top to bottom' and [the changes were designed] so that the Government could avoid blame when parts of the health service failed through lack of money, as they most certainly would. The report in a local newspaper also revealed that one third of the 3000 staff at Guy's Hospital had voted by a ratio of nine to one against becoming a self-governing hospital.[8]

I have already referred to our concern about the implementation of parts of Kenneth Clarke's proposals prior to parliamentary approval of the legislation at a time when clinical services were being restricted because of lack of resources. Subsequently we sought the advice of our lawyers on the advisability of seeking a judicial review, because the Secretary of State was undoubtedly setting up all sorts of shadow authorities without parliamentary approval. Our solicitors took counsel's opinion from Anthony Scrivener QC who said that in view of the huge parliamentary majority the Government enjoyed a judge may well rule, or probably would rule, that the Secretary of State was not acting unlawfully. We decided to take no action. Harry Keen, on the other hand, had advice from a different QC, James Goudie, and a writ for judicial review was issued and heard in early February. Unfortunately, Goudie's argument that Clarke did not have the power to spend the money was rejected by the judges and enormous costs were awarded against Harry's organisation.

MYSTERIOUS FAXES

One evening at about 11 p.m., I received a telephone call from Clare Dover, who was at that time the health reporter for the *Daily Express*. She was the same journalist who sought to justify the right-wing newspapers ignoring our campaign the previous year. She asked me to come to her home in East Ham that night, and would not say why, except that she had a document that I had to see. I put my clothes over my pyjamas and drove there. The documents she possessed were political dynamite, and how she got them was, to put it mildly, interesting. A lady who owned a local flower shop suddenly started receiving a large number of faxes, which she could not understand, and not knowing what to do with them she had contacted her local newspaper. The staff there also did not know what to make of them but suggested that Clare might. She recognised them as internal faxes between lawyers in the Department of Health and the Secretary of State's office. They showed that the lawyers feared that Clarke was overstepping the mark, and that if the Association applied for a judicial review there was a distinct chance we would win. Clare's then boyfriend said that whatever happened he would take them to the press.

The following morning I took the documents to Ian Field. Having read them he said 'John are you a British subject?', to which I replied in the affirmative. He then asked, 'Are you a loyal British subject?', and I confirmed that I was. He then said words to the effect that the faxes were Government documents, improperly acquired, and it was my duty to return them. I was quite shattered, but knowing that someone else was supposedly taking them to the press I agreed. (I was told that a small paragraph appeared in a medical journal somewhere but I never saw it!) I think that was one of the great mistakes of my life. Although Harry Keen had lost his court case it had not attracted much attention, but the damage that widespread publication of the faxes in the press, and maybe even on the television, might have caused to Kenneth Clarke is a matter of conjecture.

THE OXFORD DEBATE

The Oxford Union Debating Society invited Kenneth Clarke, me and others to a debate on the 15 February 1989, the motion being 'The house believes that the Government health reforms will not work for patients'. Apart from members of the university other invitees included Michael Meacher, the Labour Spokesperson on Social Security, and Charles Kennedy, speaking for the Liberal Democrats. Shortly before it was due to take place, the President of the Union, Edmund Lazarus, announced that Kenneth Clarke would not be available that night as he had to steer the Bill through its committee stage in the House of Commons, which had inexplicably been brought forward. However he did find time that same evening to appear on BBC TV's *Question Time*.[9] The *Oxford Times*, under the headline 'Minister "scared off" by demo', reported that a huge demonstration was being planned for the night of the debate in support of the ambulance workers by a pressure group called Oxfordshire Health Emergency who were confident of getting 5000 protesters.[10]

On the night of the meeting I visited the demonstration, which was very well attended in spite of the pouring rain, and I spoke with some of the ambulance men. In the debating hall, which was crammed to capacity, the motion was proposed by Michael Meacher and opposed by my friend Jerry Hayes, who was supported by Clive Froggatt. I supported Michael Meacher and we won the vote by 291 to 100.[11]

THE BILL PROGRESSES

I continued attending meetings of the Standing Committee on the Bill, and although the opposition tabled 800 amendments, some of which we had drafted, and there were over a hundred hours of debating time, not one of them was passed. Harriet Harman attacked the government for failing to reassure critics about the reforms and I said there had been no changes apart from those the government wanted.[12] I announced that we would continue our campaigning and lobbying when the Bill went to the House of Lords, where I hoped we might achieve major changes. We had won a very minor victory – Kenneth Clarke stated that GPs who over-prescribed would not automatically be penalised.[13] On 6 March under the heading 'Health plans split Tories' the newspaper *Today* reported that 71 percent of the 836 people questioned in a poll disapproved of the NHS 'reforms', and that of the Conservative voters 37 percent disapproved and the rest of them were undecided. The assumption could be made from that report that no Conservative voters positively supported the Government, but even I found that difficult to believe. What was important was that most of those asked said that the proposals should first be tested in a pilot scheme before going nationwide – BMA policy – and to most people a self-evident truth.[14] On the last day of the committee stage Robin Cook stated categorically that if Labour won the next election they would reverse the changes. Outside Parliament, a computer study of proposed changes in the East Anglia region suggested that the system would collapse.[15]

While all this was going on we were preparing the groundwork for the debate in the House of Lords, following our established routine of sending out information packs to selected Lords, and arranging meetings with those we thought might be helpful. Lord Molloy of Ealing, a former Labour MP and Minister, made a very useful speech in criticising opted-out hospitals and expressed his belief that there was a danger in the two-tier system. He went on, 'I believe there is a very serious risk of jettisoning the superb organisation we have for consultation between members of staff and officials in the National Health Service and indeed members of the government', How right he was. He then mentioned the BMA and its opposition to the Government's reforms and continued 'the Chairman of the British Medical Council [sic], who may be a bad person in some people's eyes but I do not believe that he is, said that the Government should recognise that those untried ideas were very unpopular. That is a moderate statement.'[16]

A few weeks later we published yet another poll, our fifth, timed to coincide with the start of the committee stage of the Bill in the House of Lords. That showed that the percentage of people opposed to the Government's proposals had gone up yet again to 77 percent, while 79 percent of those polled opposed the idea of GPs having their own fixed budgets. I pointed out that even at this stage the government could accept the idea of regional experiments.[17]

At the height of all this intense medico-political activity there were two small events, which I found rather touching. My local newspaper, the *Borehamwood Times*, in its feature '25 years ago this week' reported that two familiar faces had made an appearance [in the newspaper] – Dr John Marks and Dr Shirley Nathan from the Theobald Centre. 'The two doctors had had their picture taken at the fourth annual dinner and dance of the Elstree and Borehamwood St John Ambulance Brigade (*see* Chapter 2)'.[18] The same day *Health Services Journal* reported, with tongue in cheek, that I was clearly delighted with the gift of a video library from the director of the MSD Foundation Dr Marshall Marinker

– widely credited as one of the brains behind the NHS White Paper. It then stated that my smile would fade when I discovered that the entire collection consisted of the Department of Health's video[s] launching the reforms.[19]

Just before Good Friday I received a phone call from the Foreign Office asking if I would meet two officials from the Polish embassy. They explained to me that the Polish Medical Association, a communist state organisation, was reforming itself as a liberal professional one, and they would be grateful if I would travel to Warsaw to offer them advice and assistance while I was still Chairman of the BMA. They would pay for Shirley and me to travel there and in addition they would arrange for the two of us have a day's sightseeing in Krakow. I accepted their offer but told them I would rather go to Byalistok, a large industrial town. They asked me why I wanted to make such an odd choice, and they looked at me rather strangely when I told them that my paternal grandfather had come from that city. They agreed to my request and I agreed to go. When I got home that evening and told Shirley she said that under no circumstances was she going to Byalistok, and the following morning I sheepishly phoned the embassy and changed the itinerary. We arranged to go in early May, but within days I received another request from the Foreign Office, this time asking me to visit Budapest to meet the Hungarian Medical Association. In view of the fact that I was most certainly giving up office in July, and my diary was more than full, we had to arrange that trip for mid-April.

FOOTNOTES AND REFERENCES

1 Sherman J. BMA fight to curb 'autocratic power'. *The Times.* 1990 Jan 4.
2 Quotes. *Sunday Correspondent.* 1990 Jan 7.
3 Cathcart B. Resolve dispute now. *Morning Star.* 1990 Jan 4.
4 Anaokar M. BMA plans reform lobby in Parliament. *Hospital Doctor.* 1990 Jan 11.
5 King's Fund Institute. *Competition and Health Care: a comparative analysis of UK plans and US experience.* London: King's Fund Institute; 1990.
6 Cash collected. *Borehamwood Times.* 1990 Jan 11.
7 Virginia Bottomley is married to Peter Bottomley MP. She went on to become the Secretary of State for Health, and was made a life peer in 2005.
8 Plans for the NHS come under fire. *Wolverhampton Express and Star.* 1990 Feb 9.
9 Clarke ducks heavyweight NHS debate. *General Practitioner.* 1990 Feb 16.
10 Minister 'scared off' by demo. *Oxford Times.* 1990 Feb 9.
11 Students snub health reforms. *Doctor.* 1990 Feb 22.
12 Anger as Bill leaves committee. *Health Serv J.* 1990 Mar 1.
13 BMA admits little has been done on NHS Bill. *Pulse.* 1990 Mar 3.
14 Health plans split Tories. *Today.* 1990 Mar 6.

15 Office for Public Management. *The Rubber Windmill: contracting for health outcomes*. London: Office for Public Management; 1990.

16 *Hansard*. House of Lords. col.1223. 1990 Mar 7.

17 Prentice T. More against health reforms. *The Times*. 1990 Apr 18.

18 25 years ago this week. *Borehamwood Times*. 1990 Apr 19.

19 *Health Serv J*. 1990 Apr 19.

CHAPTER 24

My last few months
in the chair

ON THE LAST WEEKEND IN MARCH 1990 I ATTENDED THE JUNIOR Members Forum in Nottingham. I had been at every forum since becoming Deputy Chairman of the Representative Body so this was to be my 12th appearance. It has no formal status within the Association[1] but it acts as a very useful safety valve for the juniors in all branches of medicine, the sole qualification for membership being that the member should be under 31 years of age. As usual the juniors treated me with great kindness, and they gave me a large farewell card and a Nottingham lace tablecloth for Shirley. I suggested to them that patients were already becoming suspicious of general practitioners because of budget-holding proposals and I told them that 'recently a patient of mine requested a completely unnecessary blood test, and when I explained why she did not need it her response was quite rapid and angry. She said, "I suppose, doctor, you want to save money to rebuild your premises".'[2] I admitted that we had not made a great deal of progress in the fight to reduce the working hours of junior doctors, but we would continue the battle in the next round of talks.

However, at their official Conference the Junior Hospital Doctors were not so friendly. A group of them alleged that their negotiating team was out of touch with grassroots opinion, and they wanted to replace them with professional negotiators. I had heard that record before. Their own Chairman, Dr Stephen Hunter from Cardiff, explained to them 'our strength is that we are practising doctors. It gives us credence in negotiating with the Department of Health, which recognises we are accountable to our colleagues.' The motion was defeated.[3]

I had a very fruitful meeting with a Labour peer, Lord Ennals, a former

Secretary of State for Health.[4] He also took the view that Kenneth Clarke's proposals were 'untried and untested'. He suggested that a system of evaluation would determine whether the government's ideas were good, bad, or worthy of being extended.

As the Executive of a trade union the BMA Council had to be directly elected by the membership and four of its members were elected in a constituency made up of the entire membership of the organisation. My membership of the Council was due to end at the close of the Representative Meeting and so I stood as a candidate in the national constituency. Although I topped the poll, the total participation in the election was just 29.71 percent. My predecessor Sir Anthony Grabham and the Labour party activist Sam Everington were also successful candidates.[5]

On 9 June Kenneth Clarke made what was described as 'a bullish speech' at the Annual Meeting of the Institute of Health Service Management at Torquay. He said, 'I have not gone through an intensive and thorough review of the NHS, published a White Paper, fought a fierce political battle with opponents lasting some 18 months and taken a major bill through Parliament in order to achieve no change. I expect to see change from the very beginning'. He boasted that 900 general practices had expressed interest in the budget holding scheme and that 70 or 80 hospitals were working on their applications to become self-governing. He did not say how many general practices there were, nor how many hospitals were not working towards self-governing status. He showed yet again how little he understood the changes that had taken place in the medical profession by harking back to the now totally irrelevant claim that, given the chance, consultants would have vetoed the initiation of the NHS in 1948. Robin Cook, commenting on the speech, said 'The danger is that Kenneth Clarke's changes are not just breaking the mould of the NHS but will break its bones as well'. I too remarked that 'this is the speech of a worried man. For him to claim that the principles of his reforms have stood up to the debate stretches credibility.'[6]

Kenneth Clarke's problems had not been helped by the fiasco surrounding his appointment of a 'public relations adviser'. It was rumoured that the whole idea came from the Tory Party Chairman Kenneth Baker, the objective being to sharpen up Clarke's act prior to the general election and to help explain the Government's controversial health service reforms to an increasingly confused and despondent public. The man appointed to this post was John Banks, Chairman of the Young and Rubicam advertising agency. (Apparently the advice to the Secretary of State came in fast: lose weight, give up smoking, stop drinking and become less abrasive.) Mr Banks was reported to have said that there was a 'yawning gap' between what the Government wanted to do to the NHS and the public's perception of the plans. The whole affair then rapidly degenerated into farce as in twenty-four hours Mr Banks was gone and all request for comments were referred by Mr Banks to his own PR man.[7]

THE ANNUAL REPRESENTATIVE MEETING OF 1990

The meeting opened on 24 June in the beautiful modern conference centre at Bournemouth with my review of the previous year's work. The Agenda Committee had arranged for the detailed discussions of the National Health Service reforms to take place as late as the Wednesday morning, thus giving me, and the media, two bites of the cherry.

I started my main address with an outline of the events before and after the publication of the White Paper and then said, 'like the confidence tricksters in Hans Christian Anderson's story *The Emperor's New Clothes*, the Government had hoped that speed and a conspiracy of silence would have allowed them to get away with their so-called reforms without fuss. Like the same boy in the story, the BMA looked and saw the reality: less choice for patients, fragmentation of the service, lower standards, and continued under-funding. For exposing the government's duplicity we have been denigrated, abused, and labelled as scaremongering.'[8]

I reminded the meeting that I had had dealings with seven Secretaries of State for Health – Keith Joseph, Barbara Castle, Patrick Jenkin, David Ennals, Norman Fowler, John Moore and Kenneth Clarke. The first six had all listened courteously to what we had to say even if they didn't agree with it and had no intention of acting on it. It was only the last one that had, often rudely, refused to listen to any advice or opinion, and was only interested in his own proposals.[9] The *British Medical Journal* noted that at the end of the speech I 'received a standing ovation of several minutes duration, which was followed by several motions of appreciation – all carried by acclamation – after which the President, Professor John Howell, interrupted the proceedings to present me with a pair of Staffordshire figures of behalf of all the representatives.'[10] The Staffordshire figures were significant – it was well known that Shirley was a serious collector.

I had always been aware of the importance of simple, easily remembered slogans – sound bites – and I wound up my opening address by saying that Mr Clark's 'so-called reforms' could 'ultimately lead to the letters NHS standing not for National Health Service but for No Hope Service, and ultimately for 'No Health Service'. It caught the mood of the moment and those three words 'No Hope Service' made headlines all over the country.[11,12]

Of course, the health service was not the only serious matter to be discussed at the meeting, and there were other subjects that, while not of national importance, bothered some doctors. For example, a small debate took place on the

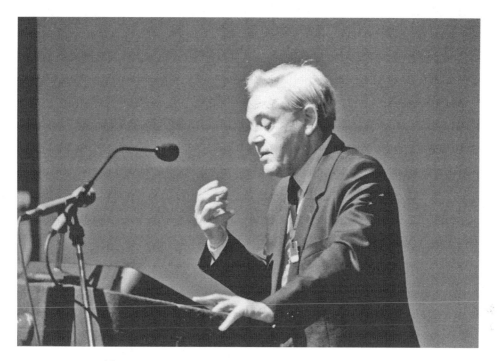

FIGURE 24.1 Addressing my last Representative Meeting as Chairman of Council, Bournemouth, June 1990.

question of whether the death certificates of smokers should record the fact that the deceased was a smoker, and another group, headed by Dr Venugopal of Cardiff, raised the issue of alternative therapies, claiming that although many patients from the Indian subcontinent used alternative medicines he had no means of evaluating them. Michael Wilson gave a report of the two-day Special Conference of LMCs, which had considered the already imposed contract, and the junior doctors again bemoaned their long working hours.

The main debate on the NHS reforms took place on Wednesday morning. Wednesday afternoon was always devoted to science and a cricket match between senior hospital doctors and junior hospital doctors, and so the morning debates received a lot of attention. My announcement that we were launching the third phase of our advertising campaign, which was to be aimed at Health Authority chairmen, NHS managers and local communities, was a major news item.[13,14] In response to many personal attacks which had been made against me by the Government and its supporters, I said that I was proud to be called a renegade and a subversive for opposing something that could damage the NHS. I received yet another standing ovation.[15]

I strongly opposed a motion calling for a 'work to rule' campaign to paralyse the health service changes, which was the policy of the National Health Service Supporters Party. One of the representatives, David Watts, a leader of that party, said 'the brave new NHS is going to dissolve into chaos. We could have slow chaos with co-operation or quick chaos if you [sic] don't co-operate. I believe we should get it over with quickly.' Dr Judy Gilley, another member of the Party and also a member of the Barnet and Finchley Division and the GMSC, who had announced her intention of standing as a candidate in the general election against her own MP, Prime Minister Mrs Thatcher, said that the BMA risked sounding boring, repetitive, and naive.[16] I opposed the proposal because I believed that to have accepted it would have played straight into the hands of Kenneth Clarke, who would have loved to label us as irresponsible militant trade unionists, concerned solely with our own problems. Furthermore, past experience showed that, even when doctors' vital self interests were at stake, including their standard of living, they refused to put patients in jeopardy. I denied that the BMA lacked vigour, and emphasised that I was neither naive nor embarrassed about taking on the Government. I asserted, 'Doctors will not work to rule. They will treat patients. If the Government wants to clobber the health service then that's too bad.'[17] The representatives sensibly decided not to have a definitive vote on the motion – passing it would have been daft and to reject it would have seemed a sign of weakness – using the long established procedural ploy of passing to the next business.

The free newspaper *Pulse*, which had long experience of reporting on general practitioner matters, agreed that I had made a correct assessment.[18] However the representatives' decision did not please the Editor of *Hospital Doctor*, a free newspaper distributed to all consultants and most junior doctors which often mirrored the policy of the Hospital Specialists and Consultants Association. He wrote:

> [The] main protagonists were bullied into allowing the debate to end inconclusively. They, and indeed all those in the BMA who seriously want to scupper Mr Clarke's plans, will certainly live to regret the day they did not have the courage of their convictions. As a result the BMA has discarded what would have been the most effective weapon in its armoury as it seeks somehow to prevent this government from causing irreparable damage to the health service.

It continued:

> only concerted action by the medical profession will do that [avert the Government from its stated aims] if doctors refuse to play ball there will be no game. The

BMA may be going soft on the NHS reforms; *Hospital Doctor*, most assuredly is not.[19]

Easy to write such stuff – not so easy to carry it out.

The 28 July 1990 was my last day in office. From a mobile studio outside the Bournemouth International Conference Centre Brian Redhead interviewed me on the *Today* programme. He also interviewed Kenneth Clarke. I spoke my piece, Kenneth Clarke denied all that I had said, and in an unprecedented move Brian, who had shown where his sympathies lay when he chaired the conference in BMA House early in the campaign, gave me the last word. The last serious debate in which I was involved as Chairman was, appropriately, on the question of AIDS. I issued a warning that Britain was facing a heterosexual AIDS epidemic because people believed that it couldn't happen to them. One representative warned the Association that AIDS would become like 'tuberculosis in the last century'.[20]

A NEW CHAIRMAN OF COUNCIL

That afternoon the BMA Council met to elect its new Chairman. There was a tradition in the Association then that the chairmanship should alternate between the consultants and the general – at that time it never dawned on anyone that the most suitable person might be an academic, a public health doctor, or a representative of some other minority group.

Dr Jeremy Lee-Potter, a haematologist from Poole General Hospital and Deputy Chairman of the Consultants Committee was elected unanimously. During an interview with Tony Delamothe of the *British Medical Journal* he revealed that he thought that his main contribution would be as a negotiator adding that 'most negotiators are pragmatists'. Asked about his attitude to reforms, he said that doctors 'had got to get the Secretary of State off the horns he had impaled himself on', exactly the same phrase that had been attributed to 'some consultants' at Swansea the previous year, when members of Council were discussing whether I should do a sixth year as Chairman. He also thought that doctors should co-operate with Kenneth Clarke to limit the damage caused by his reforms.[21] I, and many others, found that statement almost unbelievable. In an interview with the *Health Service Journal* I was asked whether the change of chairmanship would change the BMA. I replied 'the policy will continue – the BMA is not one-man.'[22]

Under the heading 'The right horse for the course?' *Pulse* expressed the view that many general practitioners would instinctively fear that their interests would no longer be represented as robustly as they were by Dr John Marks, 'the very model of a working GP'. It suggested that Dr Lee-Potter should make it clear to the Health Secretary that the BMA under his leadership 'would not scruple to campaign [sic] against reforms even if it meant opposing a small group of its own members'. It continued 'if Dr Lee-Potter messes this one up the consequences may be nothing less than the slow erosion of the NHS. Only time will tell whether the profession's leaders have put their money on the right horse.'[23]

WE LOSE

The day after I demitted office the National Health Service and Community Care Act 1990 received the Royal assent. I believe the profession, the NHS, and the community as a whole had lost out to a brutal Secretary of State and a Government with a huge majority. Even Alain Enthoven had been concerned over the absence of pilot projects, was unclear how the proposals would work out in practice, and saw the timetable as being amazingly fast.[24] It was not until years later, when Nick Timmins published his book *The Five Giants: a biography of the welfare state*, that I became aware of how close we had been to winning.

In March 1990 the Conservatives suffered a massive by-election defeat in Mid Staffordshire, and April 1990 was not a very happy time for the Government with riots over the poll tax taking place in Trafalgar Square and elsewhere. In June Mrs Thatcher sent Sir David Wolfson, who had been head of her Political Office from 1979 to 1985, along with Lord Rayner, the Chairman of Marks & Spencers, and Sir Robin Ibbs, to various NHS sites to make an assessment as to whether the reforms would work or not. They came to the conclusion that they would not. Mrs Thatcher had a meeting with Kenneth Clarke and the three top NHS executives and, according to Nick Timmins, Clarke said '[she] wanted to scrap the health reforms – put them off, or postpone them until after the election – taking much longer over it and spending much more time on costing systems and management techniques'. However, in the end the changes went ahead on time because Clarke absolutely refused to have them stopped.[25]

FOOTNOTES AND REFERENCES

1   Turner EG, Sutherland FM. *History of the British Medical Association (Volume II)*. London: British Medical Association, 1982.

2   Patient backlash feared over GP budget holding. *Doctor*. 1990 Apr 12.

3   Rebel juniors failed to sack their leaders. *Hospital Doctor*. 1990 Jun 21.

4   Lord Ennals, formerly David Ennals, served as Secretary of State for the Department of Social Services from 1976 to 1979. He was made a life peer in 1983 by Prime

Minister Margaret Thatcher, and died in 1995.

5 BMA notices: Council election results 1990–2. *BMJ*. 1990; **300**: 1403.

6 Clarke vows to 'break the mould' for NHS. *Dundee Courier and Advertiser*. 1990 Jun 9.

7 Smith H. Why PR failed to make Clarke in its own image. *Doctor*. 1990 May 17.

8 Knight M. Reform leads to a 'no hope service'. *Coventry Evening Telegraph*. 1990 Jun 25.

9 O'Sullivan J. Clarke 'intransigence' attacked. *Independent*. 1990 Jun 26.

10 'Scrutator.' The week in Bournemouth. *BMJ*. 1990; **301**: 47.

11 Woodman R. Doctors warn of NHS 'no hope service'. *Western Daily Press*. 1990 Jun 26.

12 Hunt J. NHS to become no-hope service doctors are told. *Birmingham Post*, 1990 Jun 26.

13 BMA step up reforms campaign: *Colchester Evening Gazette*. 1990 Jun 27.

14 Sherman J. BMA renews attack on health service reforms. *The Times*. 1990 Jun 28.

15 'Scrutator.' The week in Bournemouth. *BMJ*. 1990; **301**: 61

16 Another member of the party, Chris Tiarks, stood as the party's candidate in the Vale of Glamorgan by-election and got over 600 votes.

17 O'Sullivan J. Doctors reject work-to-rule in health service. *Independent*. 1990 Jun 28.

18 Editorial. *Pulse*. 1990 Jul 7.

19 BMA blows its offensive. *Hospital Doctor*. 1990 Jul 5.

20 Webster M. Heterosexual AIDS epidemic warning. *Bournemouth Evening Echo*. 1990 Jun 29.

21 Delamothe T, Lock S. New Chairman of Council for BMA. *BMJ*. 1990 Jul 7.

22 Sheldon T. News Focus: the divisive nature of the marketplace. *Health Serv J*. 1990 Jul 5.

23 The right horse for the course. *Pulse*. 1990 Jul 7.

24 Smith R. Words from the source: an interview with Alain Enthoven. *BMJ*. 1989; **298**: 1166–8.

25 Timmins N. *The Five Giants: a biography of the welfare state*. London: HarperCollins; 1995: 471–2.

CHAPTER 25 .... I am a past
Chairman

WHEN I GAVE UP OFFICE I HAD MANY LETTERS OF APPRECIATION BUT
the one I probably valued most was from Lord Richardson, who as a newly
appointed consultant at Wembley Hospital had met his new houseman,
the recently qualified John Marks, 42 years earlier in August 1948.[1] Lord
Richardson was President of the BMA and President of the GMC while I was
deeply involved in both organisations and he had always treated me with great
kindness, although he could be rather sharp with others.

I BECOME INVOLVED IN THE LIFE ASSURANCE INDUSTRY

I was introduced to Silverwood, a company in Lincoln that had started a computerised agency for the provision of life assurance medical examinations. The
concept was brilliant: a life assurance company would request an examination
from Silverwood on a computer link. They in turn would contact a general
practitioner on their list by another computer link, and the doctor would
arrange an appointment, carry out the examination using a standard form, and
return the completed form to Silverwood, all within a few days. Unfortunately
the software did not work, and so the arrangements were conducted by
telephone between the insurer, Silverwood, and the doctors. Even so the system
worked much quicker than the existing one where delays of a month were not
unusual.

David Jones, their Managing Director, asked me to advise the company on
such matters as medical ethics and the standards required of doctors seeking to
join their panel, and to become their medical advisor[2] and deal with complaints

made by examinees against their doctors. I agreed to do so on a fee-for-service basis.

On 30 October the Managing Director of Definitech Ltd, Eddie Caplin, announced that his company had taken over the medical examination system run by Silverwood, and I had been appointed as the company's Medical Director. The business began to thrive under Eddie's management, more and more insurance companies and other companies that require personnel to have medical examinations joined the network. For potential clients the company's reputation was enhanced by the knowledge that I was a past member of the General Medical Council; that I was a stickler for high standards; and that deviations from those standards could, and did, lead to doctors being removed from our panel. Within 12 years Definitech became a financial success, and it was taken over by a larger company. Unfortunately, as the new owners and I did not see eye to eye on certain matters I soon ceased to have any relationship with the company, losing my last contact with clinical medicine in the process.

I TAKE UP WRITING

Over the years I had been commissioned to write articles in medical magazines and newspapers, and I had appeared fairly frequently on television and radio. Just before I gave up the chairmanship I was approached by the magazine *Doctor* and asked to write a monthly medico-political article. The first one began: 'Today is a date of great significance in my life. I qualified when the NHS opened its doors on this day in 1948 and was also elected BMA Council Chairman on 5 July 1984.' I then gave a resume of the struggle over *Working for Patients* and the reforms and warned potential budget holding general practitioners that 'He who sups with the devil needs a long spoon'. I predicted that my successor Jeremy Lee-Potter could look forward to an interesting time ahead.[3]

A month later my second article reminded readers that Jeremy Lee-Potter had at one time represented the hospital doctor's interests on the GMSC, and 'he is a kind physician and looks it, but he has an underlying toughness, considerable negotiating skills and a deep suspicion of the government's proposals. I have complete faith in his ability to represent the whole profession in the difficult years ahead.'[4] Unfortunately events led to my changing my mind within a very short time.

Jeremy Lee-Potter was settling into his new job, holding meetings with the CMO Donald Aitcheson, Kenneth Clarke, and my old friend Dr Clive Froggatt. Needless to say that meeting took place at an expensive London restaurant, and Clive had made it very clear, as he had to me, that he had the ear of Kenneth Clarke and Mrs Thatcher. Jeremy reports in his book *A Damn Bad Business*,

'Clive was unflattering about John Marks, who he claimed was less than suppor-tive of the BMA consultant leaders, although he had apparently never denigrated me'.[5] The history of my relationships with consultant leaders in the past, my nomination for Chairman of Council, and my total endorsement of Jeremy in the quotations above are incompatible with Clive Froggatt's allegations.

A NEW COUNCIL AND NEW POLITICAL LEADERS

The first meeting of the Council under Jeremy's chairmanship was not a par-ticularly happy one. There was obvious concern at the new approach towards reforms, described by one newspaper as 'softly-softly' and the Council unani-mously approved a motion put forward by Tony Grabham and me that the BMA should continue its opposition at a national and local level. Only two members of the Council spoke in favour of Jeremy's new approach: Dr Ian Bogle, the Chairman of the GMSC, and Dr Mac Armstrong, a GP negotiator.[6,7] At that same meeting Stephen Lock and I were awarded the Association's highest honour, the Gold Medal for Distinguished Merit. The medals would be presented at the Annual Meeting in Inverness in July 1991.[8]

On the evening of 9 November I was enjoying myself at a party in a London restaurant when I was called to the telephone. A government reshuffle had taken place: William Waldegrave had replaced Kenneth Clarke at the Department of Health, with Clarke being shifted to Education. No senior BMA officer could be found – they were all away at a brainstorming weekend – but somehow or other the BBC found me and asked for my views on the subject. They were succinct: 'God help the teachers'. I did not know then that Mr Clarke's first words on being appointed had been that he hoped to 'ginger up' the teaching profession and that the next day he had described how he had gingered up the medical profession through a system of appraisal. These events were reported in an editorial in *Education – the Journal of Educational Administration, Management and Policy*, along with my remark that Mr Clarke's idea of reform was to do things his way, and that the battle he claimed to have won need never have been fought and was a Pyrrhic victory.[9]

A couple of weeks later Mrs Thatcher fought an election to retain her leader-ship of the Conservative Party, and also to remain Prime Minister. It is often forgotten how amazingly close she came to winning – just two more votes and she would have won on the first ballot. Asked to comment I said, 'Thatcher was a disaster for the NHS' and added that her demise had not lessened my concern about the service.[10] In my monthly column I said that to a man of Mr Waldegrave's intelligence (a first at Oxford and a fellow of All Souls) the naivety of many of the applications to be trusts would be obvious, and that he was not bound to approve them nor recognise budget-holding practices. My hope that he would deal with them appropriately did not materialise – hospitals teetering on the brink of bankruptcy were granted trust status completely inappropriately.[11]

The next few months were relatively quiet. I did take part in a televised debate on the NHS reforms with Clive Froggatt on the BBC's *Around Westminster* and appeared in a discussion about the GMC and its press coverage on *Hard News*. As Chairman of the BMA Foundation for AIDS I attended many meetings and I also got involved in an exchange of correspondence in the columns of *The Times* on the subject of mass screening for HIV infections. I pointed out that routine testing pregnant women would not necessarily prevent the birth of infected babies, and that to test all patients undergoing major surgery would not be cost-effective since the age group in which HIV infection was most prevalent was different from the group most commonly undergoing surgery.[12]

At the meeting in Jamaica of the Commonwealth Medical Association I had been appointed as Chairman of its Council. A meeting of that Council was held in London in January 1991. I had also been appointed to the Board of Action on Smoking and Health (ASH), where I continued my involvement in the anti-tobacco lobby and its attempts to involve the Government in active measures to curtail smoking.

BACK TO MEDICAL POLITICS

The Annual Representative Meeting of 1991 held in Inverness in July turned out to be one of the most unpleasant meetings I had ever attended – even worse than the meetings in Liverpool and Swansea. At the May meeting of Council the members became very angry with their Chairman because of what they perceived to be his lack of action against the reforms, and allegations were made that he was sympathetic towards the Government's position. I personally did not believe that, but I was convinced that he either had to change his ways or go.

The rot started on the Sunday night before the ARM started when Jeremy gave a TV interview that was generally interpreted as a weakening of the Association's opposition to the reforms. When Council member Simon Fradd expressed anger at Jeremy's remarks it was widely reported, and a group of doctors from Sheffield sent a fax demanding that Jeremy be sacked. By the time the meeting opened on Monday morning the atmosphere was electric. The first major event at the ARM is the speech by the Chairman of the Council, and in his book Jeremy says that his opening speech was not a bad one.[13] Sadly, I beg to differ: it was a very bad one. I could see support for him in the hall draining away, and the members of the Council looking more and more uncomfortable and angry. The speech was described as leaden in the *Glasgow Herald*[14] while *The Times* noted that Jeremy Lee-Potter looked uncomfortable on the platform.[15] The debate after that speech was not supportive of Jeremy, and against his advice the representatives then went on to pass a resolution stating quite bluntly that the NHS was not safe in the hands of the Conservative Government and demanded that the Association campaign with more vigour to modify the changes being imposed.[16]

Reports circulated during the Representative Meeting that a motion of no confidence in Jeremy was to be moved at the Council meeting by Simon Fradd, Ruth Gilbert, and Sam Everington – three young active and leftward-leaning members.[17] *The Times* predicted that Jeremy might face a vote of no confidence and that several Council members were ready to support Sir Anthony Grabham, 'who is willing to stand'.[18] In Jeremy's account of 'one of the most determined attempts to unseat its Chairman that the BMA had ever seen', his statement that Tony Grabham and I were among the ringleaders was not strictly true.[19] Both of us knew that Jeremy had failed to carry out the Association's policy, and we both knew that he should be replaced, but we also knew no one who could replace him. The two of us therefore agreed to support a motion of confidence in Jeremy, which was passed unanimously with the clear implication was that he was on probation.

During the debate in Council hostility had been shown by some members to Simon Fradd and the other young doctors who I described as 'having the guts to say publicly what others had been saying *sotto voce*'. I went on to remind 'those [council members] who had accused Dr Fradd and his supporters of sub-version, mischief-making and putting their own interests ahead of those of the Association' that 20 years earlier exactly the same had been said of me by the BMA 'establishment' and that if I had kept quiet we would not have reformed the GMC, the Chamber's proposals would have torn the Association apart, and abortion for social factors would be legal but 'unethical'.[20]

At the formal adjourned Annual Meeting on the Wednesday evening the Chairman of Council had to introduce Stephen Lock and me to the President, who presented each of us in turn with our gold medal. The full text of the citation was printed in the programme, and reading it still causes me embarrassment. Reporting the event, the *Jewish Chronicle* said that the Association's President had praised me for having helped to restore the BMA's reputation as a campaigning organisation,[21] while my local newspaper interviewed me at length on the reforms and quoted some of the more embarrassing parts of the citation that Jeremy had had to read.[22]

WE BECOME INVOLVED IN REAL POLITICS

Two days before the October Council meeting Jeremy Lee-Potter and Ian Field were invited to breakfast with the Prime Minister. When Council met it approved the BMA document *Leading for Health* described by Jeremy as a 'manifesto' on the future of the NHS.[23] Simon Fradd proposed that the document should go to a Special Representative Meeting in February, but the voting resulted in a tie. In such a situation the Council rules provided for it to be re-debated at the following meeting, which would be held in January. A few members of the Council thought we were being political but Tony Grabham said that our deafening silence could be construed as supporting the Tories. Fortunately the next item on the agenda was a report on the existing reforms, and an amazing litany of cuts and chaos it was. I knew the procedures of the BMA, and I therefore proposed that an SRM be convened in February, not to discuss the manifesto, which would have contravened standing orders, but to discuss the reforms and the manifesto. I argued that that was not the same proposal as Simon Fradd's and was therefore new business. Unbelievably, the Chairman allowed the motion to be put to the vote and it was passed. There was a strong possibility of a general election in early 1992 and I knew that a Representative Meeting in March would guarantee that health would remain at the top of the agenda when politicians were at their most vulnerable.[24]

Commenting on these matters in a long editorial entitled 'The doctors' anodyne prescription', *The Guardian* reported Jeremy's meeting with John Major five months after Mr Waldegrave had agreed that such a meeting should take place 'fairly soon'. It suggested that the meeting had been arranged hurriedly to save Dr Lee-Potter's bacon and to prevent the Government from facing a more confrontational leader, and that without such a meeting the Council might well have got rid of its Chairman. It said that the Chairman of Council had stressed that he did not want to be drawn into politics and that he did not want to rock the boat. The editorial ended 'Dr Lee-Potter should stop worrying about which political party should benefit from the exposure of the deficiencies in the health service and its under-funding. His concern should be NHS. Ministers are fully aware of just how key an issue the NHS has become. Strategically, the BMA has rarely been in a more powerful position to extract vital concessions from Whitehall. But to win them, it will have to add leadership beef to the breakfast menu.'[25]

In November the *Sunday Telegraph* reported that ministers were planning a hard-hitting election campaign to conquer public scepticism over their handling of the NHS, something that could hold the key to election success. It reported that the BMA believed that the Government could succeed only if it slowed the pace of reform or put them on hold. It quoted me as saying, 'they have got themselves into a terrible mess because of Mr Clarke's, Mrs Thatcher's, and to some extent Mr Waldegrave's arrogance. The reforms are unsellable.'[26]

In November the MSD Foundation organised a meeting entitled 'Demographic change – is time running out?'. The speakers included Baroness Cumberlege, Chairman of the South West Thames Regional Health Authority, and David Willetts of the right-wing Centre for Policy Studies. General practitioners who attended the meeting claimed that the speakers were picked for their loyalty to the Tory reforms and used the opportunity to heap praise on trust hospitals and fundholding. I was a member of the Board of the Foundation and I expressed the view that the meeting was out of touch with reality.[27]

Dr Peter Holden, a Derbyshire GP and a member of BMA Council, announced that he was tabling a motion for the January Council meeting demanding that the SRM be called off if it fell between the announcement of a general election and the polling date. Revealing the fact that he was a member of the Conservative Party, he claimed that his sole interest in the matter was the good name of the BMA. I retorted: 'I should have though the Conservative party would have welcomed the meeting, as they tell us that most doctors are behind the NHS reforms'.[28]

FOOTNOTES AND REFERENCES

1 Letter from Lord Richardson. 1990 Jul 7.
2 Marks J. The checkups doctors love to hate. *Doctor.* 1990 Jun 28.
3 Marks J. Tory record bodes ill for budgets: GPs budget holders giving Government a propaganda victory. *Doctor.* 1990 Jul 5.
4 Marks J. NHS Act was never a case for compromise. *Doctor.* 1990 Aug 2.
5 Lee-Potter J. *A Damn Bad Business.* London: Victor Gollancz; 1997: 149–155.
6 BMA splits in thinking on anti-reforms drive. *General Practitioner.* 1990 Oct 19.
7 Dr Mac Armstrong later became the first medical politician to be appointed as Secretary of the Association, and after that he was appointed as Chief Medical Officer for Scotland.
8 Two gold medallists. *BMJ.* 1990 Oct 20: 933.
9 Mr Clarke will put appraisal back on the agenda. *Education.* 1990; **176** (19): 385.
10 Thatcher was a disaster for the NHS. *General Practitioner.* 1990 Nov 30.
11 Marks J. All change on political front. *Doctor.* 1990 Dec 6.
12 Marks J. (Chairman of Trustees, BMA Foundation for AIDS). Testing for AIDS. *The Times.* 1991 May 31.
13 Lee-Potter J. op. cit.: 194.
14 MacDermid A. BMA chief fends of charges of 'going soft'. *Glasgow Herald.* 1991 Jul 1.
15 GPs prescribed dose of strong medicine for BMA chief. *The Times.* 1991 July 2.

16 Sherman J. Doctors demand tougher stand on health service reforms. *The Times*. 1991 Jul 2.
17 Doctors drop BMA coup bid. *Health Serv J*. 1991 Jul 11.
18 BMA chief in confidence vote. *The Times* 1991 Jul 4.
19 Lee-Potter J. op. cit.: 194.
20 Marks J. Leader misjudged doctor's fury. *Doctor*. 1991 Jul 25: 21–3.
21 BMA awards top honour to its ex Chairman. *Jewish Chronicle*. 1991 Jul 5.
22 Jezzard K. Gold Medallist doctor attacks NHS reforms. *Borehamwood Times*. 1991 Jul 11.
23 British Medical Association. *Leading for Health: a BMA agenda for health*. London: BMA; 1991.
24 Marks J. Health will top the election agenda. *Doctor*. 1991 Oct 17.
25 The doctor's anodyne prescription. *Guardian*. 1991 Oct 5.
26 MacDonald V. Spin doctors prescribe NHS remedy. *Sunday Telegraph*. 1991 Nov 17.
27 Charity attacked for pro-reform bias. *General Practitioner*. 1991 Nov 22.
28 BMA rows over party politics. *General Practitioner*. 1991 Nov 22.

CHAPTER 26

A variety of activities including boxing and lecturing and a disputed SRM

ALTHOUGH I WAS NOW AN EX-CHAIRMAN MY VIEWS WERE STILL SOUGHT on a variety of subjects. In October 1991 the boxer Michael Watson was seriously injured in a professional match with Chris Eubank. I called for the 'obscenity' of professional boxing to be banned, rejecting the argument that banning the barbaric business would drive it underground. Watson sustained a subdural haemorrhage and Dr Adrian Whiteson, the British Boxing Board of Control's Chief Medical Officer, said there had only been 14 such cases in British boxing since 1948. I described that as a 'disgrace', and quoted from a 1984 BMA report that expressed doubt about whether the participants or others fully appreciated the risks of delayed cumulative brain damage resulting from boxing.[1]

As Chairman of the Commonwealth Medical Association I was the lead signatory in a letter to *The Times* urging the heads of government of the Commonwealth, who were meeting in Harare, to take a global lead in upholding human rights. The other signatories were acting on behalf of the Commonwealth Lawyers Association, the Commonwealth Legal Education Association, the Commonwealth Trade Union Council, and the Commonwealth Journalists Association. We pointed out that there was an unprecedented concern for human rights in Eastern Europe, the Gulf, and Africa and that it would be an abdication of our aspirations if the Commonwealth now ignored the needs of its own citizens.[2]

I was invited to lecture at the Centre for Medical Ethics of Jews' College, part of the University of London. My subject was 'Ethical battles I have fought', the main one of course being the struggle to maintain David Steel's Abortion

Act of 1966. I also raised the issue as to whether it was ethical for doctors to take industrial action against their employers, given patients might well suffer. I maintained, and I still maintain, that doing nothing in certain circumstances, such as the crisis in general practice in the mid-60s, would do far more damage to patient care in the long term. Resignation from the National Health Service would not deny patients medical care – alternative methods of financing it would have to be made.

A week later I spoke in Dublin at a meeting of the 'Club Avenir de la Santé', chaired by Dr Niall Tierney, Chief Medical Officer of the Republic of Ireland's Department of Health. I chose as my subject 'Health services: reformed or deformed?'

My sister Sheila suggested that I give a talk to the Edgware Branch of the Jewish Association of Cultural Societies (JACS) of which she was Secretary. I prepared a lecture with slides and I called it 'The NHS – beginning, middle, and end?' I explained the origins of the service going back to 1911 and its developments after 1948. Then I described Kenneth Clarke's Limited List and 'so-called reforms' and suggested that they were the beginning of the NHS's end – hence the question mark in the title. It must have gone down well because I started receiving lots of requests to speak at meetings from Richmond to the eastern suburbs of London. I soon realised that there was a network of society secretaries who handed on the names of voluntary speakers to their colleagues in similar organisations. Over the next few years I gave countless repeats of the same show to various groups of people, many of whom were of my own generation and remembered how bad things had been before 1948. I was particularly pleased to give one to my own Branch of U3A (The University of the Third Age) in Harrow.

In December my younger daughter Laura married Dan Patterson, a man she had met and ignored as a teenager, then met again as a young woman. Daniel had become a very successful television producer, and earlier in the year he had won a British Academy of Film and Television Award for his programme *Whose Line Is It Anyway*.[3]

THE SRM

In December the GMSC voted to recommend the Council to postpone the SRM.[4] The *Sunday Express* claimed that doctors were set to boycott the BMA's Special Conference amid claims that it was a waste of money. It described how the meeting was called by 'left-wingers' and that 'moderates' feared it was being staged just to embarrass the Government. It listed five hardliners who masterminded the politically explosive conference, including Sir Anthony Grabham!

(I wondered how Barbara Castle would have responded to the claim that Tony Grabham was a left-winger!) The allegation was completely fictitious – I had used my knowledge of committee procedure, and others' ignorance of it, to ensure a debate took place in Council, and a majority of the Council had voted with me.[5]

In the spring of 1992 elections were held for the Council of the BMA. As a result of the constitutional changes all the voting members were to be elected for three years. I decided to stand for election and my election address was quite simple:

> I believe that the 'so-called reforms' are the greatest threat to the NHS since its formation, and that the Association's policy of opposing them and publicising their failings is correct. Council has not pursued these policies effectively, and the public are unaware of the true situation. Doctors' demoralisation and apathy is being portrayed as acquiescence! I'm proud of my past record and I ask you to vote for me again to represent you and to demonstrate the need for a more vigorous response from our leaders.

I headed the list of first preferences by a reasonable margin.

An article in the *Daily Telegraph* attempted an analysis of how the medical profession would act in the run-up to the general election. It reported that Paddy Ross, the Chairman of the BMA's Consultants Committee and a lifelong supporter of the Conservative Party, had resigned over the Government's health service reforms. It noted my insistence that our campaign against reforms was inspired not by politics but by concern for patients' welfare. It said that the Socialist Health Association claimed its membership had risen, while the Conservative Medical Society admitted that its membership, merely 500 doctors, had fallen significantly. The article finished with details of two previous polls in *Doctor* and the *BMA News Review* which suggested that doctors were leaving the Conservatives 'in droves'.[6]

THE SPECIAL REPRESENTATIVE MEETING 26 MARCH 1992

Far from doctors boycotting the meeting the hall was packed and the motion that the meeting should be abandoned was moved right at the start. In opposing it I used some of the words that I had used in my election address, 'Doctors' demoralisation and apathy is being portrayed as acquiescence', adding 'there has been a thunderous hush from the BMA'. I asked the representatives if they really thought that their constituents had sent them to the meeting just to pack up and go home after five minutes – the wrecking motion was crushed.[7] The meeting voted overwhelmingly in support of a motion that the reforms had failed.[8]

After finishing my speech I had been asked by a BBC television reporter to meet her during the lunch interval to broadcast on the *One O'clock News*. Unfortunately there was confusion over the venue and the broadcast took place without me. The Labour Party held a press conference at the same time. It presented a film *Jennifer's Ear* which attempted to show the difference in treatment between the private and public sector. Unfortunately, the delay in Jennifer's NHS treatment turned out to be the result of a simple administrative error. Neither political party emerged from the 'war of *Jennifer's Ear*' with much credit, but the Labour Party still went ahead proclaiming that the election would be a referendum on the health service. Sam Everington, who had sat beside me on the Council for many years, tried to persuade me to support the Labour Party publicly, and maybe even help in their campaign against the 'reform' of the NHS. I declined, mainly because I did not wish to place the BMA in jeopardy if a serious attack was made on it under trade union laws related to political funds.

Looking back I think that was a mistake, because I would have been acting in a personal capacity and not representing the Association, but equally I doubt if anything I did would have made any difference to the election result. The Sheffield debacle had sealed that.

During the general election campaign there was speculation as to what would happen if the Tories lost, and the *Yorkshire Post* ran a series of articles on key personalities, analysing the potential candidates for the leadership if Mr Major were to be forced to fall on his sword. When asked to comment I described Kenneth Clarke, an obvious contender, as 'facultatively deaf' while an unnamed source in the field of education said it was quite staggering 'what he doesn't know, but he has a very clear overview of what he wants to do'.[9]

Soon after the general election, when the Conservative government was re-elected, rumours began to circulate about Jeremy Lee-Potter's future.[10]

A SERIOUS DIGRESSION – CIGARETTES AND STAMPS

In September 1950 Richard Doll and Dr Austin Bradford-Hill published a preliminary report that suggested a link between cigarette smoking and lung cancer[11] and four years later they produced their study of the smoking habits of doctors and the link with lung cancer.[11,12] In 1957 the Medical Research Council announced that there was a direct causal connection between smoking and lung cancer[13] and five years later a report by the Royal College of Physicians reached the same conclusion and also suggested a link between smoking and coronary heart disease.[14] At the time I was a very heavy smoker and completely addicted.

The only time I was free of the problem was when I had infective hepatitis in Egypt. However, after I recovered from that, cigarettes became more and more attractive, and as they cost next to nothing in the Forces, I was back to my 20-a-day habit in no time at all.

After the 1957 report I tried to give up the habit, and bought a radiogram, which we could otherwise not have afforded, using the money I was going to save by not smoking. Within weeks I had lapsed. In January 1961 we went for a day trip to Winterton in Norfolk to see whether we would spend a summer holiday there. My daughter Laura was then nine months old and I looked at her and decided I would like to live long enough to see her grow up. I realised that if I continued smoking 20 cigarettes a day I probably would not. I determined to stop.

A few days later a patient consulted me about a problem and I noticed that he was carrying the magazine *Stamp Collecting*. I told him of my problem with smoking and he suggested that I might like to take up stamp collecting and pay for it by putting aside each day the amount of money that I would have spent on tobacco. He took me to a stamp auction where I bought a collection of British Commonwealth stamps issued during reigns of King George VI and Queen Elizabeth II. I soon discovered that serious philatelists concentrated on a very small range of stamps. I cannot remember when or why I decided to collect printing errors relating to the current reign, but I did. I also joined the Wembley Philatelic Society.

That society, like most philatelic societies, held competitions for its members. A collector submits a number of album sheets which are then judged by experts using criteria such as knowledge, interest, and presentation. My handwriting is barely legible and I would have scored zero marks for presentation and so I decided to type all my entries. What I did not know was that the philatelic elite frowned upon typed pages.

An entry I submitted to the Wembley Society in 1967 was awarded the Members Cup which was restricted to beginners in competitive philatelic. Later that year I entered the British Philatelic Exhibition, where to my surprise I was awarded a bronze medal.[15] In the next three years I obtained another bronze medal and two silver ones.

In 1985, when I was Chairman of Council of the BMA, a medical journalist interviewed me about my hobby. I pointed out that although I had not stopped collecting stamps I did not have time available to do justice to them.[16] Ten years later another journalist asked me whether I had any ambitions left in life. I said just one – that I would like to win a national silver gilt medal for my stamp collection, and a few weeks later I achieved it.[17]

More important than stamps, in 1984 I lead a deputation to Norman Fowler in an attempt to influence the Government's negotiations on sports sponsorship by tobacco companies, due to be negotiated the following year.[18] A Private Members Bill was introduced which was hoped would lead to the banning of sports sponsorship by tobacco companies. On 7 February 1985 the BMA organised a delegation that included Sir Raymond Hoffenberg, President of the Royal College of Physicians, to meet the Sports Minister and seek support for the Bill. There were at the time various 'voluntary agreements' whereby tobacco firms agreed to control the advertising of tobacco, but they were honoured in the breach. The Minister would only agree to consider further evidence, nothing more, but by chance the meeting took place just 24 hours after Buckingham Palace announced a review of its policy of granting 'Royal warrants' to tobacco companies, which was prompted by Princess Margaret having had an operation for lung cancer the previous month. These events received widespread publicity and comment in newspapers all over the country, under glaring headlines such as 'Black clouds for tobacco giants' in Glasgow,[19] 'New blow to tobacco firms' in Wolverhampton,[20] and 'Tobacco – a new blow' in Edinburgh.[21]

The following year I led yet another delegation, which included Sir Douglas Black and others, to the Treasury. We wanted the Chancellor to raise taxation on tobacco well above the level of inflation, claiming that a 15 percent rise in the price of 20 cigarettes would be expected to cut smoking by 5 percent and save 183 000 lives.[22] We did not succeed.

I JOIN A PICKET LINE

On 25 June 1992 Lady Thatcher was ennobled as Baroness Thatcher. When it was announced that she had accepted a post as a consultant to Philip Morris, the world's biggest tobacco company, there was an immediate outcry within the medical profession at the deal[23,24] which *Evening Standard* priced it at $1 million (£510,000) a year.[25]

Sam Everington had the brilliant idea of preparing a 'heraldic shield' which showed a dead body, two people shaking hands above a pile of money and two smoking cigarettes, which he and I tried to hand into Lady Thatcher's office on 31 July in the presence of a large number of reporters and photographers. Sam accused her of 'promoting death' and I said it was a tragedy that a lifelong public servant could end up promoting one of the world's greatest producers of poison. Although both of us insisted, correctly, that were attending as individuals the reporters persisted in their assertion that as we were members of the BMA Council we represented that organisation. We did not. It was also reported, correctly, that I was an executive member of ASH but that organisation too had no involvement in the stunt.[26]

Photographs of the shield, and Lady Thatcher's office's refusal to comment[27] were published all over the country.

A PUBLISHING ERROR

On the morning of Sunday 2 August 1992 I received a telephone call from Dr David Williams in Anglesey asking me when I had become friendly with Kenneth Clarke, and later I received several similar calls. I was advised to buy the current copy of the *Independent on Sunday*. On page six there was an interesting article on education in which it was described how the right-wing of the Tory Party was tightening its grip and how Kenneth Clarke had poked fun at the School Examination and Assessment Council when he was appointed as Secretary of State for Education and had then set out to 'rout' the education establishment. The article went on to explain the White Paper issued by John Patten, Kenneth Clarke's successor, who wanted a new national body to oversee schools that 'opted out', thereby gradually taking responsibility for education away from local education authorities.[28] Accompanying the article was a series of photographs and one of them had a caption: 'Dr John Marks, member of both Standing Education Advisory Committee (SEAC) and now the National Curriculum Council (NCC) co-author of *Whose Schools?: a radical manifesto* and bogeyman of the education "trendies"'. The photograph was a very good one – of me.

I spoke to my friend and solicitor Clive Woolf, and he wrote a stern letter to the Editor calling for the publication of an appropriate letter from me to be published in the next issue of the paper. Under the heading 'Political insult added to injury' a letter from me was published in which I pointed out that I was completely out of sympathy politically with both the right and the left, and believed in centralist moderation. I reminded the readers that although I had been called a 'left-winger' when I was opposing Kenneth Clarke's 'so-called reforms', I had been equally strenuous in my opposition to Barbara Castle's proposals [to remove private beds from the NHS] in 1974 for the same reason – both were introduced for purely doctrinaire reasons unrelated to the real problems of the National Health Service. The Editor had the last laugh – the paper published an appolgy – to both men![29]

In November I flew to Jamaica to chair a meeting of the Council of the Commonwealth Medical Association at which I was presented with a beautiful commemorative mug. Later that month we took a holiday in South Africa. I had been invited to South Africa several times in the past but I had declined because I could not be associated in any way with apartheid, and had demonstrated my opposition to it by supporting Sir Anthony Grabham when he had persuaded the

BMA to leave the WMA a couple of years earlier. However, by the end of 1992 things were moving, and when we went on safari to Londaloza National Park one of the other guests was Nelson Mandela, who had not yet been completely rehabilitated but was, in effect, 'out on licence'. He was treated with great honour by all those there, and he mixed freely with all of us. It was a completely unexpected historical occasion, one which we never forgot.

In May 1993 I received a letter from Nicholas Timmins, who I had first met many years earlier when he was the health and social services correspondent of *The Times*. His letter told me that 'in a moment of madness', *The Independent* had given him six months sabbatical leave to write a history of the welfare state from Beveridge onwards, and that health played a large part in the story. He commented on 'all those wonderful battles of the 1980s' and suggested that we meet together to talk about the health service from its foundation onwards. I was delighted to be asked and I invited him to lunch in Elstree a few weeks later when we had a long chat about health matters starting with what was available before the NHS and continuing through some of the early crises in the service, advances in medicine and above all the struggle over Kenneth Clarke's 'reforms'. The interview included items that were discussed 'on and off the record'. In September we had a second meeting, and the book was published in 1995.[30] It was immediately recognised as an authoritative work on the subject, David Willetts describing it as 'the best and most authoritative account of what happened to the welfare state in the 80s, and why'. In 1996 Nick became the Public Policy Editor of the *Financial Times* and in 2001 a second edition of his book was published. As far as I was concerned I was faithfully reported, I had no quarrel with any of his comments, and I learned a lot.

THE COUNCIL CHAIRMANSHIP – AGAIN

Jeremy Lee-Potter's three years in office ended at the close of the 1993 ARM, when he would have to be re-elected or replaced. In my view he had to be replaced. There was nothing personal about it – he had failed to carry out the Association's policy. The reforms were charging ahead and the profession was demoralised. The problem that we had faced in Inverness two years earlier had to be faced again – who would replace him? As far as I was concerned the only likely candidate to succeed was Sandy Macara, who had enjoyed a successful professional career in academic public health in Bristol, had chaired the BMA's Ethical Committee, and was a very good Chairman of the RB. His three-year term would come to an end a few hours before the election. Although Jeremy Lee-Potter says in his book that Sandy had long coveted the job[31] he had hidden his ambitions from me so successfully that long before the RB I had to spend a considerable time persuading him to stand and convincing him that there was more than sufficient support in the Council to ensure his election. I had done my homework.

Jeremy was to be proposed by Ian Bogle, Chairman of the GMSC, and Brian Lewis, a consultant who had been Chairman of the RB. For various reasons neither of these two men was popular with members of the Council who were not deeply involved with their craft committees. On the other hand I knew that the votes of the 'odds and ends', that is the representatives of the smaller branches of medicine, were vital. I canvassed vigorously and openly for Sandy who was proposed and seconded by Ruth Gilbert and Chris Tiarks, two doctors Jeremy had dismissed as 'left-wingers' but who were known by the rest of the Council as being passionately opposed to the reforms. Jeremy expressed surprise at the size of his defeat, but I had got the figures about right – Sandy was successful by a majority of two to one.

I continued with my insurance work, and the various committees on which I still served, and above all I was available to sit on the Professional Conduct Committee of the GMC, which often ran for a fortnight. These hearings reinforced what I had known for many years – that there was a handful of doctors who were a disgrace to their profession, and that there were patients who would complain with the least possible justification. The standard of proof required against a doctor appearing in front of the Professional Conduct Committee of the GMC was the criminal standard of 'beyond reasonable doubt'. Although there was a feeling among the general public that doctors looked after their own, it was almost always the layman that 'let off' doctors whom the professionals would have hung drawn and quartered, because the case against them failed to reach the required level of proof.

In the early 1970s, when I negotiated the reorganisation of the GMC, I insisted that members should retire at the age of 70. Elections for the Council took place every five years and 1994 was the year when the statutory election would take place and as I was only 69 years of age I was eligible to stand. However if I were elected my memership would last one year or less. I did not stand.

In April 1994, three years after Kenneth Clarke's reforms had been put in place, *BMA News Review* asked a number of doctors, patients, politicians and opinion-formers for their views on them. Interviewees were also asked to rate the success of the changes on a scale of one to ten. The results were unsurprising. David Tod, President of the National Association of Fundholding Practices not unexpectedly gave it ten out of ten, while I gave it a measly one. Interestingly, Linda Lamont, the Director of the Patients Association, gave the reforms a rating of just three, and Alan Maynard, the Director of the Centre for Health Economics at York University scored it at three to five. He commented

'Ministers have no coherent strategy and refused to evaluate the reforms for fear of being confused by facts'. Clive Froggatt gave it eight out of ten, Harry Keen two, while Virginia Bottomley and her shadow David Blunkett both declined to give an evaluation.[32]

A month later I was invited to write an analysis of the progress of the reforms under the heading 'Galloping major heads towards initial change'.[33] I reminded the readers that the NHS was not about acute medicine and surgery – it was supposed to be 'comprehensive' – and that in spite of Mrs Thatcher's promises charges had been introduced for eye tests, and the manipulation of NHS dentists' fees was forcing many dentists to provide NHS treatment to priority groups only. There was also evidence that some trusts and fundholders were refusing treatments to uneconomical patients or discriminating arbitrarily against the elderly, and in one case allegedly discriminating against a blind patient. I pointed out that the Merger and Monopolies Commission's report on the supply of private medical services, published in February, had called for the BMA scale of recommended specialist fees to be banned on the grounds of price-fixing, but it was all right for insurance companies to produce a set of fees that they were willing to pay consultants. I wondered whether the Government's wholehearted endorsement of the MMC's report and its concern about the private medical insurance industry stemmed from its seeing the industry as the Messiah who would provide the answer to ever-increasing spiral of health care spending. I pointed out that Virginia Bottomley had told the Tory Bow group 'we now need to look at the private finance option for NHS projects as the rule, rather than the exception'.

On 12 June 1994 Shirley and I held a garden party for our friends and relatives at Brown Gables to celebrate our Ruby Wedding Anniversary. We had much more exotic plans for the real day. Our attention had been drawn to an advertisement by Swans Hellenic cruises offering a 40 percent discount on their 40th anniversary cruise for anyone celebrating a significant 40th anniversary, which was an offer we could not refuse. Because I was in the Mediterranean I missed the broadcast of Michael Cockerell's 'film portrait' of *The Bloke Next Door – Kenneth Clarke*[34] to which I had contributed.

On 28 September 1994 the *Daily Telegraph* reported that the Tory Party's 'favourite doctor' had been arrested.[35] The doctor was of course Clive Froggatt, who had been arrested for offences related to the misuse of controlled drugs. The article gave a glowing report of his relationships with the Conservative Party and how he had come to the notice of a Norman Fowler. That same article quoted me as saying that Clive was 'a Tory first and foremost, above everything else. He's blue to the core, and he is pleasant. That's why Conservative Secretary of State like him.' His arrest led to questions being asked in the House of

Commons. Mr Bayley asked the Secretary of State if she would list the dates on which she had met Dr Clive Froggatt, in what capacities Dr Clive Froggatt had given advice to the NHS Executive, the Department of Health or to Health Ministers, and whether he was paid for that advice, and of which official committees of the NHS Executive or the Department of Health Dr Froggatt was a member. For the Government Mr Sackville replied that there was no record of Dr Clive Froggatt serving on any official committees.[36] I felt desperately sorry for Clive as a person, but I felt that his arrest was a serious indictment of the Conservative Government's reliance on advice from unelected individuals at a time when ministers were refusing to listen to those who had been properly elected to represent their colleagues.

The matter did not end there. Following the 1997 general election the new Government announced its own reform of the NHS. During the debate in Parliament, Secretary of State Frank Dobson said:

> Their [the last Government's] reorganisation of primary care was based on advice from a Tory doctor who was a smackhead, Dr Clive Froggatt. He advised Margaret Thatcher and successive Tory Health Secretaries, ending up with the Right Honourable Member for South-West Surrey (Mrs Bottomley). He told the *Observer* that he was taking heroin every day. Conservative Members may be interested to know how he financed his heroin habit. He did it through prescription fraud, obtaining pure heroin in the names of dead or terminally ill patients. He ended up being convicted for fraud. Therefore, the Tories were advised on their major reorganisation of the NHS by a junkie and a fraudster. No wonder it is in such an organisational mess. No wonder we need a review.[37]

In October the BBC produced *A Public Eye Special* on 'The Health Business' by Donald McCormick, which showed how the distinction between public service and private enterprise was becoming increasingly blurred, and raised the question as to whether the NHS could survive its dose of market medicine.[38] The following month I wrote an article in *General Practitioner* to mark the 10th anniversary of the Limited List. The article included a miniature representation of the front page of the issue of *General Practitioner* dated 16 November 1984, which carried the banner headline 'How Fowler conned the public'. Under the subheading 'First blacklist was the start of NHS decline' I pointed out that my predictions of gloom in the NHS had come true and a pattern had been established for NHS transmutation. I noted that Labour had promised to abolish fundholding, and I warned fundholders that their bonuses would go the way of group practice allowances, which had been introduced 20 years earlier to encourage general practitioners to set up group practices. As soon as there were enough of them the allowance disappeared.[39]

In the late spring of 1995 I was interviewed for the Jimmy Young show on the subject of the National Health Service,[40] and a few weeks later I gave an interview on ITN as part of yet another profile of Kenneth Clarke. I attended two functions honouring my siblings – a party at Edgware infant's school to celebrate the retirement of my sister Sheila and a lecture and dinner at the University of Surrey to celebrate the retirement of my brother Vincent. Although I had been Chairman of the Council of the BMA for an unprecedented six years, and although I had been awarded its Gold Medal, the Council never bothered to hold a dinner in honour of my retirement. I think that distinction is unique, certainly within the last 40 years. Whether it was an accident, incompetence, or even a 'deliberate mistake', it should not have happened. I was never particularly bothered, but Shirley was, and remains, deeply hurt on my behalf.

In general, life was much more relaxed. We went for a long weekend to Prague and did not have to visit any doctors, hospitals, or organisations. When I got home I could really concentrate on my stamps and at the autumn Stampex – The British National Stamp Exhibition – I finally won a small silver gilt medal for an exhibit entitled 'GB QEII Photogravure Stamps: Perfection – an impossible aim'.

FOOTNOTES AND REFERENCES

1 Levitt L. Top doctor urges ban on 'barbaric' sport. *Jewish Chronicle*. 1991 Oct 11.

2 Marks J, Chogwe R, Ghai Y, *et al*. Human rights at Harare Summit. *The Times*. 1991 Oct 14.

3 Sacks A. Whose wife is it anyway? *Jewish Chronicle*. 1992 Jan 3.

4 O'Sullivan J. Senior GPs try to delay conference on NHS changes. *Independent*. 1992 Jan 24.

5 Bale J, Salmon J. The rebel doctors: hardliners behind BMA health revolt. *Sunday Express*. 1992 Feb 9. In addition to Tony Grabham and me, the article listed Sam Everington, who was openly left-wing (being an adviser to Robin Cook the Labour Shadow Health Secretary), Simon Fradd, who had been a member of the Hospital Doctors Association, and Chris Tiarks, who had founded in the National Health Service Supporters Party and who stood in the bye-election in the Vale of Glamorgan constituency.

6 Weaver M. A case of second opinions. *Daily Telegraph*. 1992 Feb 2.

7 Laurence J. BMA special conference – Doctors oppose reforms to NHS. *The Times*. 1992 Mar 27.

8 O'Sullivan J. BMA leaders urged to get tough on 'reforms'. *Independent*. 1992 Mar 27.

9 Neville S. Pugilist who packs a paunch is poised for tilt at the leadership. *Yorkshire Post*. 1992 Apr 8.

10 Brown C. Tories root for Lee-Potter victory. *Doctor*. 1992 Jun 25.

11 Doll R, Hill AB. Smoking and carcinoma of the lung: preliminary report. *BMJ*. 1950; **4682**: 739–48.

12 Medical Research Council's statement on tobacco smoking and cancer of the lung. *Lancet*. 1957; **272**: 1345–7.

13 Doll R, Hill AB. The mortality of doctors in relation to their smoking habits; a preliminary report. *BMJ*. 1954; **4877**: 1451–5.

13 Medical Research Council's statement on tobacco smoking and cancer of the lung. *Lancet*. 1957; **272**: 1345–7.

14 *Smoking and Health*. London: Royal College of Physicians; 1962.

15 Supplement to the catalogue of the British Philatelic Exhibition 1967.

16 *Pulse*. 1985 Nov 16.

17 *Health Serv J*. 1995 Aug 31.

18 New deal on tobacco and sport? *Pulse*. 1984 Nov 10.

19 Black clouds for tobacco giants. *Glasgow Evening Times*. 1985 Feb 7.

20 New blow to tobacco firms. *Wolverhampton Express and Star*. 1985 Feb 7.

21 Tobacco: a new blow. *Edinburgh Evening News*. 1985 Feb 7.

22 Doctors ask Lawson to raise tobacco tax. *General Practitioner*. 1986 Feb 28.

23 Protest over Thatcher tobacco deal. *Press and Journal (Aberdeen)*. 1992 Aug 1.

24 Maggie tobacco 'deal' under fire. *Western Daily Press*. 1982 Aug 1

25 Rogers L. Doctors fume over Thatcher's tobacco deal. *Evening Standard*. 1992 July 31

26 Doctors in office protest. *Western Daily Mail*. 1992 Aug 1.

27 BMA balks at Morris role for Thatcher. *Brand News*. 1992 Aug 6.

28 Judd J, Crequer N. The right tightens grip on education. *Independent on Sunday*. 1992 Aug 2.

29 Political insult added to injury. *Independent on Sunday*. 1992 Aug 9.

30 Timmins N. *The Five Giants: a biography of the welfare state*. London: HarperCollins; 1995.

31 Lee-Potter J. *A Damn Bad Business*. London: Victor Gollancz; 1997: 228–9

32 The NHS reforms three years on. *BMA News Review*. 1994 Apr.

33 Marks J. Galloping major heads towards initial change. *Young Principle*. 1994 May.

34 BBC. *The Bloke Next Door: a film portrait of Ken Clarke*.

35 Tory Party's 'favourite doctor' arrested. *Daily Telegraph*. 1994 Sept 28: 3.

36 *Hansard*. House of Commons. col. 1268. 1994 Nov 3.

37 *Hansard*. House of Commons. col. 917. 1997 Jun 25.

38 BBC. *Public Eye Special – The Health Business*.

39 Marks J. First blacklist was the start of NHS decline. *General Practitioner*. 1994 Nov 18.

40 BBC Contract dated 15 June 1995.

CHAPTER 27 .... *Doctors*
in the Dock

IN FEBRUARY 1995 EMMA WALKER, A QUALIFIED DOCTOR WHO WORKED
as a producer for the BBC, asked me to meet her to discuss a problem. If I had
had even the most vague inkling of the anxiety, stress and sheer misery that I
would suffer later as a result of that meeting I would have run a mile when she
called.

Emma was involved in a series entitled *Doctors in the Dock*, which was about
six doctors who had been struck off the Medical Register. Every one of them
believed that they were victims of injustice. I was asked to advise on the case of
one of the doctors, Dr Patrick Hickey. The BBC could not understand why Dr
Hickey had appeared in front of two different statutory bodies that appeared
to have reached different conclusions, and needless to say Dr Hickey wanted to
use that as evidence of his allegedly unfair treatment. I was presented a sheaf of
papers about 8 inches thick. These included the report of an inquest, a transcript
of a Misuse of Drugs Tribunal hearing, the hearing in front of the Professional
Conduct Committee (of the GMC) and the appeal to the Privy Council against
the GMC ruling. I agreed to read them and to give the production team the
benefit of my opinion for a modest fee.

It took me a long time to read the documents but the explanation I gave
to Emma Walker was quite simple. Each body had well-defined powers. The
Misuse of Drugs Tribunal considered Dr Hickey to be negligent but it could not
stop him practising. Furthermore, as he persisted with his intention of carrying
on as a single-handed general practitioner he had to be in a position to prescribe
controlled drugs in an emergency. The Tribunal therefore restricted him to
such prescribing. The Professional Conduct Committee of the GMC, where he

appeared a year later found him guilty of serious professional misconduct and struck him off the Register. That meant that he could no longer practise medicine and his appeal to the Privy Council against the GMC's ruling was rejected.

I AGREE TO APPEAR ON THE PROGRAMME

I had several meetings with Emma and her team and finally she asked me if I would appear on the programme, but at no time was it suggested by me that I should be paid for appearing. I was interviewed on camera in my study at Brown Gables for the best part of two hours, and at the end I was asked to sum up. I did so in the following words: 'Dr Hickey got out of his depth through ignorance. He was using dangerous, potentially lethal drugs with no idea how to handle them. That's how he got into trouble. He put ideas, which are unorthodox, ahead of the hard facts: that drugs are dangerous'.

I did not see any of the rushes, nor did I play any part in the editing of the programme. The series *Doctors in the Dock* was shown on BBC 2 in November and December 1995. The programmes had emotive titles like 'Kidneys for Sale', 'Lethal Injection', 'Unfit to Operate', and in Dr Hickey's case, 'A Fatal Prescription', which was transmitted on 7 December 1995.[1]

THE BROADCAST

The programme opened with a shot of Dr Hickey unlocking his unused surgery and lamenting that he had not been there for five years because he found it too painful. The narrator explained that Patrick Hickey had practised for 23 years using a form of medicine based on his unusual medical belief; a theory of 'primal therapy' related to a concept of 'psychic pain'. In a highly dramatic voice the narrator said that these beliefs were to be his downfall when in 1987 a drug he prescribed caused the death of a young addict.

I then appeared for the first time and was shown making the dogmatic but completely accurate statement with which I had ended my recorded interview. I gasped in horror when I saw it. My remarks were followed by a caption in black block lettering, 'A Fatal Prescription' after which a brief history of Patrick Hickey's medical career was given. He had become disillusioned with conventional medicine and had read a book on 'holistic medicine', meaning 'whole person medicine' – something that many conventional doctors, including me, try to practise. He set up a centre in Newquay which provided what the programme described as 'all sorts of exotic treatments, many derived from Oriental and Asian medicine'. His receptionist, Diana Truscott, said that Dr Hickey had become completely isolated from his local professional colleagues and that his unusual approach led to two-thirds of his patients leaving his practice. Dr Hickey then remarked that it was impossible to do holistic medicine unless the doctor had undergone a spiritual conversion and had been directed by God into that way of life.

The next contributor was Dr David Peters from the British Holistic Medical Association, who said he had to remind himself constantly that he was still a conventional doctor with all that that implied. This was followed by my second contribution: 'If you have unorthodox ideas you have to discuss them with other doctors, to make sure you're staying within some reasonable guidelines and limits'. The narrator then described how Newquay had become a centre for drug addicts, after which another of my statements was inserted: 'Every doctor knows that drug addicts will do anything to get drugs. So it's difficult, you need an expertise. There are well-known guidelines to help doctors who are not used to treating them, and there's always specialist advice available'. The next contributor was Dr Philip Robson, a 'drug misuse specialist' who agreed that any general practitioner could help a drug addict, but it would be difficult to continue issuing prescriptions without special training or at least specialist support. The narrator said laconically that Dr Hickey had no such training.

The programme then described in detail the story of Martin Scholes, a drug addict who consulted Dr Hickey on 10 September 1987 when he was obviously high on the amphetamines that he regularly injected. He told Dr Hickey that he was due to appear in court in a few days as he had been stealing money to feed his habit. He had been a patient of Dr Hickey many years before, but the doctor made no attempt to find out whether he was still on the list – he was not – or whether he had another doctor. Dr Hickey spent an hour and a quarter with him but during that time he did not take a proper clinical history nor did he carry out any form of conventional examination. Although Scholes showed classical signs of amphetamine intoxication – sweating, agitation and aggression – Dr Hickey decided that he was suffering from amphetamine withdrawal and offered him holistic treatments such as re-birthing and dynamic medication, and recommended that he attended church on Sundays. He also offered some Valium, whereupon Scholes became aggressive and demanded something stronger. Whether he specifically requested Diconal or not was never resolved because Dr Hickey kept no notes, but he was certainly given 30 tablets of Diconal, a controlled drug with special restrictions on its prescribing because it was well known as being in demand by drug addicts who crushed the tablets and injected the suspension into their veins.

Five days later Scholes appeared again having used up all the Diconal and Dr Hickey gave him a further supply. The next day he appeared yet again, giving what Diana Truscott described as a 'cock and bull story' that he had left the prescription in his jeans when they were washed. In spite of his receptionist telling him that he was an idiot, Dr Hickey issued yet another prescription, and even when the local pharmacist telephoned him to query the script, he insisted that the Diconal be dispensed. He then told the television interviewer that he had no idea that drug addicts would abuse Diconal in the way that Scholes had. Commenting on these events I said:

> You have an absolute duty, when you prescribe, to know what you are prescribing, what the effects of it are, what the side effects and risks are. It is inconceivable that in 1987 a doctor did not know that addicts used Diconal. And the only way a doctor could get in that position was by deliberately, or unintentionally, isolating himself from medical thought and from the community as a whole.

The narrator said that the following day Scholes was found dead with a syringe loaded with Diconal suspension still in his arm, that an inquest was held when a verdict of death by misadventure was recorded. The coroner was so concerned that he reported the case to both the Home Office and the GMC. Home Office drug inspectors looking at Dr Hickey's prescriptions over a six-month period and found 48 cases of irregular prescribing. Later that year he appeared before a Misuse of Drugs Tribunal which found that he had completely ignored the guidelines that had been issued by the Chief Medical Officer and other publications on the use of Diconal by drug addicts. In addition he had prescribed irresponsibly and the committee considered there was a risk that he would continue to do so. He was barred from prescribing controlled drugs save in an emergency.

The programme then described how Hickey appeared before the Professional Conduct Committee of the General Medical Council and was found guilty of serious professional misconduct, whereupon his name was erased from the Register. I explained to the viewers how the powers of the two bodies were different, but that there was no conflict between them: both considered Dr Hickey to be negligent and dangerous. Subsequently, Dr Hickey appealed to the Privy Council and his appeal was rejected, as was an attempt to secure reinstatement on the Register at a later date.

Subsequently I remarked that I did not know of any doctor or textbook that would recommend giving Diconal to treat amphetamine abuse, because it could convert an amphetamine abuser to a Diconal abuser, which is much worse. For good measure I added the remark that Dr Hickey was using his position as a registered doctor 'to take powerful conventional drugs and use them on the way out theory in a way that no doctor in this country would support'.

My last contribution to the programme was based on my reading of the

Misuse of Drugs Tribunal's views of the possible future if Dr Hickey continued his irresponsible prescribing. I said, 'Scholes was a disaster waiting to happen. This man put his own narrow ideas in front of the weight of medical opinion on the management of drug addicts. If Scholes hadn't come, sooner or later somebody similar would have come, with the same outcome'. The programme ended with Dr Hickey explaining to his solicitor how he proposed to handle his second application for reinstatement to the GMC, showing a video of himself in a long white gown in an oriental country being shown how God created matter. His final words were: 'Jesus Christ was a healer; he did not need to take histories or do physicals'.

The programme lasted for half an hour and my eight small contributions lasted in total less than four minutes. I forgot all about it and in February Shirley and spent three very pleasant weeks in New Zealand.

I GET A WRIT

When we returned home and opened our mail I found a writ for slander issued on behalf of Dr Hickey. It had to be acknowledged within 14 days of its delivery. I had just one day left and I was in a panic.

I phoned my solicitor, who said that as it was a matter affecting my professional career I should contact the Medical Protection Society (MPS). They were very helpful and in view of the time restrictions offered immediate help in dealing with the emergency of the writ, but the Assistant Secretary involved explained to me that she would need to seek guidance from the Society's Council as to whether they could take the case on. It might be argued (and it was argued later) that Dr Hickey was using me to attack the GMC in what the lawyers call a 'collateral attack on the decision of a lawfully constituted quasi-judicial tribunal'. Although I had been a member of the GMC I had no knowledge of the case prior to my meeting with Emma Walker.

The MPS instructed Counsel Mr G Bishop QC and Ms A Copeland and during the next few weeks I had several consultations with them. On 24 July 1996 an application was made to Mr Justice Popplewell to strike out the claim, but he rejected the application saying that plaintiff's case was very thin and the chances of succeeding were not great but not impossible.

WE GO TO COURT

When the trial in the Queen's Bench Division at the Royal Courts of Justice opened three years later Mr Bishop again applied to have the case struck out but Mr Justice Gray, who was hearing it without a jury, again rejected the

application.[2] The trial lasted for a total of eight days, Dr Hickey being represented by Mr F Reynolds QC and Mr J Crystal. After a whole series of legal
submissions Dr Hickey gave evidence on the first day when it came out quite
clearly that he had no knowledge of Regulations concerning controlled drugs,
nor that addicts crushed Diconal and injected themselves with it. He was
questioned as to why he had not taken proceedings for libel against the BBC or
the other two doctors who had appeared in the programme. He said it was too
expensive to sue the BBC, a view that Mr Bishop disputed as they could have
been be linked to my case, and the other doctors had not been motivated by
malice as I was! In response to the question 'Do you consider that Dr Marks
did not honestly believe what he said which was broadcast in the programme?',
Hickey replied 'yes'. He tried to justify his management of Scholes and went on
to claim that every single statement that I had made was false.

The sole medically qualified witness appearing on Dr Hickey's behalf was
another Dr John Marks – Dr John Angus Marks – who had been involved in
research and treatment of drug problems in Northwest England but had recently
emigrated to New Zealand. To avoid confusion Mr Justice Gray insisted that
he be called Dr John Angus Marks at all times so that 'Dr Marks' would apply
only to me.

When I was sworn in my examination by my counsel Mr Bishop was just
one question – to confirm that a large bundle of papers in front of me was the
statement that I had made on the 19 March 1998. I was then cross-examined
at length by Mr E Reynolds QC on behalf of Dr Hickey. I confirmed that I
did not treat drug addicts in my practice, save in an emergency, and that apart
from my insurance work I had had no contact with patients since 1989. I was
then questioned for a couple of hours about how I became involved in the
case, my relationships with the BBC, my expertise on drugs, why I came to the
conclusions that I did and so on. I was treated in reasonably humane manner.

After the lunchtime adjournment Mr Crystal took over the cross-examination
and the whole atmosphere changed. He went back over many of the points that
had been raised in the morning but with short sharp questions. At one stage Mr
Bishop intervened and asked that I be allowed to answer the questions being put
to me, to which Mr Justice Gray said, 'Yes, a little more latitude for the witness'.
Mr Crystal also asked me if I accepted that the views I was advancing about
another doctor were extreme, to which I replied, 'No, they weren't extreme
views. They are logical views. They are sad views actually'. He then said in a
very sarcastic voice, 'Anybody who saw the programme can see your complete
sympathy for Dr Hickey. Leaving that to one side, you accept that if you do not
have sufficient facts at your fingertips then you would have been irresponsible?'
I replied that when I had dozens and dozens of pages of questions and answers

that Dr Hickey had given on at least three separate occasions, those were facts on which I could make a comment. Mr Crystal then went on to suggest that 'I could have no reasonably honest belief in the extremity of the statements that I had made which were broadcast in the BBC programme'. I told him that I totally rejected that.

Mr Crystal then said, 'As a former member of the General Medical Council and as a dominant political figure in the medical world, your approach to what you did not know about was to describe it as no more and no less than orthodox. It is unorthodox because Marks does not know it?' I replied that there was nothing to suggest that and I had never said that.

I pointed out how I had been involved in reforming the GMC in the 1970s. I reminded Mr Crystal that the panel hearing Hickey's case included lay members like Jean Robinson, at that time one of the leaders of the Patient's Association and another participant in the television programme. There were also least four general practitioners. I continued, 'If you're going to suggest, Sir, that those people would not listen to the facts and the evidence and come to a reasonable conclusion, and that I would not be beholden to respect their findings, I really must reject that'.

Mr Crystal then returned to the theme that 'unorthodox' meant 'Marks does not know'. 'Would it be fair to say that your approach to anybody who does not practise your kind of medicine is one of distaste?' he asked. I replied 'No, Sir. I have no problems with unorthodox medicine as I practised hypnotherapy, which a lot of people think is gaga. I practised it extensively and some patients got great benefit from it. However, before using it I went on a course, I read books and I joined the relevant medical society. I knew that if one of the patients I was hypnotising jumped out of a window, and they do, I would have a problem and I would be prepared to answer it because I could produce evidence that I knew what I was dealing with'.

Watching Mr Crystal's face as I was talking gave me a little pleasure. He had allowed me to distinguish between what I and any other reasonable doctor would do before embarking on the unorthodox management of patients with the irresponsible behaviour for which Dr Hickey had rightly been removed from the Register.

Mr Crystal then referred to the 'damage' I had done to Dr Hickey and asked if I accepted that the words I spoke were broadcast to a considerable number of people to which the straight answer was 'yes'. He then asked me if it was correct that I had been asked to apologise and had refused to which I replied 'of course'.

I then stuck my neck out saying, 'If what I've said is not fair comment on what Dr Hickey did, if what I said is without reasonable justification, then I understand that I must lose'. Mr Crystal started his next question when Mr Justice Gray intervened again saying, 'All that is not really a question for any witness, it is a question for me is it not?'

I was then is re-examined by Mr Bishop, who took me through Dr Hickey's management of the Scholes case and asked me how I would have dealt with it. He then took me through the report of the Misuse of Drugs Tribunal, which included an assessment that Dr Hickey's prescribing was so irresponsible that they feared that something like it would happen again.

When Dr John Angus Marks gave his evidence on behalf of Dr Hickey he agreed that he would have taken a history on the same lines as me, and that he would have performed an examination along the lines that I had set out. He expressed the view that Dr Hickey complied with the minimum requirements of conventional practice. When Mr Justice Gray asked him about Dr Hickey's not making records of Class A drug prescriptions he replied, 'I think that is not responsible'. I still feel it was highly significant that he could not use the single word 'irresponsible'.

The last person to enter the witness box was my sole expert, Professor Griffith-Edwards, Emeritus Consultant Psychiatrist at the Bethlem Royal and Maudsley Hospitals and Emeritus Professor of Addiction Behaviour at the University of London. When asked about the prescription of Valium in the circumstances in which Dr Hickey found himself he suggested that he would probably have given five tablets each of five milligrams, and certainly would not have gone beyond ten tablets.

Mr Bishop then asked him about prescribing Diconal in those circumstances to which he answered, 'I think – and I'm using the word very factually – that is indefensible.' After Professor Griffith-Edwards there was a certain amount of legal argument among the lawyers, and then Counsel on each side made their final submissions. By then the trial had lasted eight days.

THE JUDGMENT

Mr Justice Grays's judgment ran to 43 pages, with the important bits coming fairly late. He concluded that Dr Hickey's knowledge of the properties and dangers of prescribing was seriously deficient. He accepted that Dr Hickey did not know that addicts crushed tablets for injection purposes, but that was due to his deliberate decision not to keep himself up to date with medical literature.

He then gave his reasons for finding that, although what I had said in the programme consisted of defamatory statements of fact, they were substantially justified. He dealt specifically with my remarks that Scholes was a disaster waiting to happen and said that Dr Hickey had equipped Scholes with a sufficient quantity of Diconal to kill himself accidentally or deliberately, and that Professor Griffith-Edwards' evidence had supported my statement. He rejected without hesitation the contention that I had acted maliciously. Then came the vital words, 'the claim must fail and judgment would be given in the defendant's favour'. We had won.[3]

The relief I felt was short lived because in no time at all Dr Hickey appealed against the judgment, but the appeal was not heard until 6 July 2002, almost seven years after I first met Emma Walker. When we went to court I noticed that Mr Reynolds QC was absent, the whole case being conducted by Mr Crystal. To my consternation the three judges left the court after Mr Crystal had given his arguments. However, Mr Bishop was grinning all over his face and advised me to calm down. When the judges returned the one announcing their decision gave me one of the few pleasurable moments I had in my dealings with Dr Hickey and Mr Crystal. He was scathingly critical about Dr Hickey's appealing against Mr Justice Gray's judgment, and went even further saying that the case should never have been brought in the first place. There was then a long discussion about exemplary costs, which was far above my head, and I never knew the outcome.

FOOTNOTES AND REFERENCES

1 BBC. *Doctors in the dock: a fatal prescription.*
2 The following account of the hearing in the Royal Court of Justice, which started on 4 May 1999, is based on the official transcript *1996-H-No.108.* The original documents comprise 504 pages of A4 paper and cover the eight days of the hearing and the judgment.
3 Dyer C. GP loses libel action. *BMJ.* 1999; **318:**1510.

CHAPTER 28   A quiet retirement, a general election and a question mark

THE ANNOUNCEMENT IN 1996 BY THE HEALTH SECRETARY OF YET another review of primary care led to my commenting that it was merely a 'device to get doctors off the Government's backs', and I expressed the hope that the pressure on the Government of a looming general election would help the profession's case.[1] Elections were also to be held for the Council of the BMA, and I decided to stand again. My appeal to voters was the usual mantra – the Government has got it wrong, vote for me to show you agree. I had already served twenty-three years on the Council and another spell of three years would take me past the quarter-century mark – although I would still be well short of Solly Wand's thirty-seven years.[2] Once more I topped the poll. At about the same time, Laura and Dan produced our second granddaughter, Sarah Esther Patterson, always known as Sally, a sister for Louis.

The 5th anniversary of the imposition of Kenneth Clarke's reforms promoted a certain amount of comment and I wrote a critical article in which I emphasised that the two-tier system that I had predicted had indeed arrived. I claimed that workers and patients were confused and demoralised because the situation in the NHS was as parlous as it had been before the unnecessary upheaval and because the real problem that led to Mrs Thatcher's panic reaction, chronic under-funding of the NHS, had never been faced. I concluded that 'one day it will have to be'.[3] Jeremy Lee-Potter was equally scathing.[4]

In the spring of 1997 preparations were being made for a general election and I realised that if the Tories were re-elected there would never be any hope that the market-orientated changes could be reversed. I asked Sam Everington[5] if I could be of any use to the Labour Party and it was arranged that I would take part in one of their press conferences. I prepared a suitable short address and on the morning of the press conference I had a briefing meeting at the Labour headquarters in Milbank with Peter Mandelson, Tony Blair and Gordon Brown. I sat in the front row of the press conference while the politicians pontificated. Tony Blair said, 'First of all we must get rid of that Conservative internal market that has caused so much damage to the NHS. We've had enough of running it like a supermarket – it's not a supermarket, it is a public service.' After they had had their say I spoke my piece, parts of which were broadcast on most of the news channels later in the day: 'My name is John Marks, and I qualified as a doctor on 5 July 1948, the day the NHS started. I spent the whole of my working life in the service and for over 30 years I was a family doctor in Borehamwood, and I was proud of the service I delivered.' I then gave the history of the reforms and why the profession opposed them, including my predictions that fundholding would lead to a two-tier service and that the treatment patients received would depend on the financial clout of their GP and their post code rather than their clinical needs; that staff would be demoralised and that there would be an explosion in the number of managers and accountants needed to maintain the system; and that 'the army of bureaucrats [generated] would be assailed by the very party that spawned them – the Tory Party', I continued 'It gives me no pleasure to say that in each case I was right . . . I am now sure that if re-elected just 14 days from now the Tories will continue downgrading NHS from "National Health Service" to "No Hope Service", and finally to "No Health Service"'.

A few days later I received an invitation to a post-election rally to be held at the Royal Festival Hall by the Labour Party. Shirley and I had invited some of our close friends to Brown Gables to watch the election results, so I ignored the invitation. One of my friends spotted it lying in the hall and asked what it was about. When I said that I was not going and would rather spend the evening with them they suggested that I had gone mad and that I should leave home immediately and head for the South Bank, which I did.

There was an excited, noisy atmosphere in the hall, which got louder and louder as more and more seats swung to Labour and a landslide victory seemed certain. When it was announced that there was to be a recount in Michael Portillo's constituency the cheers were enormous, and when the seat was won the noise nearly took the roof off. I met several interesting people that evening, Chris Smith, Frank Dobson, Richard Branson, Richard Wilson and others. At dawn I joined the massive crowd welcoming Tony and Cherie Blair outside the hall to the strains of the Labour Party's theme tune 'Things can only get better'.[6] When Tony Blair presented his first Cabinet, Frank Dobson, not Chris Smith, was named as Health Secretary.

I have already referred to my lecturing to groups of retired people who wish to keep their minds stimulated in organisations such as Jewish Association of Cultural Societies (JACS)[7] and the University of the Third Age (U3A). In 1997, for the first time, the talk I gave often ended on a hopeful note with the suggestion that the Labour Party might in fact save the NHS.

That same year Hilary gave birth to Jules, our seventh grandchild. His elder brothers doted on him – Shirley and I used to say jokingly that he had four parents. In the following year our eighth and last grandchild Raphael arrived, we enjoyed a fabulous trip to Southern India, and the National Health Service had its 50th anniversary. The *British Medical Journal* published a small volume, *Our NHS: a celebration of 50 years*, to which I contributed a chapter entitled 'Medicine and medical politics: a personal saga'.[8]

A well-attended reunion was held in Edinburgh in July to mark our 50th year of graduation, but unlike our 40th anniversary no great fuss was made in the media. I was coming to the end of my medico-political life and I left the reunion to attend my last Annual Representative Meeting, which opened on 5 July 1998 in Cardiff. I took part in my last major debate, the subject being euthanasia and assisted suicide. Both of these activities are illegal, but the juniors felt that there was a need for a conference to re-examine the whole situation, and the establishment wanted no part of it. Thus the last speech I made to the Representative Body had a strong link with one of my earliest ones on an ethical matter. According to the *Guardian*[7] I made an impassioned call for the representatives to listen to the voices of youth and reminded them of the previous ethical dilemma that we faced in 1968 when I was booed off the platform for suggesting that the Association's attitude to social abortion was hypocritical not Hippocratical. I continued, 'In over 40 years, I have never deliberately killed a patient, but I have given them increasing doses – sometimes huge doses – of drugs to ease their pain in their final weeks, knowing that it might shorten their lives. Perhaps I am being hypocritical, I don't know. I just know that when the time comes, I want a doctor who will give me a lot of assistance. It is just possible that the young Turks are light years ahead of the fuddy-duddies, as they were 30 years ago, but only full and open discussion can tell us.' By a narrow majority the junior doctors motion that a major conference should be held to discuss the subject was carried on a card vote.[9]

From then onwards I did no gainful work, instead I concentrated on gardening, collecting stamps, playing bridge, and going to the cinema and the theatre. I continued to be involved in the Harrow Branch of the University of the Third Age (U3A) current affairs group, and I also attended courses at the Workers Education Association (WEA) history at the Finchley Branch and Music Appreciation at Edgware.

On a more serious note, as a mere observer I watched Mr Blair's 'New Labour' Government introduce almost all of Kenneth Clarke's ideas. I made a conscious decision to say and do nothing until 19 February 2007, when I read an article in *The Times* by Nigel Hawkes. He claimed that few doctors could remember now why they hated the Conservatives so much.[10] I remembered! I wrote to *The Times* in response: 'I certainly "remember why I hated Tories so much"'. Not only did I welcome Labour as the saviour of the NHS in 1997, I also took part in one of its electoral press conferences. In 1989–90 the Labour Party and the BMA had fought against the internal market, and had rightly condemned the Tory idea of Private Finance Initiative (PFI), with the private sector providing facilities which the NHS would use. The present Administration regurgitated PFIs as Public Private Partnerships (PPP). To add to the confusion New Labour Party PPPs encompass PPIs, which are 'patient and public involvement forums'. The amount of money New Labour has wasted on failed projects, and the chaos from untried, untested and often unworkable reforms introduced without pilot studies makes even Mr Clarke's efforts appear almost benign'.[11]

A day or two later I received a phone call from Victoria Lambert, who asked if she could interview me for the *Daily Mail*. The article appeared under [their]

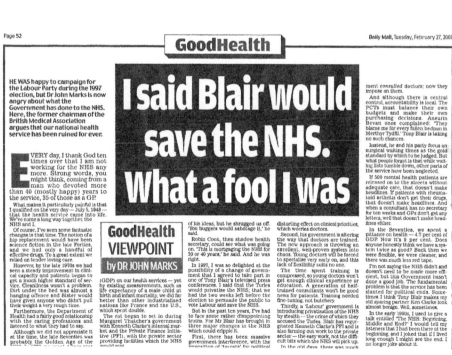

FIGURE 28.1 Interview with Victoria Lambert of the *Daily Mail*, 'I trusted Tony Blair', 22 February 2007. © *Daily Mail*.

banner headline, 'I said Blair would save the NHS. What a fool I was.' I said that Mr Blair had brought about three major changes in the NHS which would cripple it. Firstly the massive government interference imposing 'targets' for political not clinical reasons, which distorted clinical priorities. Secondly his Government is altering the way that doctors are trained which led to chaos in 2007. Thirdly a 'Labour' Government was introducing privatisation of the NHS by stealth – the crime of which they accused the Tories.

I ended the article 'In the early 1990s I used to give a talk entitled "The NHS: Beginning, Middle, and End?"'. I would tell my listeners that I had been in at the beginning, and I joked that if I lived long enough I might see the end. I no longer a joke about it.[12]

On 3 November 2007 along with the Chairman of the BMA, Dr Hamish Meldrum, I took part in a march organised by 'NHS Together' a coalition put together by the TUC which included the BMA, the RCN Union and others. About 7000 people participated. The main speaker was David Prentis, President of the TUC, who said, 'We're here today to tell the world that we will not allow our health service to be sold off to private companies on the altar of profit'.[13] He was referring to a New Labour government, not a Conservative one. I remarked to my colleagues that Aneuran Bevan would be turning in his grave!

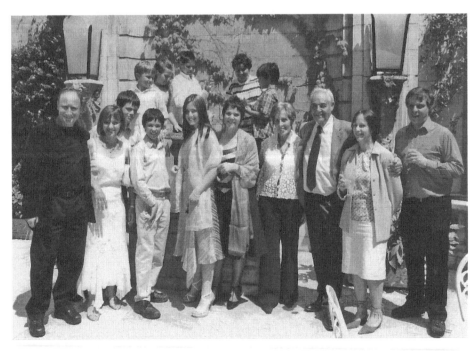

FIGURE 28.2 Our family celebrating our Golden Wedding Anniversary, June 2004.

My involvement in Keith Joseph's first reorganisation of the NHS is proof that I believed that changes in the service were necessary. However governments – Labour and Tory – have introduced countless radical changes in the NHS without proper evaluation, merely to meet timetables and political objectives and in the process have paid lip service to patients' needs and choices and avoided proper consultation. I believe now that the health service that Bevan introduced in 1948, a service in which the state provided health care for all its citizens free at the time of use, is doomed. I suspect that it will be replaced by a service in which the state commissions health care to be provided by many different organisations, some of which may be independent private companies and others whose names will link them with government or quasi-governmental organisations. Whether or not they will be free at the time of use remains to be seen.

This would seem an appropriate time to finish. I have had a long and interesting life, having been involved in almost every major change in the National Health Service and medical practice in Britain for almost 60 years. I have often had to make a conscious effort to remind myself that it really was Rose and Lew Marks' little boy sitting in my seat. I have been asked on many occasions what was the most important thing I did in my life. The answer is still the same: I married Shirley Nathan.

FOOTNOTES AND REFERENCES

1 GPs demoralised as never before. *Pulse*. 1996 Feb 10.
2 Marks seeking a medical record. *Jewish Chronicle*. 1996 Feb 9.
3 Marks J. Five years of reform: to what end? *Hospital Doctor*. 1996 Apr 11.
4 Reforms have turned off NHS altruism. *BMA News Review*. 1996 Apr: 34
5 Sam had worked part time at the House of Commons as adviser to Robin Cook, Dawn Primarolo, Margaret Beckett, Harriet Harman and Chris Smith.
6 The song 'Things Can Only Get Better' was written by Peter Cunnah and Jamie Petrie. As a result of its being used by the Labour Party in 1997 it rose to number 19 in the charts that year. The same name was given to a book by John O'Farrell, *Things Can Only Get Better: eighteen miserable years in the life of a Labour supporter*, which was published by Black Swan in 1998.
7 Letter from the Jewish Association of Cultural Societies, 9 January 1992.
8 McPherson G, editor. *Our NHS: a celebration of fifty years*. Oxford: Wiley-Blackwell; 1998.
9 Boseley S. BMA moves on suicide. *Guardian*. 1998 Jul 8.
10 Hawkes N. Few remember why they hated Tories. *The Times*. 2007 Feb 19.
11 Marks J. *The Times*. 2007 Feb 21.
12 Lambert V. Good health viewpoint. *Daily Mail*. 2007 Feb 27.
13 NHS staff protest against reforms. Available at: www.bbc.co.uk/2/hi/uk_news/7076231.stm

Index

'JM' refers to John Marks

Abbott Mead Vickers 182, 192, 206–7
abortion law reform 43–9
   background 43–4
   case of 'Betty H' 43–4
   1967 legislation 44
   medical profession's response 44–6
   ongoing opposition 47–9
   Rabbinical intervention 48–9
   see also Gillick case
acupuncture practices 107
Admani, Dr Karim 130
Agenda Committee representations
  (BMA) 59, 66–7
AIDS/HIV and the BMA 117–22, 227
   early decisions 117–18
   educational leaflets 118, 119
   policies on testing without consent
    (Bristol ARM 1987) 118–21
   reversing test policies (Norwich ARM
    1988) 121–2
AIDS and You (BMA 1987) 118, 119
Air Call 139
Aitken, Ian 167
alcohol advertising 154–5, 161–2
Alexander, Dr Benny 58, 59, 66–7, 105,
  120, 121, 143–4, 216

Alton, David 47
ambulance service, industrial action
  (1989) 213
amphetamine ban (1971) 55–6
ampicillin studies 71–2
Annual Representative Meetings (ARMs)
  1966 University of Exeter 59
  1981 Brighton Centre 112
  1983 Dundee 134–5
  1984 Manchester 141–2
  1985 Plymouth 153–5
  1986 Scarborough 161–2
  1987 Bristol 118–20, 166
  1988 Norwich 121–2, 171–2
  1989 Swansea 196–201
  1990 Bournemouth 224–8
  1991 Inverness 233–4
  1998 Cardiff 262
Appleyard, Dr James 122
ARMs *see* Annual Representative
  Meetings (ARMs)
arms spending 141–2
Armstrong, Dr Mac 232
ASH organisation 243
Association of the British Pharmaceutical
  Industry (ABPI) 55

Association of Panel Committees 101
Association of Scientific, Technical and
  Managerial Staffs (ASTMS) 108
Atkinson, Air Marshal Sir David 14, 31,
  131
audit activities 156

Baker, Kenneth 223
Balen, Malcolm 183, 186–7
Ball, Dr John 58, 137, 150
Banks, John 223–4
bar mitzvah 6–7
Barber, David 167
Barber, Dr Geoffrey 70
Barnes, Dame Josephine 109, 114
Barnet Division of the BMA 52–3,
  108–10
Barnet General Hospital 72, 157
Batchelor, Grant 24
BBC
  Around Westminster 233
  Doctors in the Dock (1995) 251–5
  Hard News 233
  Jimmy Young Show 249
  Money Programme (1970) 63
  Newsnight programme (1985) 149
  One O'clock News 241
  Panorama (1988) 167–8
  Pillars of Society (1988) 172
  A Public Eye Special 248
  Today programme (1989) 186
  Today programme (1990) 227
  Watchdog (1987) 164
  World This Weekend (1988) 167
Bedding, Mrs 8–9
Beevers, Dr 15–16
Bennison, Ishia 195
Benyon, William 45
Bernstein, Dr 17, 20
Bethell, Lord 133
Betnovate 73
'Betty H' case 43
Bevan, Aneuran 94
Bickerstaff, Rodney 195
Biko, Steve 112–13
Birmingham Children's Hospital 167
Biting Rubber Estates 67

Black, Sir Douglas 149, 243
Blair, Andrew 110, 158
Blair, Henry 35–6
Blair, Tony 261–4
Bloom, Dr Harold 34–5
Bloomfield, Eileen 10
Blunkett, David 247
BMA (British Medical Association)
  background history and constitution
    83–5, 124
    Chambers Report 86–8
    Council chairmanship elections
      227
    establishing the Medical Guild 85
    industrial relations legislation 85–6
    presidency arrangements 124
    role of Representative Body 181
  'block' voting practices 57
  influence of local representatives 102
  influence of minority groups 129–31
  JM's career appointments 53, 57,
    60–7, 95
    Deputy Chairmanship of the
      Representative Body 66–7, 108
    Chairmanship of the Representative
      Body 112–13
    Chairmanship of the Council 142–
      228
    re-election as Chairman 200–1
    end of tenure as Chairman 227–8
  1985 new library opening 160–1
  150th anniversary year (1982) 124–31
  overseas clinical meetings 106–7, 113–
    15, 135–6, 209–10
  performance reviewed in *The
    Economist* 204–5
  post-1990 council and leadership
    232–6
  Special Representative Meeting – 1992
    (SRM) 239–41
  splinter groups 101–2
  Treasurer appointments 143
  white tie dinner (1988) 169
  women representatives 59, 129–30
  on alcohol advertising 154–5, 161–2
  on confidentiality 47, 117–22
  on drink-driving 169–70

on GMC reforms 64–6
on GP advertising 170–1
on GP deputising services 139–40
on HIV/AIDS testing 117–22
on human fertilisation and embryology
    153–4
on NHS funding (IHSM/RCN
    collaboration 1985) 157, 166–7, 168
on nuclear defence 134–5, 155
on pay and conditions
    direct reimbursement scheme 51–3
    Review Body recommendations
    (1970) 62–4
on prescribing lists 146–9
    on seat belts 184
    on surrogate mothers 154
    on Working for Patients (1989) 170–1,
    180–1, 184–7, 189–94, 196–201
    poster campaigns 203–4, 206–7
    on world arms spending 141–2
    see also Annual Representative
    Meetings (ARMs)
BMA News Review 143, 148, 180–1,
193, 199–200, 246–7
BMA Services Ltd (BMAS) 141–2, 159
Board of Deputies of British Jews 144–5,
158
Boehringer Ingleheim 96–7
Bogle, Dr Ian 232, 246
Bolt, David 93, 104–5, 198
Borehamwood Post 53–4
Borehamwood Practice (Hertfordshire)
36–42
Borehamwood Times 219
Borney, Gordon 195
Borrie, Dr Peter 72
Bose, Dr Deb 135
Bottomley, Virginia 213, 216, 247
'Bourne Case' 43
Bowman, Dr 39
boxing 238
Boyson, Rhodes 121
Braine, Sir Russell 47
Brain, Margaret 211
Bremner, Norrie 14
British Association for the Advancement
of Science 95

British Journal of Clinical Practice 73
British Life Assurance Trust (BLAT)
180
British Medical Journal (BMJ) 76, 94,
143, 155
Brown, Gordon 261
Brynmor Jones Working Party 62–7
Buck, Mr 111–12
Buckingham Palace, Royal Garden Party
111
Buckman, Laurence 41, 186, 209
BUPA (British United Provident
Association) Ltd 103
Burrows, Maurice 93, 137, 142–3, 149
Bushey Maternity Hospital 39

Callcut, John Shirley 24
Cameron, Dr James 52, 90–1, 97, 104–5
Campbell, Captain 30
Campbell, George 8
Canada, BMA overseas meetings 135–6
capitation fees 50–2
Caplin, Eddie 231
Carlton Club 183–4
Carne, Dr Stuart 148–9, 183, 184–5
Cashman, Michael 118
Castle, Barbara 92–3, 95, 102, 180
Central Advisory Service Committee
    (CAC) 139
Central Committee for Hospital Medical
    Services (CCHMS) 84–5, 92–3, 102
cephalexin 73
Chambers Report (1972) 86–8, 108
Chambers, Sir Paul 74, 86–8, 108
Channel 4
    News (1988) 121
    Stitching up the NHS (1989) 195
Chapman, Sydney 108–10, 200–1
Charing Cross Hospital 20
Charles, Judith 143
Charles, Leo QC 120
A Charter for the Family Doctor Service
    (BMA 1965) 52
Chawner, John 196
China and Hong Kong
    BMA's Overseas Clinical Meetings
    106–7

China and Hong Kong (*continued*)
  Commonwealth Medical Association
  Council – 1984 145
civil defence measures, BMA policy
  134–5
Clarke, Dr Alistair 86
Clarke, Kenneth 157, 172, 204–5, 247
  becomes Secretary of State 172
    moved to Dept of Education 232
  on the BMA 178–9, 181, 183–4, 197
  on GP deputising services 139–40
  on GPs 183
  on junior doctors' working hours 173
  on NHS IT systems 208
  on prescribing lists 146–9, 218
  on White Paper reforms 172–3, 178–9,
    181, 183–5, 204–5, 207–8
    misses Oxford Union Debate 218
    and pace of change 223
    performance reviewed in *The
      Economist* 204–5
Clay, Trevor 15
Cockerell, Michael 247
Cohen, Dr Brad 114
Collier, Matthew 167
Collins, Dr Joseph 70
Commonwealth Medical Association
  (CMA) 162
computer systems 208
*The Conference of Local Medical
  Committees and its Executive* (Marks
  1979) 74–6
Conservative Party Conferences 209
consultant contracts 92–3, 101–2
Cooke, Alistair 114–15
Cook, Robin 174, 180, 182, 213, 219,
  223
Coombe Hospital (Dublin) 18–19
Corfu, working holidays 103
Cormack, Dr George 57
corporal punishment 2
Corrie, John 45–6
coterminosity issues 80–1
Crossman, Richard 63
'Cullompton principle' 93
Cumberlege, Baroness 236
Current Practice 136

Cyprus, Commonwealth Medical
  Association (CMA) meeting 162

Daily Express 46, 121, 142, 207
Daily Mail 187, 263–4
Daily Telegraph 187
A Damned Bad Business (Lee-Potter)
  231–2
Danckwerts, Mr Justice 51
Davey, Rosemary 20
Davidson, Dr Keith 66, 90–2
Dawson, Dr John 118, 182
Definitech Ltd 230–1
Delamothe, Tony 227
deputising services for GPs 91–2, 139–40
dermatology appointments 72–3
Diana Princess of Wales, opening of the
  BMA library 160–1
Dimbleby, David 167–8
'dipensary practice' 17
direct reimbursement schemes 51–3
disciplinary proceedings, patient
  complaint against JM 103–4
District Management Teams (DMTs)
  79–81
Dixon, Dr Maureen 195
Dobson, Frank 248, 261
Doctor magazine 137, 149, 150, 211–12
  JM's contributions 231–2
Doctors in the Dock (BBC) 251–5
Domestos Health Education Awards
  (1987) 168
Dover, Claire 189, 207
Draper, Jill 158
drink-driving and breath tests 169–70
Dublin, undergraduate clinical
  experiences 18–19
Duke of Edinburgh 198
Duke-Elder, Sir Stewart 41
Duncan, Nigel 216
Dundee, ARM – 1983 134
Dunwoody, Dr John 62

The Economist 179, 204–5
Edgware General Hospital 39
education
  early schooling 5

grammar school years 5–11
    entering university 11–12
    university and pre–registration training
        13–20
Egypt
    JM's military postings 25–32
    returning as BMA chairman 157–8
El-Kirsh (Egypt) 27–8
Elian, Dr 102
Elliott, Dr Arnold 58, 94
Ellis, Prof. Harold 91, 106, 157
Elstree Rural Council 53
Elton, Sir Arnold 183–4
embryo research 153–4, 155
Empire Windrush 25
Endhoven, Prof. Alain 168, 179
    on timescale for reforms 179, 228
endocarditis, use of penicillin 17
Ennals, Lord David 65, 222–3
Etherington, Ruby 168
evacuee experiences 7–11
Everett, Dr Wynn 50
Everington, Sam 223, 234, 241, 243,
    260–1
eye problems
    initial infection 31–2
    management problems 41, 64

Fairburn, Joan 144
Feldman, Dr Stanley 106
Field, Dr Ian 174–5, 196–7, 208, 217–18,
    235
Filer, Roy 5
Financial Times 245
The Five Giants (Timmins) 228, 245
flying experiences 9–10
Ford, Dr Angus 198
Fowler, Norman 131, 155, 157, 185,
    242–3, 247
Fradd, Simon 233–5
France, Boehringer Ingleheim invitation
    96–7
Fraser, Sir James 47, 131
Froggat, Clive 168, 193–4, 195, 209,
    218, 231–2, 233, 247
    addictions uncovered 247–8
    on JM 231–2

Fry, Dr John 94, 200
fund-holding general practitioners
    179
    Labour promises 248–9

Garrett, Dr Ray 73
General Practitioner 66, 101, 102, 108,
    124, 196
general practitioners
    advertising services 170–1
    deputising services 91–2, 139–40
    fund-holding 179, 248–9
    reforming pay and conditions 50–5
        1975 proposals 91–2, 93–5
        1986–8 proposals 173–4
General Practitioners Association
    101–2
Generic Substitution (National Health
    Service) Bill 148
Gilbert, Ruth 234, 246
Gilchrist, Dr A Rae 16–17
Gilley, Dr Judy 226
Gillick case 46–7
Gillis, Dr Annis 71
Ginsberg, Alec 29
Glaister, J. & Brash, J. 11
Glasgow Herald 87
GMC (General Medical Council)
    composition reviews (Brynmoor Jones)
        62–7
    constitutional reform 60–2, 62–7
    elections 105, 144, 201
    1975 Merrison Committee 65
    Professional Conduct Committee
        246
    professional fees 60–2
    on confidentiality 47
GMS Voice 51–2
GMSC (General Medical Services
    Committee)
    background history and introduction
        84–5
    constitutional reforms 59–60
    JM's career 57–60, 90–2, 93–9
    on NHS structure
        1962–9 changes 78–9
        1988 reform proposals 173–4

GMSC (General Medical Services Committee) (*continued*)
  on pay and conditions
    direct reimbursement scheme 51–3
    Review Body proposals 51–2, 58–60, 93–4
    1986–88 proposals 173–4, 203
  on prescribing lists 146
Godber, Sir George 60–1
Goldbaum, Binya 1–2
Goldbaum, Julius 1–2
Goldman, Teddy 40
'Goodman proposals' 93
Goodman, George 23, 35
Goodson-Wickes, Dr Charles 193
Goodwin, Shirley 195
Goudie, James QC 217
Gover, Ken 8–9
Grabham, Anthony 93, 97, 104–5, 110–13, 129, 131, 134, 137, 150, 196–7, 223, 232, 235, 239–40, 244–5
Graham, Bill 14, 35
Grahame, Dr Rodney 212
Grand Junction Arms (Harlesden) 4, 5–6
'Green Papers', introduction 78
Greenfield Committee 146
Greenwood, Dick 134
'Grey Book' (*Management Arrangements for the Reorganised NHS* 1972) 81
Grey-Turner, Dr Elston 66, 85, 95, 104
Griffith-Edwards, Prof. 258
Griffiths Report (1983) 144
Gryn, Rabbi Hugo 145
The Guardian 62, 197, 235
Guy's Hospital (London) 180, 212–13

Hainbach, Mark 141
Hampstead Medical Society 184–5
Hancock, Christine 195
Hancock, Stephen 129
Hardman, Rev. Leslie 37
Harkess, Jimmy 14–15, 33, 35
Harman, Harriet 182, 218
Harwen, Dr Cynthia 74
Hastings, Dr Charles 83, 161

Havard, Dr John 66, 110, 126, 127, 129, 161–2, 180, 183, 194
Hawaii, WMA council meetings – 1982 129
Hawkes, Nigel 263
Hayes, Jerry 193, 218
Hayhoe, Sir Barney 157, 205
Head, Peter 96
Heads of Professions meeting (1984) 145
'Health Index' 167
Health Service Act–1976 99
The Health and Social Services Journal 155–6
Heath, Edward 90–1
hepatitis infections 30
Hertfordshire Local Medical Committee 58–60, 63–4, 86
Herts Advertiser 53
Hickey, Dr Patrick 252–9
History of the British Medical Association – Volume II (Grey-Turner and Sutherland 1982) 66
HIV/AIDS and the BMA 117–22, 227
  early decisions 117–18
  educational leaflets (Dawson 1987) 118, 119
  policies on testing without consent (Bristol ARM 1987) 118–21
  reversing test policies (Norwich ARM 1988) 121–2
Hodes, Carl (Charles) 36–7, 39, 42
Hoffenberg, Sir Raymond 243
Holden, Dr Peter 236
holidays, family 102–3
Hong Kong, BMA's Overseas Clinical Meetings 106–7
Hopkins, John 194
Horner, Stuart 134–5
Horus 157
Hospital Consultants and Specialists Association (HCSA) 102
Hospital Doctor 143–4, 226–7
hospital organisational reforms *see* self-governing hospitals
The House Magazine 156–7, 212
Howell, Prof. John 224

HRH Prince of Wales, presidency of the BMA (1982) 124–31
human fertilisation and embryology, BMA debates (1985) 153–4
Human Fertilisation and Embryology Act (1990) 49, 155
Hunter of Newington, Lord 209
Hunter, Dr Stephen 222
Hunter, Paul 41
Hunt, Lord John 65–6, 70
Hunt, Philip 195
Hussein, Dr Hamid 102, 130
hypnosis, BMA working party 136

Ibbs, Sir robin 228
Illman, John 108
Independent 192, 206
Independent on Sunday 244
Independent Review Body see Review Body reports
India, exploratory visits (1985) 158–9
industrial action, ethical considerations 238–9
Industrial Relations Act – 1971 85–6
inquests 22–3
Institute of Hospital Administrators, Annual Conference – 1970 62
internal market
  concept origins 168, 179
  see also Working for Patients (DoH 1989)
International Congress on Group Medicine 97
international politics and meetings
  China and Hong Kong 106–7
  France 96–7
Ireland
  meetings and presentations 239
  undergraduate clinical experiences 18–19
Irish Medical Association 111
Irish Medical Organisation 144
Irvine, Dr 140
Irving, Dr Donald 96
Isaacs, John (Jack) 3, 4
Israel, working holidays 102–3
IT systems 208

Jacobovitch, Sir Immanuel 48
Jamaica
  CMA meetings 244–5
  1987 exploratory visit 162–3
  JM appointed Chairman of Council 233
  Joint Clinical meetings 209, 209–10
James White Bill (1975) 43
Jamieson, EB ('Jimmy') 13–14
Jamplis, Dr 110
Jarrold, Ken 157
Jay, Maurice 6
Jenkin, Patrick 99
Jennifer's Ear 241
Jewish Association of Cultural Societies (JACS) 239, 262
Jewish Chronicle 48, 112, 234
Jewish heritage and observances 1–4, 134
  meetings and discussions 200, 239
Joint Consultants Committee (JCC) 84–5, 92
Jones, David 230–1
Joseph, Sir Keith 64, 65, 79–81, 85
junior doctors, hospital working hours 173, 222
Junior Members Forum (BMA) 222

Kaput Holim (Israel) 102–3
Keable-Elliott, Dr Tony 66, 90–1, 93–4, 97, 99, 104–5, 122, 126, 130, 137, 141–3
Keen, Prof. Harry 212, 217, 218, 247
Kennedy, Charles 218
Kennedy, Prof. Ian 47
Kindersley, Lord 51
King, John 16
Kings fund, report of US healthcare 216
Kinnock, Neil 159
Kitchinski, Lewis Myer see Marks (formally Kitchinski), Lewis Myer
Kitchinski, Mottrel 1–2, 3
Knight, Dr Geoffrey 39
Knight, Jill (Baroness Knight of Collingtree) 209
Kopelowitz, Dr Lionel 48, 140, 158
Kumar, Dr Surendra 122
Kyle, James 120, 122, 143, 205–6

Lambert, Victoria 263–4
Lamont, Linda 246
Lawrence, Dr Ralph 66
Lawson, Nigel 168
Leach Wilkinson, Mr 34
Leading for Health (BMA 1991) 235
Learmonth, Prof. Sir James 17–18
Lee-Potter, Dr Jeremy 103, 173, 196,
  227–8, 231–6
  attempts to unseat 233–4, 241, 245–50
  on outcome of Conservative reforms
    260
Lester, James 193
Lewis, Dr Brian 137, 246
Limited list 146–9, 156, 218, 239
Links, Mrs JG 160
LMCs *see* Local Medical Committees
  (LMCs)
Local Medical Committees (LMCs)
  background history and introduction
    84–5
    first conference 84–5
  John Marks' career 50, 52, 58, 86
  on pay and conditions
    direct reimbursement scheme 52–3
    Review Body implementations 52–3,
      58–60
  published histories (Marks) 74–6
Lock, Stephen 110, 232, 234
Lutton, Dr Clifford 87–8, 108
Lyons, Dr Thomas 114

Macara, Sandy 121, 245–6
McColl, Ian 180, 195
MacCormack, Mike 143–4
McCormick, Donald 248
McDonald, Victoria 187
McKinsey and Co. Inc. 79–81
McNaughton, Prof. Callum 154
Major, John 168, 235
Malaysia, exploratory visits (1985) 158
Malveney, Colonel 25
Mandela, Nelson 245
March (Cambridgshire) 7–10
Marinker, Prof. Marshall 155, 219–20
Marks (formally Kitchinski), Lewis Myer
  2–3, 3–6, 8

Marks, Dr John Angus 256–8
Marks, Helen (JM's daughter) 141, 209
Marks, John
  background and family 1–4
  childhood experiences 3–12
  clinical interests 72–3
  clinical work 111–12, 159, 208–9
  commercial ventures 67
  disciplinary matters 103–4
  education
    school 5–12
    university 13–20
    postgraduate 33–4, 36
  fatherhood and family matters 40, 79,
    135–6, 140–1
  first jobs 35–42
  health issues 30, 31–2, 41–2, 64, 106
  hobbies 241–3, 249
  holidays 102–3
  litigation and tribunal cases 251–9
  marriage 35–8
  medical doctorate 74–6
  medical registration 20
  political offices 53, 57, 60–7
    BMA Council member 57, 60, 62,
      95
    BMA Deputy Chairmanship of the
      Representative Body 66–7
    BMA Chairmanship of the
      Representative Body 112
    BMA Chairmanship of the Council
      142–228
    Commonwealth Medical Association
      Chairmanship 238–9
    GMC appointments 144
    GMSC appointments 57–60, 91–2
    Local Medical Committees (LMC)
      appointments 50, 52, 58, 86
    Professional Conduct Committee
      (GMC) 246
    RCGP posts 71
    St John's Ambulance Brigade 50,
      53–4
  post-Chairmanship activities 230–6,
    238–49, 251–9, 260–5
    on impact of Conservative reforms
      246–7

Labour party involvement 261–5
life assurance work 230–1, 246
writing 231–2
published works
    contributions to BMJ publications
        262
    early clinical studies 71–3
    and journal articles 101–2, 156–7
    social medical histories 74–6, 94
RCGP fellowship 71
religious and cultural meetings and
    observances 134, 200
Ruby Wedding Anniversary 247
Marks, Laura [JM's daughter] 135–6,
182, 239, 260
Marks, Lewis Myer (formally Kitchinski)
[JM's father] 2–3, 3–6, 8
Marks, Richard [JM's son] 40, 79, 140–1,
154, 155, 163
Marks, Rose (nee Goldbaum) [JM's
mother] 1, 3–5, 10, 76
Marks, Sheila [JM's sister] 5, 7, 239,
249
Marks, Sue 192–3, 216
Marks, Vincent [JM's brother] 5, 7, 10,
35, 95, 106, 212, 249
Maxwell, Dr John 60
Maynard, Alan 246
Meacher, Michael 218
media training 150
Medical Act – 1978 65–6
Medical Association of South Africa
    (MASA) 113, 129
medical audit 156
medical education reforms 60–1
Medical News 99
Medical Practitioners' Union (MPU) 94,
108
Meldrum, Dr Hamish 264
Mellor, David 173, 182
Merck Sharpe and Dohme (MSD) 155
Merrison, Dr Alec 65
Miami visit (1981) 110
Middlemiss, Barbara 110, 158
Miles, Michael 13
military service
    Senior Training Corps 14–16

Royal Army Medical Corps (1949–53)
    25–32
Miller, Dr Jack 61, 105
Miller, Stephen 41, 64
Minton, Joseph 41
Moascar (Egypt) 28–30
Molloy of Ealing, Lord 219
Moore, John 166, 167, 170–1, 172
Moran, Lord 71
Morning advertiser 162
Mount Vernon Hospital 72
MSD Foundation 155, 219–20, 236
Murley, Reginald 102

Nathan, Alec 35–6
Nathan, Esther 35–6
Nathan, Shirley
    career 35, 40, 71
    family 35–6
    influence and advice 87–8, 105, 140,
        265
    interests 42
    marriage and honeymoon 36–8
    medical politics 45–6, 140
        on abortion reform 45
        on ambulance service pay claims 216
        on Working for Patients 197
    motherhood 40
    photographs 38, 54
    public offices 71, 108
    RCGP fellowship 71
    Wedding Anniversaries 247, 264
National Association of Doctors in
    Practice 101
National Medical Guild 101
Neuberger, Rabbi Julia 155
Newman, Dr Lotte 154
Newnes, Dr George 40
Newton, Tony 167
NHS organisation
    background and origins 19
    early reform proposals 78–9, 79–81
    Griffiths Report (1983) 144
    industrial action and funding shortfalls
        (1986–87) 157, 166, 168
    insurance-based proposals (1982/1985)
        168, 179

NHS organisation (*continued*)
  internal reviews (1988) and BMA
    responses 168, 170–1, 172
  see also Working for Patients (DoH
    1989)
NHS Reform Group 194
NHS Support Federation 212, 217, 218,
  226
Noble, Dr John 61, 105
North Middlesex Hospital (Edmonton)
  33
nuclear war, BMA policy on medical
  implications 134–5, 155
nursing profession
  1988 industrial action 168
  pay reviews 133–4

obstetrics
  surrogacy and embryo research 153–4,
    155
  training and qualifying 33–4, 36
O'Donnell, Dr Michael 64
Offences Against the Persons Act of 1861
  43
Ogilvie, Clare 179
Outwin, Dr Ray 61, 120
overseas doctors 129–30, 134
Overseas Doctors Association (ODA)
  129–30
Owen, David 92
Oxford Union Debating Society 218

Pallot, Peter 185
Parkinson, Cecil 111, 186–7
Patten, John 244
Patterson, Dan 239, 260
Pavitt, Laurie 99, 148
pay beds crisis 92–3, 101–2
Payne, Professor Jimmy 136, 142–3
penicillin, heart disease studies 17
personal health issues
  eye problems 31–2, 41–2, 64
  suspected melanoma 106
Petronius, Gaius 168
Pfizer Lecture (1975) 76
Pickersgill, Dr 122
poker games 114

Poland, official visits 22
Poole, Roger 213
Porritt, Sir Arthur 78
Post Newspaper 157
Postgraduate Medical Journal 73
Practitioner 72
Prentice, Thomas 207
Prentis, David 264
prescribing lists (1984–5) 146–9, 156,
  218, 239
presidency of the BMA 124
Price, Sir David 193
*Primary Health Care: an agenda for
  discussion* (DHSS 1986) 174
Prince of Wales, presidency of the BMA
  (1982) 124–31
Princess of Wales, opening of the BMA
  library 160–1
private practice and the NHS 92–3, 99
'pro-life' lobbyists 45–6, 47–8
Public Expenditure and the NHS (IHSM/
  BMA/RCN 1985) 157, 166–7
published works of JM
  early clinical studies 71–3
  journal articles 101–2, 156–7
  social medicine histories 74–6, 94
Pulse newspaper 60, 65–6, 93, 137, 155,
  213, 226, 227–8

Quinn, Sheila 133–4
Quo Vadis restaurant (London) 34

racism concerns, medical conferences
  134, 135
radio discussions, 'The Politics of Choice'
  164
Rae, Alan 31
RAF experiences 9–10, 11
Rasen, Timothy 193
Rayner, Lord 228
Reay, Lieutenant General Sir Alan 131
Redhead, Brian 186, 227
Redwood, John 168
Rees-Mogg, William 97–8
Rees, Dr Michael 131
research studies undertaken by JM 72–3
resource management initiatives 157, 179

Resource Management Initiative (RMI) 179

Review Body reports 51–2, 58–60, 62–4, 93–4

Richard Scott Lecture (Edinburgh) 216

Richardson, Dr John 24, 97, 127, 230

Riddell, Alistair 181, 192, 198

Riddle, Dr Gyles 58, 59, 66–7, 105

Ridge, Dr Ben 60, 90–1

Ridley, Nicholas 184

Ripley, Godfrey 50

River Nile trip 157–8

Robinson, Kenneth 53, 78

Rose, Dr Fraser 70

Ross, Dr Jimmy 74

Ross, Paddy 172–3, 179, 196, 240

Roundwood College 5

Royal Army Medical Corps (RAMC) 25–32

Royal College of General Practitioners (RCGP)
  background and origins 70–1
  on GP deputising services 139–40
  Presidential Dinner (1989) 182–3

Royal College of Nursing (RCN) 149
  on nursing auxiliaries and pay 133–4

Royal College of Surgeons, on the White Paper reforms 184

Royal Commission on Doctors and Dentists Remuneration 51

Royal Dance Hall (Tottenham) 16

Royal Festival Hall, BMA's 1982 AGM meting 124–9, 130

Royal Society of Health 90

St John's Ambulance Brigade 50, 53–4

St Leonard's Hospital (Shoreditch) 17, 20

St Martin's Hospital (Bath) 33–4

Sammy Davis Jr 114

San Diego, BMA's Overseas Clinical Meeting 113–15

San Francisco visit 110

Sattin, Philip 36–7, 42, 50

Scally, Dr Gabriel 141

Scarman, Lord 47

Schneider, Prof. 195

Scholes, Martin 253–5, 258–9

school food campaigns 168

Scott, Dr Melvyn ('Beardy Scott') 53

Scrivener, Anthony QC 217

'Scrutator' 118

seat belts 184–5

self-governing hospitals 179, 180, 212–13, 216
  criticisms and concerns 216, 219, 232–3

Senior Training Corps (STC) 14–16

'septic abortion' 44, 45

Seven Sisters Hotel (South Tottenham) 6

Shangri-La hotel 158

Shapiro, Henry 29

Shcharansky, Anatoly 133

Shearer, Anne 62

Sherman, Jill 197

Shevlin, Dr Bernard 136

Shrodells Hospital (Watford) 17

Sidel, Prof. Victor 195

Silverwood 230–1

Simmons, Dr Norman 102

Simmons, Stanley 44–5

Sim, Myer 45

Sinclair, Bernard 163

Sinclair, Hilary 154, 163

Singapore, Commonwealth Medical Association Council – 1984 145

Sissons, Peter 121

Sky Television, *Target* programme (1989) 191

Slack, William 184

Smith Kline and French radio award 149

Smith, S. 11, 17

South Africa, case of Steve Biko 112–13

Soviet Government, case of Anatoly Shcharansky 133

Special Report on the Government's White Paper – Working for Patients (BMA 1989) 189–91

Special Representative Meeting – 1992 (SRM) 239–41

Spens Report (1946) 50–1

sports sponsorship 242–3

SRM *see* Special Representative Meeting

stamp collecting 241–3
  winning silver gilt medal 249

Standing Medical Advisory Committee (SMAC) 148–9
Steel, David 44, 46
Stevenson, Dr Derek ('Docker Stephenson') 51, 53, 62–3, 95
Stevenson, John 93
Stevenson, JW 154
Stitching up the NHS (Channel 4 1989) 195
Stone, Dr Richard 200
Stroh, Sylvia 34
Styles, Dr Bill 140
The Sun 167, 189
Sunday Telegraph 235–6
Sunday Times 81
surrogate motherhood 154

Taj Palace Hotel 158
Taylor, Mary 6
Taylor, Pamela 150, 181, 192, 216
Tebbit, Norman 191
Tel-el-Kabir (Egypt) 30
television appearances 45
    on the AIDS testing crisis 121
    on NHS funding deficits (1988) 167
    on prescribing lists 149
    on public healthcare concerns 164
    on 'Working for Patients' 191, 195
    see also individual channels; programmes
Thatcher, Margaret 108–9, 133, 149, 168, 226, 228, 243–4
Theobald Street surgery 111–12
Thomas, Dr 'Bert' 6, 8, 11
Tiarks, Chris 246
Tierney, Dr Niall 239
The Times 51, 62, 87, 95, 97–8, 120, 130–1, 133, 148–9, 156, 197, 207, 233, 234
Timmins, Nicholas 47, 148, 184, 206, 228, 245
Today newspaper 200
The Todd Report (RCME 1968) 60–1
Tod, David 246
Todd, Sir Ian 184–5
Tottenham County School 6–11
trainee assistantship schemes 34–5

transplant surgery 79
Trist, Sylvia 24, 96
Trumpington, Baroness 156–7

United States
    1981 visit 110
    1987 visit 162–3
University of Edinburgh 11–12, 262
    JM's undergraduate experiences 13–20
    award of MD to JM 74–6
        lodgings 13–14
University of Exeter, ARM meetings 59
University of the Third Age (U3A) 262
University of Windsor (Canada) 135–6

Vaughan, Dr Gerry 65, 145
Veil, Simone 97
Venugopal, Dr 225
Vickers, Dr Paul 96–7
Vogt, Dr Marthe Louise 76

Waldegrave, William 232–3, 235
Wales, BMA council meeting (1989) 180
Walker, Emma 251–5
Walker, Isobel 104–5
Walton, Sir John 114, 124, 126, 155
Wand, Dr Solomon 145
war-time experiences 7–11
Ward, Dr Dorothy 130
Warden, John 197
Ware, 'Eggy' 10
Warnock Report (1984) 153–4
Washington, 1987 exploratory visit 162–3
Watford Evening Echo 64
Watford General Hospital 72
Watson, Michael 238
Watson, Prof. Jim 195
Watts, David 226
Weizman, Rabbi Malcolm 134
Weller, Dr 58
Wells, Dr Chris 80–1
Wells, Dr Frank 55
Wembley Hospital (London) 20–5
Wess-Pessel, Lord 65
Westbury, Gerald 106
Western Infirmary (Edinburgh) 17, 18

Westerway, Dawn 144
Wexford (Ireland) 111
'The White Paper' *see Working for Patients* (DoH 1989)
White, Dr Mary 114, 130
Whitehorn, Katherine 186
Whitelaw, William 117
Whiteson, Dr Adrian 238
Whowell, Dr Brian 58
Wilkinson, Mr 40
Wilkinson, Paul 197
Willesden County School 5
Willetts, David 168, 187, 205, 236
Williams, Dr David 244
Williams, Prof. Sir Dillwyn 183, 211
Williams, Dr Morgan 61
Williamson, Mrs 14–15
Willink, Sir Henry 70
Wilson, Harold 63
Wilson, Michael 146, 149, 172–4, 185, 203, 207, 225
wine tasting 161
Winterton, Nicholas 117–18, 205
Wolfson, Sir David 228
women in medicine
    BMA debates and conferences 114, 129
    BMA representation 59
Women's Medical Federation (WMF) 129–30
Woolf, Clive 244
Woolf, Mr Justice 46–7
Working for Patients (DoH 1989)
    concept origins 168, 179
        projected implementation costs 211
        public opinion 218–19
        timescale concerns 179, 183–4, 194, 205, 228
    the approaching storm 166–75
        disputes over NHS funding 166–9
        the Government Review is announced 168
        BMA response 170–1
        smear campaigns 171–2

White Paper leaks 174–5
    the storm breaks 178–87
publication day 178–9
    BMA's response 180–1
    public relation gaffes 182–3
    Carlton Club dinner 183–4
    BMA 'War Party' goes public 184–7
professions reject reforms 189–201
    SRM report and meeting 189–94
    ongoing opposition 194–6
    Swansea ARM meeting and JM's re-election 196–201
the campaign continues 203–10
    media and advertising 203–4, 206–7
    independent analysis 204–5
    Scottish dissent 205–6
    meetings with Government 207–8
publication of the NHS and Community Care Bill 211–13
    press conference 211
    reactions and analysis 211–13
progression of the Bill 215–20
    decisions over judicial reviews 217–18
    discovery of mysterious faxes 217–18
    the Oxford Union Debate 218
    preparations for House of Lords debate 219–20
    third phase of BMA campaign 225–7
    calls for strike action 226
    Bill gains Royal assent 228
    post-Act opposition 232–6
    outcomes and evaluations 246–7
World Jewry 149
World Medical Association (WMA)
    Council Meeting – 1982 Hawaii 129
    Council Meeting – 1983 Venice 136–7
    General Assembly – 1981 Lisbon 112–13

Yellowlees, Sir Henry 180–1, 182, 200
York University, Centre for Health Economics 157, 166–7